RAPID REVIEW SERIES

BEHAVIORAL SCIENCE

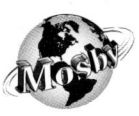

Visit our website at **www.mosby.com**

RAPID REVIEW SERIES

Series Editor

Edward F. Goljan, MD

BEHAVIORAL SCIENCE

Vivian M. Stevens, PhD
Professor of Behavioral Sciences
Oklahoma State University Center for Health Sciences
College of Osteopathic Medicine
Department of Psychiatry and Behavioral Sciences
Tulsa, Oklahoma

Susan K. Redwood, PhD
Associate Professor of Behavioral Sciences
Oklahoma State University Center for Health Sciences
College of Osteopathic Medicine
Department of Psychiatry and Behavioral Sciences
Tulsa, Oklahoma

Jackie L. Neel, DO
Associate Professor of Psychiatry
Oklahoma State University Center for Health Sciences
College of Osteopathic Medicine
Department of Psychiatry and Behavioral Sciences
Tulsa, Oklahoma

Richard H. Bost, PhD
Associate Professor of Behavioral Sciences
Oklahoma State University Center for Health Sciences
College of Osteopathic Medicine
Department of Psychiatry and Behavioral Sciences
Tulsa, Oklahoma

Nancy W. Van Winkle, PhD
Associate Professor of Behavioral Sciences
Oklahoma State University Center for Health Sciences
College of Osteopathic Medicine
Department of Psychiatry and Behavioral Sciences
Tulsa, Oklahoma

Michael H. Pollak, PhD
Professor of Behavioral Sciences
Oklahoma State University Center for Health Sciences
College of Osteopathic Medicine
Department of Psychiatry and Behavioral Sciences
Tulsa, Oklahoma

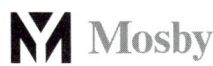

Mosby

An Imprint of Elsevier Science

St. Louis   London   Philadelphia   Sydney   Toronto

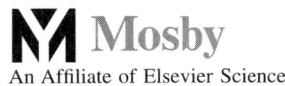
Mosby

An Affiliate of Elsevier Science

The Curtis Center
Independence Square West
Philadelphia, Pennsylvania 19106

NOTICE

Behavioral science is an ever-changing field. Standard safety precautions must be followed, but as new research and clinical experience broaden our knowledge, changes in treatment and drug therapy may become necessary or appropriate. Readers are advised to check the most current product information provided by the manufacturer of each drug to be administered to verify the recommended dose, the method and duration of administration, and contraindications. It is the responsibility of the licensed health care provider, relying on experience and knowledge of the patient, to determine dosages and the best treatment for each individual patient. Neither the publisher nor the editor assumes any liability for any injury and/or damage to persons or property arising from this publication.

The Publisher

International Standard Book Number 0-323-02007-0

Acquisitions Editor: Jason Malley
Managing Editor: Susan Kelly
Developmental Editors: Donna Frassetto, Martha Cushman, Marjorie Toensing, Mary Durkin
Publishing Services Manager: Patricia Tannian
Senior Project Manager: Anne Altepeter
Senior Designer: Kathi Gosche
Cover Designer: Melissa Walter
Illustrator: Matt Chansky

Printed in the United States of America

Last digit is the print number: 9 8 7 6 5 4 3 2 1

To my husband, Craig, my partner in science and in life, and our children, Nina and Nathan, and to my parents, Lawrence and Angela –VMS

To my husband, Greg –SKR

To my patients, who inspire me with their courage and determination to overcome mental disorders –JLN

To my wife, Diana, for her loving patience and support during my evenings and weekends of writing –RHB

To my husband, Gary, and our daughters, Debbie and Jenny, who have been extremely supportive during this project –NVW

To my wife, Maura, for always being there –MHP

Preface

The *Rapid Review Series* is designed for today's busy medical student who has completed basic sciences courses and has only a limited amount of time to prepare for the United States Medical Licensing Examination (USMLE) Step 1. With a commitment to meeting the needs of these students, we conducted numerous focus groups throughout the United States, trying to learn what would better prepare students for the Step 1 examination. Each book in the *Rapid Review Series* offers a visually integrated approach to review and is packaged with a CD-ROM to help students practice for the actual USMLE Step 1.

Special Features

BOOK

- **Target topics:** summary of major topics discussed in the chapter
- **Two-color, easy-to-follow outline:** concisely organized need-to-know information integrating basic science and clinical correlations
- **High-yield margin notes:** recall topics most likely tested on Step 1
- **Visual elements:** computer-generated two-color schematics, summary tables, and clinical boxes
- **Bold and color text:** highlights key words and phrases
- **Practice examinations:** two sets of 50 clinically oriented multiple-choice questions in current USMLE Step 1 format, including complete discussions (rationales) for all options
- **Table of normal laboratory values**

CD-ROM

- **Full-color: 450 clinically oriented multiple-choice questions** in current USMLE Step 1 format and content
- **Test mode:** 60-minute timed test of 50-question block by science, system, or random selection
- **Tutorial (review) mode:** customize your review (questions and discussions) by science, system, or random selection with immediate feedback
- **Bookmark capability**
- **Table of common laboratory values**
- **Scoring function:** instant statistical analysis showing your strengths and weaknesses; print capability

Authors' Preface

Behavioral science is a discipline that is applicable in almost all medical encounters. Knowledge of behavioral science theories helps physicians to foster positive relationships with patients, thus enhancing patient adherence. Knowledge of epidemiologic concepts helps physicians to interpret medical findings and to guide patient care more skillfully. Scientific understanding of mental disorders enables physicians to identify psychiatric symptoms, so treatment can begin and recovery can be hastened. As students study each medical discipline, they will find that some aspect of behavioral science is involved.

The review of behavioral science topics in this book is to aid students as they prepare for the United States Medical Licensing Examination Step 1. The material is presented in a concise but thorough fashion. Seventy-five tables are included to help access information quickly and are useful to compare and contrast specific information. Fifty-two clinical case boxes are presented throughout many chapters to help students integrate behavioral science within a clinical context. There are 450 questions, many with clinical vignettes and all with detailed discussions for all answer choices, that emulate the USMLE Step 1 format.

The book is organized in a logical and sequential manner. Introductory sections review fundamental topics, such as interviewing skills and human development. The sections that follow present the more clinical topics, such as psychopathology. Students who wish to review specific topics will find that each chapter is comprehensive enough to stand on its own.

We hope that you will find this book helpful in preparing for the USMLE Step 1 examination and in your future endeavors. We wish you success!

Vivian M. Stevens, PhD
Susan K. Redwood, PhD
Jackie L. Neel, DO
Richard H. Bost, PhD
Nancy W. Van Winkle, PhD
Michael H. Pollak, PhD

Acknowledgment of Reviewers

The publisher expresses sincere thanks to the medical students and faculty who provided many useful comments and suggestions for improving both text and questions for the book and CD-ROM. Our publishing program will continue to benefit from the combined insight and experience provided by your reviews. For always encouraging us to focus on our target, the USMLE Step 1, we thank:

Ellen K. Carlson
University of Iowa College of Medicine

John D. Cowden
Yale University School of Medicine

Barbara A. Cubic
Eastern Virginia Medical School

Stephen M. Dolter
University of Iowa College of Medicine

Melissa Jordan
University of Iowa College of Medicine

Melanie Santos
Virginia Consortium Program in Clinical Psychology

Lara Wittine
University of Iowa College of Medicine

Julie Zurakowski
Northeastern Ohio Universities College of Medicine

Acknowledgments

We wish to acknowledge and thank Vivian Stevens for her invaluable contributions and dedication to the production of this book. In addition to authoring and coauthoring many chapters, she spent countless hours organizing and focusing us, negotiating for and with us, and attending to the myriad details surrounding this book.

Susan K. Redwood, PhD
Jackie L. Neel, DO
Richard H. Bost, PhD
Nancy W. Van Winkle, PhD
Michael H. Pollak, PhD

We extend our deep appreciation to Susan Kelly, Managing Editor. Her expertise, vision, and tireless efforts greatly enhanced the quality of this book. Special thanks to Donna Frassetto and Martha Cushman, whose skillful editing clarified the original chapters. Thank you to Marjorie Toensing and Mary Durkin, question editors, and to Matt Chansky, illustrator. We are grateful to Jason Malley, Acquisitions Editor, and the publishing team at Elsevier for giving us the opportunity to write this book.

We are greatly indebted to Edward Goljan, a colleague, for his support and guidance throughout the writing process. His dedication and enthusiasm for teaching continue to inspire us. We thank colleagues who reviewed portions of the manuscript and took time to give us valuable feedback. Sincere thanks to the many medical students we have taught and the patients we have served who have helped us with our understanding of the behavioral sciences. Thank you to Sheila Mayes and Sandra Arnett for word-processing early drafts of the manuscript.

Thank you to our spouses and our children for their constant support as we worked on this project.

Vivian M. Stevens, PhD
Susan K. Redwood, PhD
Jackie L. Neel, DO
Richard H. Bost, PhD
Nancy W. Van Winkle, PhD
Michael H. Pollak, PhD

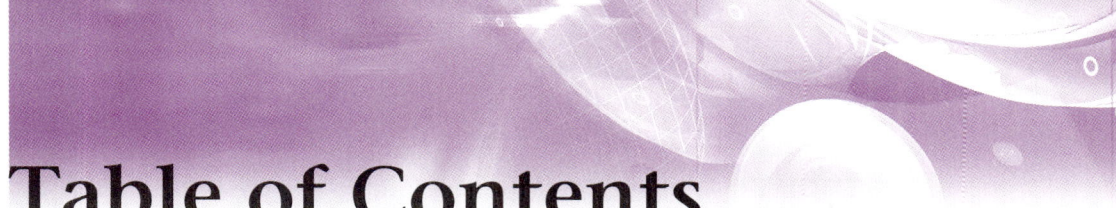

Table of Contents

Psychosocial Influences on Health

1

The Physician-Patient Relationship

Target Topics

▶ Developing the physician-patient relationship
▶ Interviewing and communication skills
▶ Responding to challenging patient behaviors and personality styles

I. **Dynamics of the Physician-Patient Relationship**
  A. **Physician factors**
    1. Effective **interviewing** and **rapport-building** skills lay the foundation for establishing a positive physician-patient relationship.
    2. Promoting a **positive physician-patient relationship**
      a. Foster a **collaborative** relationship with the patient (e.g., value the patient's input).
      b. Behave in a manner that builds **trust** (e.g., be genuine, instill hope but do not give "false" hope by creating expectations that may not be realistic).
      c. Show **respect** for the patient (e.g., call the patient by name, be nonjudgmental).
  B. **Patient factors**
    1. Personality style
    2. Cultural background
    3. Personal history
    4. Social support

> Build a positive physician-patient relationship with trust, respect, and collaboration.

       5. Personal meaning of illness (e.g., viewing illness as a punishment)

C. **Social factors: the "sick role"**

    1. **Talcott Parsons** proposed the concept of the "sick role," which describes the societal expectations and responsibilities that apply to the ill patient.

       a. The **societal expectations** of the sick role include **exemption from the patient's usual responsibilities** and **absence of blame for being ill.**

       b. The **societal obligations** of the sick role include **motivation to get well** and **willingness to cooperate** with health care advice.

    2. The **concept of the sick role may *not* be well-suited for all medical conditions** (e.g., a patient with a chronic illness whose goal is to optimize his or her level of functioning).

II. Interviewing and Communication Skills

A. **Interviewing goals**

    1. Establish **rapport** and foster **trust** in the physician-patient relationship.

    2. **Obtain information** necessary to make an appropriate diagnosis and develop a treatment plan.

> Physician-patient rapport aids data-gathering, improving diagnostic accuracy and treatment outcomes.

B. **Benefits of effective interviewing and communication skills**

    1. Greater **patient satisfaction**

    2. Improved patient **adherence** with medical recommendations

    3. Increased **diagnostic accuracy**

    4. Improved **medical outcomes**

C. **Effective interviewing skills**

    1. **Building rapport with the patient**

       a. Upon entering the room, introduce yourself and **address the patient by name.**

       b. Engage in brief **nonmedical conversation.**

       c. Use appropriate **nonverbal behaviors** (e.g., smile, eye contact).

       d. **Sit**, if possible.

       e. Be sensitive to the **patient's comfort and privacy.**

    2. **Collecting data**

> Open-ended questions encourage the patient to provide complete information.

       a. **Open-ended questions** are effective in the early stages of the interview and allow the patient to freely describe symptoms and concerns.
         Example: "What brings you here today?" Or, "How would you describe the pain?"

       b. **Direct**, or **close-ended, questions** are designed to obtain specific information and often require a "yes" or "no" reply.
         Example: "Have you had thoughts of suicide in the past?"

> Direct questions help to elicit specific information.

      c. Facilitating responses, such as nonverbal behaviors (e.g., nodding) or verbal statements encourage the patient to elaborate on his or her concerns.
      Example: "Tell me more about that."

      d. Paraphrasing or reflecting on what the patient has said, by taking a portion of the patient's statement and repeating it in the form of a question, encourages the patient to elaborate on a topic.
      Example: "The pain started 5 days ago?"

  3. Clarifying information

      a. Confrontation can be used to address inconsistencies in a patient's responses or physical presentation.
      Example: "You say you feel fine, but you look as if you're having trouble breathing."

      b. Summary statements are useful for reviewing the pertinent points, demonstrating an understanding of what the patient has said, and for correcting misinformation.
      Example: "Let me review what you've told me to this point. Your back started hurting 2 days ago when you picked up the laundry basket. The pain is in your lower back, it hasn't responded to over-the-counter medications, and it has been getting worse."

D. Barriers to effective interviewing

  1. Using medical jargon
  Example: "Your labs show an elevated creatine."

  2. Asking leading questions
  Example: "You've been taking your medication twice a day, haven't you?"

  3. Offering premature reassurance
  Example: "Everything will be fine."

  4. Making patronizing remarks
  Example: "You just relax. I'll handle this."

  5. Asking multiple questions
  Example: "Have you had any problems, such as poor appetite, insomnia, fatigue, or difficulty concentrating?"

III. Challenging Situations in the Medical Encounter

A. Recognizing emotional reactions in the physician-patient relationship

  1. Transference (Box 1-1)

      a. Transference is an **unconscious process** in which the **patient** brings feelings and attitudes from previous experiences, either positive or negative, and applies those feelings to the physician.

      b. A **transference reaction** is often signaled by an **unexpected response** from the patient or a response that is disproportionate to the situation.

      c. Transference is more likely to occur when a patient is seriously ill or under increased stress.

> Transference: when the patient applies feelings from past experiences to the physician.

BOX 1-1	The Patient Who Is Displaying Transference

The developmental history of a 46-year-old woman indicates that her mother withheld food from her as a child because the mother believed her daughter was overweight. The patient is currently about 23 kg (50 lb) overweight and has recently developed hypertension. When her physician advises her to lose weight, she becomes angry and does not comply with his advice.

BOX 1-2	The Physician Who Is Experiencing Countertransference

A 33-year-old female physician is reviewing the chart of a 58-year-old man with type 2 diabetes mellitus. The physician dreads visits with this particular patient, because he constantly criticizes her and believes he knows more about diabetes than she does. She keeps her visits with him brief and feels angry with him for several hours after he leaves. Although this patient likely would be difficult for many physicians, he evokes especially strong negative feelings from this physician. While discussing the patient with a colleague, she realizes that the patient reminds her of her father, who was very critical of her and was never satisfied with any of her accomplishments.

> Countertransference: when the physician applies feelings from past experiences to the patient.

> Emotional expression is associated with positive health consequences.

    d. Physicians should maintain a respectful, empathic approach to the patient when dealing with transference reactions.

2. **Countertransference** (Box 1-2)
    a. Countertransference is an **unconscious process** in which the **physician** brings **feelings** and **attitudes** from **previous experiences,** either positive or negative, and applies those feelings to the patient.
    b. Countertransference **can affect the physician's judgment** and provision of medical care.
    c. **Strong feelings toward a patient** may be a signal that countertransference has developed.
    d. **Constructive responses by the physician** when experiencing countertransference
        (1) Acknowledge these feelings.
        (2) Strive to keep personal reactions from interfering with the quality of medical care provided. If necessary, refer the patient to another physician.
        (3) Consult with colleagues.

B. **Acknowledging patient emotions and challenging behaviors**
    1. **Expressing emotions** about stressful life events is associated with **positive health consequences,** such as improved immune functioning and fewer physician visits.

BOX 1-3	The Physician Who Is Displaying Empathy

After waiting for over an hour to be seen, a 37-year-old man, who has been pacing back and forth in the examination room, makes a sarcastic remark to the physician. The physician, believing the patient's sarcasm to be a sign of anger, quickly acknowledges how upsetting it must be for the patient to have waited so long and offers an apology for the delay. The patient becomes visibly less agitated throughout the remainder of the visit.

2. When the patient's emotions are not acknowledged and responded to in a constructive manner, they often intensify (e.g., a patient's anxiety is likely to increase if it is not recognized and addressed by the physician).
3. Increased levels of emotional arousal are likely to interfere with a patient's ability to provide an accurate history and to remember treatment recommendations.
4. **Empathic communication**
   a. Empathic statements are **effective responses to patients' emotions.**
   b. **Empathy** refers to responding to patients in a way that shows an effort to recognize and understand the patient's feelings and experiences (Box 1-3).
   Example: "You seem angry," or "It sounds like the process of recovering from your surgery has been very frustrating for you."
   c. Empathic communication requires **active listening** and attending to what the patient is expressing both verbally and nonverbally.
   d. Empathic communications can **increase rapport** between the patient and physician and can have a therapeutic effect on the patient's level of distress.
5. **Validation** reassures the patient that his or her concerns are understandable in the circumstances.
   Example: "Most people experience anxiety while waiting for the results of a biopsy."
6. Table 1-1 lists strategies for responding to patients' emotions and challenging behaviors.

Empathic responses by the physician show an effort to understand the patient's feelings and experiences.

IV. Personality Styles and the Medical Encounter
A. **Personality style** refers to the manner in which an individual characteristically responds to events and experiences in the world. It reflects a habitual pattern of how the individual thinks about, relates to, and perceives his or her own self and environment.
B. A patient's personality style often becomes **exaggerated in stressful circumstances,** such as during illness.

TABLE 1-1   Strategies for Responding to Challenging Patient Encounters

Type of Patient	Description	Possible Reasons for Emotions or Behavior	Physician's Approach to the Encounter
Reticent	Gives brief responses Reluctant to talk	Anxiety, depression	Offer encouragement and reassurance Use facilitating responses that encourage the patient to talk Use direct questions and offer response choices
Rambling	Talks excessively Repeatedly strays from topic	Lonely, anxious	Listen to a few anecdotes initially Use fewer open-ended questions Offer response choices Paraphrase and redirect topic Gently inform patient of time limitations
Anxious	Trembles Breathes rapidly Fidgets Sweats Asks numerous questions	Natural response to illness Sign of a psychiatric disorder Past unpleasant medical experiences	Acknowledge distress Explore fears Offer empathic responses Provide realistic information Avoid premature reassurance Ask if patient has any unanswered questions Expect to address concerns more than once
Sad	Tearful Sighs	Grieving Depression	Explore reasons for sadness Allow patient to cry Offer empathic responses
Angry	Speaks loudly Uses obscenities Makes critical sarcastic remarks	Natural response to illness Particular circumstances in patient's life	Acknowledge patient's anger Do not respond with anger Explore reasons behind patient's anger Offer empathic responses If patient is blaming others, remain neutral but supportive Set limits on behavior, if needed Apologize, if appropriate
In denial	Ignores symptoms Denies need for treatment Minimizes impact of illness	May be an adaptive response, particularly when given initial news of medical diagnosis Provides time to adjust to medical situation	If denial does not interfere with treatment, do not pursue; can return to issue in future Elicit patient's perspective and present physician's perspective; avoid arguing Emphasize concern for patient Adhere to ethical obligation to inform about illness and treatment
Nonadherent	Does not follow treatment regimen or recommendations	Lack of belief in medical regimen Does not understand or remember medical advice	Identify barriers to adherence Customize intervention to patient's circumstance

TABLE 1-2   Strategies for Responding to Personality Styles in the Medical Encounter

Personality Style	Description	Physician's Approach to the Encounter
Dependent	Passive approach to self-care Frequent phone calls and visits Excessive need for reassurance Gives physician all the credit for patient's medical improvement	May need to see patient more frequently Give choices and encourage patient to take responsibility Emphasize patient's role in recovery Help patient establish or access social support
Paranoid	Suspicious Accusatory Angry Interpersonal sensitivity	Be straightforward in discussions about medical care Maintain formal demeanor Avoid excessive empathy, which can arouse suspicion
Obsessive-compulsive	Detail-oriented Excessive need for control	Include patient in decision-making process Provide detailed explanations of medical care
Schizoid	Socially withdrawn Emotionally detached	Respect patient's need for privacy Do not expect patient to display much emotion
Histrionic	Dramatic and emotional Sexually provocative behavior	In response to emotionality, remain calm and appropriately reassuring For seductive behavior, keep in mind that behavior may intensify if not addressed Maintain professional boundaries Set limits on behavior in a calm manner Have another staff member present during medical encounter
Narcissistic	Acts in superior manner Entitled demeanor May demand special treatment	May need to set limits, but do so in a manner that appeals to patient's perception of being special

    C. Modifying the approach to a patient, based on an understanding of the patient's personality style, is likely to lead to an improved physician-patient relationship or medical interaction.

    D. Table 1-2 lists strategies for working with a patient's particular personality style.

2

Family, Society, and Culture

I. **The Family and Its Role in Health**
   A. **General characteristics of families**
      1. **Definition of family:** two or more people who are **related biologically**, **emotionally**, or **legally**, and who function together to provide the physical, emotional, and social needs of each member
      2. **Types of family structures**
         a. **Traditional nuclear families**
            (1) The traditional nuclear family consists of a **father**, a **mother**, and their **biological children**.
            (2) Approximately **56% of children** live in a **traditional nuclear family**.
            (3) The proportion of households consisting of traditional nuclear families is declining.
         b. **Single-parent families**
            (1) The single-parent family consists of a **single parent** and his or her **biological children**. This type of family may occur as a result of the death of a spouse, out-of-marriage pregnancy, separation, or divorce.

      (2) Approximately **25% of children** live in a **single-parent household,** and the proportion of these families is increasing.

      (3) About **85%** of single-parent households are **headed by women.** These families are more likely to be **economically disadvantaged** than male-headed single-parent families.

      (4) **Single parents** are at **increased risk for physical and mental health problems,** likely related to decreased income and social support.

   c. **Blended families**

      (1) The blended family is one in which a **stepparent, step-sibling,** or **half-sibling** is present in the household.

      (2) Approximately **15% of children** live in a blended family, and the percentage is increasing.

   d. **Extended families**

      (1) The extended family includes **relatives,** such as grandparents, aunts, uncles, and cousins, in addition to **parents** and **siblings.**

      (2) The number of extended family households is increasing, especially among new immigrants to the United States and single-parent families.

   e. **Families with gay or lesbian parents**

      (1) Lesbians and gay men increasingly are **becoming parents,** either on their own or with a same-sex partner, usually following divorce from a heterosexual partner.

      (2) **Children** raised by gay or lesbian parents **show no differences in development or functioning** when compared with children raised by heterosexual parents.

3. **Family demographic data and trends**

   a. The median **age at first marriage is increasing** in the United States and currently is approximately 27 years of age for men and 25 years of age for women.

   b. **Most people marry:** 74% have married by age 35, and 95% have married by age 65.

   c. **Family size is declining.**

      (1) In the United States, the average family includes 3.14 members.

      (2) About **13%** of married couples **do not have children.**

   d. In **68%** of families with children, **both parents are employed.**

   e. **Unmarried partners** are present in 5.2% of all households, and this percentage is increasing.

      (1) About 40% of these households include children.

      (2) **Cohabitation** before marriage is associated with an **increased rate of divorce.**

> About 52% of black children live in a single-parent household with their mother.

B. Divorce
- Divorce **increases** the risk of **physical and mental health problems** among affected adults and children.
  1. **Statistics**
      a. The **United States has the highest divorce rate worldwide;** nearly half of recent first marriages will end in divorce.
      b. Divorce rates are **highest during the early years of marriage;** first marriages that end in divorce last an average of 7–8 years.
      c. Most divorces occur in **families with children under the age of 18.**
      d. About **75%** of divorced individuals **remarry** after divorcing from a first marriage. The overall rate of remarriage is **higher in men.**
  2. **Factors that increase the risk of divorce**
      a. Young age at marriage
      b. Differing socioeconomic or religious backgrounds
      c. Premarital pregnancy
      d. Low socioeconomic status
      e. Death of a child
      f. Short courtship
      g. Limited family support
  3. **Effects of divorce on adults**
      a. The rates of **death, cancer,** and **infectious diseases** are higher in divorced adults than in single, widowed, or married adults.
      b. The risk of **suicide** and **substance abuse** is higher among divorced adults than among married adults.
  4. **Effects of divorce on children**
      a. Children of divorce are reported to be more **aggressive,** to have more **problems in social relationships,** to have **lower self-esteem,** and to exhibit **lower academic performance** than children from intact families.
      b. **Adolescents** are at increased risk of **dropping out of high school,** developing a **substance abuse problem,** becoming **depressed,** and committing **suicide.**
  5. **Custody arrangements**
      a. **Sole legal custody** assigns to one parent all legal rights, including the right to make decisions about children's medical care.
      b. In **joint legal custody,** both parents retain the decision-making power.

C. Adoption
  1. Adoption is the process by which one or two **adults** who are **not the biological parent(s)** of a child **become the legal parent(s).**
  2. Approximately 50% of all adoptions involve adults unrelated to the child; the other 50% involve stepparents or relatives.

Nearly half of all first marriages in the United States end in divorce.

Adolescents whose parents divorce are at increased risk for dropping out of school, substance abuse, depression, and suicide.

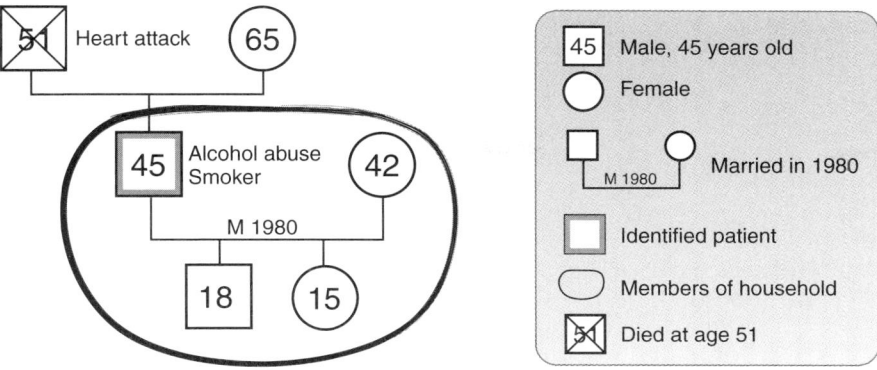

Figure 2-1   Sample genogram.

3. Rates of **emotional and behavioral problems** are higher among adopted children and **increase with the age of the child at adoption.**
D. Family health issues
   1. **Stressful life events**
     a. Several of the most significant sources of stress are related to **disruptions in family relationships** (e.g., death of spouse or child, marital separation, divorce).
     b. Stressful life events are associated with an **increased risk of illness** (see Chapter 3).
     c. The **death of a spouse** is associated with an increased rate of death for the surviving spouse during the first 6 months following the loss, especially for elderly men.
     d. **Social support systems** buffer the negative effects of illness.
       (1) The **family**, and particularly **marriage**, typically are the **most important** sources of social support for an individual.
       (2) A supportive marital relationship has a **positive** effect on **physical** and **mental health.**
   2. **Health behaviors** (e.g., smoking, exercise, eating habits) and health **beliefs** (e.g., when to consult a physician) are strongly **influenced by the family.**
   3. Medical **crises** and **chronic illness** require significant **adaptation by family** members, who are often the primary caregivers.
   4. **Family-oriented medical care** treats the patient within the context of the family.
     a. The **genogram** is a diagrammatic method of collecting information about the patient's nuclear and extended family, including family medical history (Figure 2-1).
     b. Identification of the **family life cycle stage** allows the physician to provide anticipatory guidance

Disruptions in family relationships are among the most stressful life events and are associated with an increased risk of illness.

A supportive marriage helps promote physical and mental health.

and assist families who experience problems during the transition between stages. These stages are:
  (1) Unattached young adult
  (2) New couple
  (3) Family with young children
  (4) Family with adolescents
  (5) Launching children
  (6) Family in later life

II. **Influence of Socioeconomic Status on Health**
  A. **Socioeconomic status** (SES) is measured by indicators such as **education, occupation**, and **income.**
  B. Compared with individuals in higher socioeconomic brackets, those with **low SES:**
    1. Have **shorter life expectancies**
    2. Have **higher rates of diseases** (e.g., chronic, infectious, parasitic), **death**, and **disability**
    3. Make **less frequent use of health care services**
  C. **Barriers to use of health care services by people with low SES**
    1. Decreased access
    2. Lack of health insurance or lack of money to pay for health care
    3. Lack of transportation
    4. Negative experiences with the health care system
    5. Inadequate knowledge of available health care services
  D. **Common health behaviors exhibited by people with low SES**
    1. Delay in seeking medical attention, resulting in more severe presentations
    2. More frequent use of emergency departments and clinics
    3. More frequent use of home remedies
  E. **Common risk factors** for a variety of diseases experienced by people with low SES
    1. Unsafe neighborhoods with inadequate housing
    2. Polluted environments and hazardous jobs
    3. Higher levels of stress
    4. Less healthy lifestyles (e.g., smoking, inadequate diet)

III. **Culture and Health**
  A. **Definition of culture**
    1. An **integrated pattern of human behavior** that includes thoughts, communications, actions, customs, beliefs, values, institutions, technology, goods, and structures of a group
    2. Provides an expected way of viewing the world (**world view**), acting, and thinking
  B. **Characteristics of cultural groups**
    1. Cultural groups *are **not* restricted to racial or ethnic groups** but can be based on such characteristics as religion, occupation, age, or disability.
      • Each individual is a member of many cultural groups

> Low SES is associated with less frequent use of health care services.

(e.g., African American, Protestant, female, middle-aged, physician).
2. **Differences between individuals within these groups** result from factors such as:
   a. Socioeconomic status
   b. Age
   c. Place of residence (e.g., urban, rural)
   d. Religion
   e. Acculturation level
   f. Length of time in the United States, if an immigrant
3. **Stereotyping** occurs when an individual views all individuals in a cultural group as being alike and sharing identical values and beliefs.

C. **Cultural influences on health behaviors**
   1. Culture influences how an individual defines **health and illness,** as well as his or her understanding of the **causes of illness and disease** (e.g., bacteria, evil eye, not being in harmony with nature).
   2. An individual's view of the cause of disease will determine his or her view of appropriate **prevention** and **treatment** measures for the disease, as well as **appropriate healers** to treat the disease.
      Example: Among some traditional Mexican Americans, illness is viewed as being caused by the imbalance of hot and cold in the body. Illness, medications, herbs, and foods are designated as having "hot" and "cold" properties. "Hot" illnesses are treated with "cold" medicines, herbs, or foods, and vice versa.
   3. Culture can influence help-seeking behaviors, attitudes toward conventional health care providers, dietary practices, birth rites, and death rites.
   4. **Use of traditional treatments and healers** is more common among recent immigrants and older, rural, lower income, and non–English-speaking individuals in the United States.
      • Use of traditional Southeast Asian remedies such as coining and cupping may be misinterpreted as child abuse (Box 2-1).
   5. Some patients benefit from **using more than one healing system** to treat a disease (e.g., a physician to treat the symptoms of abdominal pain and a medicine man to treat the perceived cause, which is breaking a taboo).
   6. A patient's **religious beliefs** may **prohibit** the **use of** some or all aspects of **conventional medicine.**
      Example: Jehovah's Witnesses do not allow whole blood transfusions or the use of most blood products. Christian Scientists rely on prayer for healing and reject most medical treatments.

D. **Racial and ethnic populations**
   1. **Majority and minority populations in the United States**

> Stereotyping occurs when all individuals in a cultural group are viewed as being alike.

BOX 2-1 **The Patient Who Is Using Complementary and Alternative Medicine (CAM) Therapy**

A Vietnamese-American woman brings her 2-year-old son to the emergency department because he is coughing and has a fever. When a physician asks the mother to remove her son's shirt, bruises can be seen running in a striped pattern down and across his back. The physician, who has not treated many Asian patients, wonders if the bruises are evidence of child abuse. He consults with a colleague, who recognizes that the marks may be caused by coining, a traditional healing practice. The colleague asks the mother what has been done at home to treat the boy's illness, including use of traditional remedies. She explains that the boy's grandmother tried coining, but it did not seem to help. The mother then brought him to the hospital. The physicians comment on the positive concern that the boy's grandmother showed him and support the mother's decision to bring him to the emergency department for treatment. They agree that a report of child abuse is not indicated.

a. The **majority** population in the United States is **non-Hispanic whites** and comprises **70%** of the general population.

b. The **minority** populations include African Americans, Hispanic Americans, Asian Americans and Pacific Islanders, and Native Americans (American Indians and Alaska Natives).

   (1) A disproportionate number of members of most minority populations live **below** the **poverty level**, and many **receive lower quality health care**.

   (2) Some members of minority populations experience **barriers in accessing the health care system** that are similar to those for people with low SES (see II C 1–5). They may also have **language barriers** that necessitate use of a trained medical interpreter (preferable to family, friends, or untrained clinic staff).

c. Each population includes many **different heritages** (e.g., Chinese, Japanese, and Korean among Asian Americans) as well as **different health traditions**.

d. **Values and beliefs affecting health care** that may be held more often by members of some ethnic and racial minorities than by non-Hispanic whites include:

   (1) **Family involvement** in health care decision-making

   (2) **Respect for elders** and the desire to care for sick elders at home

   (3) A **present** (as opposed to future) **time orientation**, which limits the value placed on preventive health care

2. **African Americans**
   a. One of the largest minority populations in the United States, comprising approximately **12%** of the general population
   b. **Lower life expectancy,** higher infant mortality rate (about twice that of the general population), and higher homicide rate (especially among adolescents and young adults) than the general population
   c. **Higher mortality rates** for heart disease, cancer, stroke, diabetes, influenza, accidents, and HIV than the general population
   d. Highest rate of **low-birth-weight infants** (13%), almost twice that of any other minority population or the population as a whole
   e. **Other health problems:** tuberculosis, hypertension, asthma, and sickle cell disease

African Americans have higher mortality rates for heart disease, cancer, and stroke than does the general population.

3. **Hispanic Americans**
   a. Are the **most rapidly growing minority** population in the United States, currently making up **12.5%** of the general population
   b. **Higher mortality rates** for diabetes, chronic liver disease, homicide, and HIV than the general population
   c. **Other health problems:** tuberculosis, hypertension, gallbladder disease (especially in women), and increased levels of stress for immigrants

4. **Asian Americans and Pacific Islanders**
   a. Comprise almost **4%** of the United States population, with **Southeast Asians** the **most economically disadvantaged** subgroup
   b. Have the **lowest infant mortality** rate and **longest life expectancy** of any minority population and the general population
   c. **Health problems:** tuberculosis, high levels of stress for immigrants, osteoporosis, hepatitis B, thalassemia, and some cancers in various ethnic groups

5. **Native Americans**
   a. The smallest but **most diverse minority** population in the United States, making up **almost 1%** of the general population
   b. Approximately 60% have access to health care from the **Indian Health Service**
   c. **Higher mortality rates** for accidents, diabetes, chronic liver disease, suicide (among male adolescents and young men), and homicide than the general population
   d. **Other health problems:** hypertension, tuberculosis, gallbladder disease, and alcohol abuse in some tribes

IV.   **Multicultural Diversity and Medical Practice**
   A.   **Importance to the physician**
      1.   Physicians should become **culturally competent** to effectively care for an increasingly diverse United States population.
         a.   In 2000, 10% of Americans were foreign born.
         b.   By 2050, about 47% of the population will be members of ethnic and racial minority groups, compared with 28% in 2000.
      2.   Physicians should become familiar with **common characteristics** of cultural groups with whom they interact, but they also must recognize that **each patient is unique** and may share, in varying degrees, the health beliefs, values, and behaviors of other members of his or her cultural group(s).
   B.   **Complementary and alternative medicine**
      1.   Complementary and alternative medicine (CAM) therapies are **used by people in all cultural groups** in the United States.
         a.   Studies suggest that **more than 40%** of the United States population use CAM therapies.
         b.   Most individuals **do *not* discuss** these therapies **with their physicians.**
      2.   **CAM therapies** include:
         a.   **Alternative medical systems** (e.g., traditional Chinese medicine, homeopathic medicine, and naturopathic medicine)
         b.   **Mind-body interventions** (e.g., art therapy, meditation, music therapy, and yoga)
         c.   **Biologically based therapies** (e.g., herbal therapies; diet therapies; orthomolecular therapies, such as magnesium and megavitamins; and biological therapies, such as bee pollen and shark cartilage)
         d.   **Manipulative and body-based methods** (e.g., chiropractic, massage therapy, and reflexology)
         e.   **Energy therapies** (e.g., therapeutic touch, qi gong, and magnets)
      3.   CAM therapies can be **therapeutic, neutral, or harmful;** many have not been studied sufficiently to know their effectiveness.

Racial and ethnic minority groups make up an increasing percentage of the US population.

Behavioral Medicine

I. Overview

A. **Behavioral medicine** is a multidisciplinary field that focuses on biological, social, and psychological influences on health and illness. Areas of emphasis include **health promotion**, **disease prevention**, and the **modification of disease-related risk factors**.

B. **Interventions** are directed at various health-related behaviors (e.g., tobacco use, diet), **health problems** (e.g., chronic pain, cardiovascular disease), and **psychosocial factors** (e.g., stress, social support, personality characteristics).

    1. **Commonly used interventions** include stress management training, relaxation training, psychoeducation, pain management, and cognitive-behavioral techniques.

    2. **Behavioral interventions** can lead to improved physical and emotional health as well as to reduced health-care costs and utilization.

II. Stress and Illness

• Problems associated with stress account for **more than 70% of visits to primary care physicians.**

A. Definition

    1. **Stress** is experienced when the **demands** placed on an individual **strain or exceed the individual's resources.**

    2. Stress can be viewed as a **stimulus** (e.g., noise, illness), a **response** (e.g., emotional distress), or an **interaction**

Death of a spouse is rated as the most severe stressor.

17

between the individual and the environment (e.g., an interplay between a person's perceptions and external demands).

B. Mechanisms by which stress may affect health
  1. **Behavioral effects**
     a. Changes in daily eating and sleep routines
     b. Social withdrawal
     c. Decreased help-seeking behavior
     d. Maladaptive coping responses (e.g., illicit drug use)
  2. **Influences (direct or indirect) on immune and physiologic functions**
     a. **Stress** can lead to **immune suppression.** Changes in immune function have been observed in:
        (1) Medical students undergoing examination stress
        (2) Women undergoing marital separation
        (3) Caregivers of persons with Alzheimer's disease
        (4) Bereaved individuals
     b. **Associated medical conditions linked to stress**
        (1) Asthma
        (2) Coronary artery disease
        (3) Hypertension
        (4) Irritable bowel syndrome
        (5) Rheumatoid arthritis
        (6) Tension and migraine headaches

C. Physiologic response to stress
  1. The stress response involves activation of the **hypothalamic-pituitary-adrenal axis (HPA),** which orchestrates the body's response to a threat (Figure 3-1).
  2. **Activation of the HPA** leads to the release of the following substances:
     a. Corticotropin-releasing factor (CRF) from the hypothalamus
     b. Adrenocorticotropic hormone (ACTH) from the pituitary gland
     c. Corticosteroids from the adrenal cortex
  3. **Stimulation of the sympathetic nervous system** results in the release of:
     a. Norepinephrine
     b. Epinephrine
  4. **Endorphins** are released.

D. General adaptation syndrome
  1. Introduced by **Hans Selye,** this syndrome describes **the body's response to stress,** including chronic stress.
     a. The **adaptation response** consists of three stages:
        (1) **Alarm stage,** in which the body's resources are mobilized
        (2) **Resistance stage,** in which the body resists or adapts to the stressor
        (3) **Exhaustion stage,** in which resources are depleted, resulting in illness and, conceivably, death

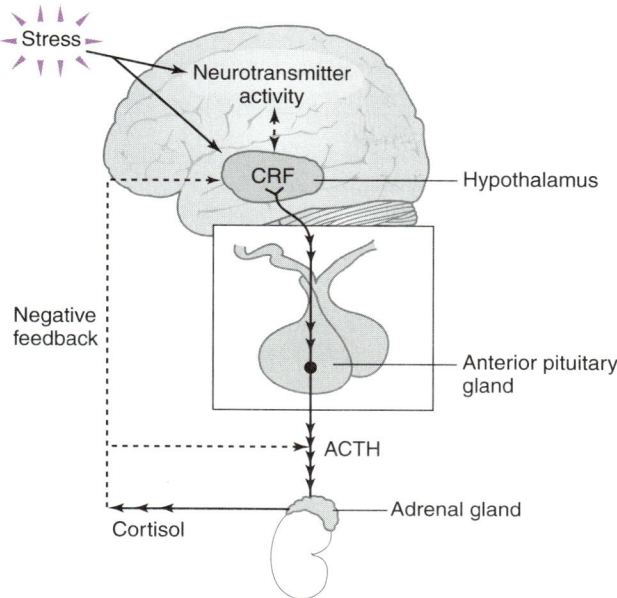

Figure 3-1   The hypothalamic-pituitary-adrenal (HPA) axis is activated during the stress response. *ACTH,* adrenocorticotropic hormone; *CRF,* corticotropin-releasing factor.

    b. This **nonspecific physiologic response** is activated regardless of the nature of the stressor.

   2. Current perspectives acknowledge the **role of psychological factors**, such as how a person appraises an event, as important in mediating the stress response.

E. **Stress and the risk of illness**

   1. Stressors include both **major life events** and **minor daily circumstances** ("hassles"), such as waiting in traffic.

   2. They may be viewed as **positive** (e.g., marriage) or **negative** (e.g., unemployment).

   3. The **Social Readjustment Rating Scale**, developed by **Thomas Holmes** and **Richard Rahe**, lists various life events and quantifies the magnitude of change (life change units) associated with these events (Table 3-1).

      • Although greater life stress is correlated with illness, **the relationship between life stress and illness is modest.**

   4. Minor daily hassles are associated with illness.

F. **Potential modifiers of the stress response**

   1. Stressful circumstances affect individuals in different ways. Two factors that influence an **individual's response to stress** are:

     a. **Appraisal of the situation**

        (1) An individual's appraisal, or **interpretation**, of a situation influences how the individual will respond to that event.

Major life events and daily hassles are linked to an increased risk of illness.

TABLE 3-1   Values Assigned to Selected Life Events in the Social Readjustment Rating Scale

Life Event	Value
Death of a spouse	100
Marriage	50
Being terminated from work	47
Retirement from work	45
Pregnancy	40
Change in residence	20
Change in school	20

(2) The appraisal process involves determining the **consequences of the event** for the individual (e.g., irrelevant, positive-benign, stressful) and the individual's **coping resources** available to manage the event.
Example: A medical school examination is postponed because a professor is ill. A student who is well-prepared for the examination views the delay as irrelevant, whereas a student who needs extra time to study views the delay as positive. A third student, who plans to be out of town on the rescheduled test date, experiences the delay as stressful.

b. **Social support**
(1) Social support is described as the **comfort and assistance an individual derives from others.** It can be of a practical nature (e.g., offering a ride, giving money) or an emotional nature (e.g., consoling a friend who is crying, providing encouragement).
(2) Social support has been shown to **benefit health**, perhaps by acting as a buffer against stress.
(3) An individual's **perception** of social support, not simply the quantity of support, **is important.**
(4) The family is an important source of support; **married** couples have **lower mortality rates** than single, divorced, or widowed individuals.

2. **Other psychosocial influences on stress and health** (Table 3-2)

a. **Personality style:** the **type A** behavior pattern is a well-known behavioral factor associated with **coronary artery disease.**

b. **Psychological factors:** perceived control, psychological "hardiness," and **optimism** appear to benefit health.

c. **Religious commitment:** studies suggest that religious commitment is associated with improved physical and mental health.

Type A behavior pattern is a risk factor for coronary artery disease.

TABLE 3-2 Psychological and Personality Factors That May Influence Health

Factor	Definition	Example
Type A behavior pattern	Characterized by competitiveness, time urgency, impatience, cynicism, and hostility (the latter associated with coronary artery disease)	A 55-year-old man becomes agitated by the slow pace in a work meeting and openly criticizes colleagues for their incompetent leadership style.
Locus of control	Internal locus of control: a belief that a person can control what happens to him or her and that these actions have an effect on the outcome	A diabetic patient diligently follows her treatment and dietary regimen, believing that her consistent adherence will greatly improve her health status.
	External locus of control: a belief that an individual *cannot* control outcomes and that good things that do happen are the result of luck or chance	A diabetic patient has little faith that anything will improve her diabetes; thus she inconsistently takes her medicines and rarely follows her prescribed diet.
Psychological "hardiness"	"Hardy" individuals show a commitment to other individuals and activities in their lives, feel a sense of control over their lives, and view stressors as challenges and opportunities for growth	A 50-year-old woman who is overweight is diagnosed with diabetes. Her physician recommends treating her condition initially with diet, exercise, and weight loss. The patient views these lifestyle changes as an opportunity to become healthier. She joins a local weight loss group and begins walking daily.
Self-efficacy	A person's belief that he or she can successfully engage in a desired behavior	A 53-year-old smoker is encouraged to quit smoking by his physician. The patient, who has quit before, believes he can successfully quit again and agrees to set a quit date.
Coping style	Problem-focused coping: actively taking steps to manage a stressful event	A woman recently diagnosed with multiple sclerosis copes by reading extensively about the disease and asking others with the illness for advice on coping with it.
	Emotion-focused coping: taking steps to modify one's emotional response to a stressful event	Another woman, given the same diagnosis, tries to avoid thinking about her disease.
	Coping strategies can be adaptive (e.g., asking for help) or maladaptive (e.g., delaying seeking care)	
Prior learning (e.g., personal experience; family models for responding to illness)	Experiences the individual has had directly or indirectly (e.g., seeing an event, or hearing about an event from someone else)	A 32-year-old woman with a lump in her breast refuses to undergo a biopsy. She relates that her mother, who died from breast cancer, underwent a rigorous chemotherapy regimen, which didn't spare her life. The patient refuses to subject herself to the same fate.

TABLE 3-3   Factors Influencing Adherence to Medical Treatment

Factor	Characteristics Associated with Decreased Adherence
Treatment regimen	Increased duration of regimen Increased complexity of regimen Increased need for lifestyle or behavioral change Lack of reinforcing events following adherence (e.g., symptoms persist despite taking medication) Presence of aversive events following adherence (e.g., unpleasant side effects)
Illness	Asymptomatic illness
Physician-patient relationship	Lack of positive physician-patient relationship Physician style that is unfriendly and impersonal
Health beliefs of patient	Low perception of vulnerability to disease Low perception of negative consequences, if illness occurred (e.g., "If I get sick, it isn't that important") Belief that costs of adherence behavior outweigh benefits Doubt about efficacy of treatment
Knowledge and attitudes	Lack of knowledge about illness Lack of knowledge about treatment rationale Lack of knowledge about how to engage in regimen or lack of skill Lack of belief (self-efficacy) by the patient that he or she can successfully engage in the desired behavior
Health care system	Poor continuity of care from visit to visit (e.g., different providers) Longer time waiting in office Lengthy interval between scheduling of appointment and actual visit
Social and cultural environment	Little or no support from family or social network to be adherent Cultural values that conflict with desired changes Limited access to care (e.g., lack of transportation, finances, child care)
Psychiatric status	Depression, substance abuse, and psychosis

III.   Adherence to Treatment Regimens
  A.   Overview
   1.   Adherence refers to the extent to which patients follow medical treatment and advice.
   2.   Adherence is often used synonymously with the term "**compliance.**" However, **adherence** denotes a more **collaborative relationship** between the patient and physician in achieving health goals.
   3.   Nonadherence is a significant problem in the clinical setting.
  B.   Factors influencing adherence (Table 3-3)
   1.   Adherence tends to decrease over time.
   2.   Patient satisfaction with the **physician-patient relationship** is strongly correlated with **improved adherence.**

3. **Psychiatric illness** can affect adherence, but its impact must be considered on an individual basis.
Example: A depressed woman, feeling hopeless about her future, sees no reason to take the antidepressant medication prescribed by her physician. On the other hand, a man with bipolar disorder is grateful for medication that has helped to stabilize his mood.
4. Adherence is *not* associated with a specific personality type or demographic profile (i.e., gender, ethnicity, marital status, intelligence, educational attainment, socioeconomic status).
C. **Strategies for improving adherence**
1. Promote a positive physician-patient relationship
2. Use good communication skills
3. Encourage the patient's participation in decision-making
4. Negotiate treatment goals whenever possible
5. Simplify treatment regimens
6. Anticipate problems with adherence in advance

IV. **Behavioral Counseling for the Modification of Health-Risk Behaviors**
A. **Overview**
1. **Behavioral factors** (e.g., tobacco use, excessive alcohol use) contribute to **morbidity** and **mortality** from many diseases; changes in these health-risk behaviors prevent many deaths each year.
2. **Physicians** have an important role in helping patients reduce their health-risk behaviors. Specific **counseling techniques** are available to help patients make behavioral changes (see Chapter 11).
3. Behavioral change usually occurs over time.
B. **Patient factors affecting behavioral change**
1. **Readiness for change**
a. A patient's stage of change is an important consideration in planning an intervention for behavioral change.
b. **James Prochaska** and **Carlo DiClemente** described **readiness for change** as occurring on a **continuum** with several stages:
(1) **Precontemplation:** *not* thinking about change
(2) **Contemplation:** considering change in the near future
(3) **Preparation:** planning for change
(4) **Action:** actively having made the desired change
(5) **Maintenance:** sustaining changes over time
c. **Interventions** that **correspond to** an individual's **readiness** for change are more likely to succeed (Box 3-1).
2. Knowledge of relevant **health information** (e.g., knowledge of one's illness, rationale for treatment)
3. **Motivation** for change and **confidence in ability to change**

BOX 3-1	The Patient Who Is in the Precontemplation Stage of Change

A 54-year-old man, who recently had a myocardial infarction, is counseled by his physician about the health benefits of quitting smoking and is advised to quit. Despite this feedback, the patient does not believe that his smoking is a problem and does not want to quit. The physician asks the patient to give further thought to quitting, indicates a willingness to help the patient when he feels ready to quit, and makes a note to ask the patient at the next visit about his interest in quitting smoking.

BOX 3-2	The Patient Who Is Ready to Quit Smoking

A 44-year-old woman, who smokes two packs of cigarettes per day, wants to quit smoking by her 45th birthday. She has been delaying smoking for brief periods whenever she feels the urge to smoke and has reduced her daily consumption to about 15 cigarettes a day. Her physician supports her decision to quit smoking and discusses treatment options to help with cessation. The patient agrees to set a quit date in 2 weeks and to try prescribed medication. The physician briefly counsels the patient about coping strategies for cessation, provides literature, and makes a follow-up appointment. He arranges for the nurse to call the patient several days after the scheduled quit date to provide support and address any problems.

    4. Social support
    5. Knowledge of **behavioral strategies** (Box 3-2; see Chapter 11)
        a. Strategies that promote behavioral change can include goal-setting, self-monitoring, and use of rewards.
        b. **Relapse prevention skills** aid in maintaining desired changes over time.

V. **Psychosocial Aspects of Pain**
    A. Overview
        1. **Pain** is a common complaint in the clinical setting.
        2. It is a **subjective phenomenon**, described as a sensory and emotional experience.
        3. An individual's **perception of pain** is influenced by the degree of tissue damage and by psychosocial factors (e.g., depression, anxiety, expectations about pain, the personal meaning an individual attributes to pain, and sociocultural factors).
    B. Types of pain
        1. Acute pain
            a. Acute pain is associated with an **injury** or a **disease** process, **sympathetic arousal**, and **anxiety**.

Depression and anxiety can augment pain.

BOX 3-3	**The Patient With Chronic Pain**

A 48-year-old man with chronic low back pain is reassured by his physician that all appropriate medical measures are being used to manage his pain. The physician suggests that the patient gradually resume some of his usual activities, as best he can, despite the continued pain. At a follow-up visit, the patient is asked about whether he has been able to engage in some of these activities and about his family's response to his pain. The patient responds that his family is "wonderful," stating that they insist that he rest at the slightest "hint" of pain and that they take over his responsibilities at those times. Upon hearing this, the physician wonders whether the family, although well-intended, is inadvertently reinforcing the patient's pain-related behaviors. He suggests a family meeting to discuss ways in which the family can help the patient with his recovery.

      b. **Interventions** focus on **diminishing pain** and removing the noxious stimulus.
  2. **Chronic pain**
      a. Chronic **pain persists beyond** the **typical healing time** or for **more than 6 months.**
      b. It is associated with **excessive disability.**
      c. **Interventions** are aimed at reducing suffering and **optimizing functioning**, even if pain cannot be directly diminished.
C. **Psychiatric comorbidity and chronic pain**
  1. Chronic pain is frequently associated with **depression** and is an independent risk factor for **suicide.**
  2. It may be comorbid with anxiety, substance use, somatoform disorders, and personality disorders.
  3. In **women**, a history of **abuse** is associated with chronic pain.
D. **Theories of pain**
  1. The **operant model** of pain highlights the role of **external consequences** (e.g., increased attention from others, avoidance of unpleasant activities) in influencing pain behavior (Box 3-3).
  2. The **cognitive model** of pain highlights the role of **cognitive factors** (e.g., an individual's belief in his or her ability to manage pain) in influencing pain.
  3. The **gate control theory**, developed by **Ronald Melzack** and **Patrick Wall**, describes a "gating" mechanism at the spinal cord that modulates the flow of information from peripheral and descending pathways. This theory describes a manner by which psychological influences can modulate the perception of pain.
E. **Pain assessment**
  1. **Direct inquiry** about the severity of a patient's pain aids in the assessment of the patient's pain status.

Chronic pain is a risk factor for suicide.

2. **Self-report methods of pain assessment** include:
    a. **Numeric rating scales,** in which pain is rated on a 0–10 scale
    b. **Visual analogue scales,** in which pain is rated by placing a mark reflecting pain intensity on a horizontal line
    c. **Faces scales** for **pediatric patients,** in which pain is rated by choosing among faces ranging from sad to happy

F. **Management of chronic pain**
    1. **Various modalities may be used:**
        a. **Nonsurgical** (e.g., transcutaneous electrical nerve stimulation, physical therapy)
        b. **Surgical** (e.g., nerve blocks)
        c. **Psychological and behavioral** (e.g., cognitive-behavioral therapy, biofeedback)
        d. **Pharmacologic**
            (1) **Analgesics, antidepressants,** and other pharmacotherapies (see Tables 10-3 and 10-5)
            (2) Patients experiencing pain may be **undermedicated** for various reasons, such as a stoic attitude toward pain or concern about addiction. In the clinical setting, however, patients with pain seldom become addicted to opioid analgesics.
            (3) **Scheduled administration of analgesic medication,** rather than pain-contingent administration, can help minimize the association between the presence of pain and the delivery of medication.
    2. **A multidisciplinary approach** can yield significant clinical benefits:
        a. Increased functional status
        b. Improved physical conditioning
        c. Decreased medication usage
        d. Enhanced coping skills
        e. Possibly decreased pain complaints
    3. **Reinforcing wellness-oriented patient behavior,** such as when a patient appropriately increases activity levels, is also an important component of care.

VI. **The Placebo Effect**

About 33% of subjects respond to placebos.

A. The placebo effect refers to **an improvement in health that occurs in conjunction with an inactive treatment** (e.g., an inert substance is given).
B. The placebo effect is believed to be **mediated by endogenous opioids.** The expectations of the patient are believed to influence the response.

4

Biological Basis of Behavior

Target Topics

▶ Anatomic and physiologic aspects of neurotransmission
▶ Classification and actions of neurotransmitters
▶ Psychiatric manifestations of neuroendocrine dysfunction
▶ Genetic component of psychiatric disorders

I. Neuroanatomy

A. The **central nervous system** (CNS), which consists of the brain and spinal cord, integrates incoming physiologic and environmental stimuli to coordinate a behavioral response.

    1. The **two cerebral hemispheres** are functionally lateralized but connected by commissures that are highly interactive.

        a. The **dominant hemisphere** controls **language organization** and **meaning.**
            • The **left hemisphere** is the dominant hemisphere in 95% of the population, including 70% of left-handed individuals.

        b. The **nondominant hemisphere** controls **visual-spatial organization** and **prosody** (i.e., emotional inflection of language).

        c. **Each hemisphere** controls **contralateral movement** and **sensory input.**

    2. **Dysfunction of specific CNS structures** has been linked to several behavioral symptoms (Table 4-1).

TABLE 4-1   Central Nervous System Structures and Associated Dysfunctions

Structure	Function	Dysfunction
Frontal lobes	Executive thinking Language Voluntary motor action based on interpretation of sensory input	Depression Mood lability Amotivation Disinhibition Broca's aphasia
Temporal lobes	Auditory and language comprehension (dominant hemisphere) Memory	Wernicke's aphasia Hallucinations associated with temporal lobe seizures
Limbic system (cortical and subcortical structures, consisting of hippocampus, amygdala, anterior nucleus of thalamus, mamillary body, cingulate gyrus)	Memory formation Assignment of emotional response to experiences and sensations	Korsakoff's amnesia (alcohol and thiamine deficiency related to bilateral hippocampal damage) Dementia Personality and mood changes Klüver-Bucy syndrome (hyperorality, reduced aggression or rage, increased sexual behavior resulting from lesions of amygdala)
Parietal lobes	Somatosensory and symbol perception along with motor integration	Right-sided lesions: apraxia, left-sided neglect Left-sided lesions: agraphia, acalculia; no right-left discrimination
Occipital lobes	Sight and visual perception	Cortical blindness Agnosia Inability to recognize objects
Reticular activating system	Alertness Sleep-wake cycles Rapid eye movement (REM) sleep	Altered mood and other psychiatric disorders, including attention-deficit/hyperactivity disorder
Basal ganglia (substantia nigra, caudate nucleus, putamen, globus pallidus)	Extrapyramidal motor system, which prevents extraneous movements and behaviors	Disorders of repetitive movement, behavior and thought (obsessive-compulsive symptoms, choreoathetotic movements, tics, parkinsonian symptoms)

> **B.** The **peripheral nervous system** (PNS) includes all **sensory** and **motor pathways** to and from the CNS.
> **C.** The **autonomic nervous system** controls involuntary functions.
>> **1.** **Two types of efferent nerves** modulate visceral responses through inhibitory and excitatory actions.
>>> **a.** **Sympathetic fibers** mediate peripheral effects pri-

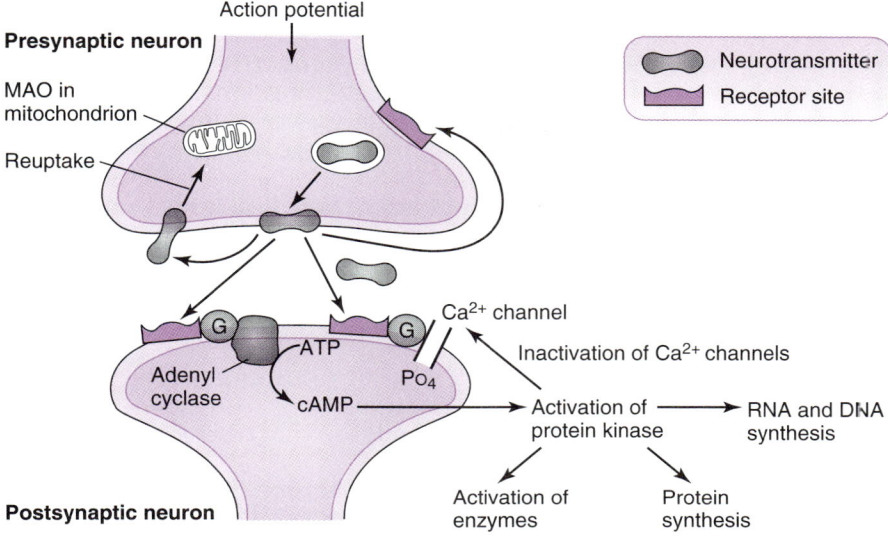

Figure 4-1   Schematic representation of neurotransmitter and second messenger activity involved in neurotransmission. *ATP,* adenosine triphosphate; *cAMP,* cyclic adenosine monophosphate; *Ca²⁺,* calcium; *G,* G protein; *MAO,* monoamine oxidase; *Po₄,* phosphate.

        marily through the release of **norepinephrine** (e.g., increasing blood pressure and heart rate).

    b.   **Parasympathetic fibers** inhibit sympathetic responses through the release of **acetylcholine** to end organs (e.g., decreasing heart rate).

  2. The autonomic system translates emotional information to visceral responses, and this interplay may induce or exacerbate illness (e.g., increasing bronchoconstriction in asthma).

II.   Neurotransmission

  A. **Physiology of neurotransmission**

    1. **Nerve cell bodies** originate in CNS structures, and their **axons** branch to distribute information to other neurons through neurochemically created **action potentials.**

    2. Neurotransmission occurs when **depolarization** triggers electrical stimulation, which in turn causes the **release of neurotransmitters** into the synaptic cleft, the space between the presynaptic axon and the postsynaptic nerve cell process (dendrite). There are trillions of such synaptic connections throughout the body.

    3. **Neurotransmitters** cross the synaptic cleft and **bind to specific receptor sites,** causing conformational changes through G proteins at the site and initiating one (of two) type of response (Figure 4-1).

        a. **Changes in ion channels:** in this response, receptor binding may change the cellular ion channels, making the cell more polarized (Cl⁻ entering, K⁺ leaving) or less polarized (Na⁺ and Ca²⁺ entering),

Messages are transmitted by action potentials modulated by neurotransmitters.

Neurotransmitters act on ion channels or on second messenger systems linked to their specific receptor sites.

thereby **inhibiting or initiating electrical transmission,** respectively.

b. **Responses by second messengers:** in this response, receptor binding may lead to responses by second messengers, producing a cascade of intracellular events that result in long-range, genetically based changes.

   (1) **Activation of adenyl cyclase** leads to phosphorylation, via adenosine triphosphate (ATP), of protein kinases, thereby changing their conformation and activity.

   (2) **Phosphorylated enzymes** activate synthesis of neurotransmitters.

   (3) **Phosphorylation of ribosomal proteins** controls protein synthesis.

   (4) **Calcium channels** are **inactivated,** also by phosphorylation.

   (5) **Phosphorylation of transcription factors** leads to control and synthesis of DNA and RNA.

B. **Classification of neurotransmitters**
   • The **three major classes** of neurotransmitters are **biogenic amines, amino acids,** and **neuropeptides.** Characteristics of the major neurotransmitters within each class are summarized in Table 4-2.

   1. **Biogenic amine neurotransmitters:** dopamine, norepinephrine, serotonin, acetylcholine, and histamine

   2. **Amino acid neurotransmitters:** gamma aminobutyric acid (GABA), glutamate, and glycine

   3. **Neuropeptides:** enkephalins, endorphins, dynorphins, substance P, cholecystokinin, neurotensin, vasopressin, and oxytocin

C. **Regulation of neurotransmission**
   1. **Neurotransmitter levels and activity** at the synapse are regulated through coordination of the following mechanisms:

      a. **Initial synthesis** of neurotransmitters is subject to the intracellular availability of precursors.

      b. Neurotransmitters may be taken back into the presynaptic cell **(reuptake)** to be **degraded by monoamine oxidase** (MAO) or to be re-released into the synapse.

      c. Neurotransmitters can **bind to autoreceptors** on the presynaptic neuron from which they were released. This action serves as a **negative feedback** mechanism, leading to a reduction in further release of the neurotransmitter.

   2. Various **pharmacologic agents** may act at receptor sites to **block** or **enhance neurotransmitter binding.**
      Example: Haloperidol blocks D_2 receptors, resulting in antipsychotic actions.

Alteration in the level or activity of neurotransmitters is linked to specific psychiatric symptoms and disorders.

D. **Effects of altered neurotransmission** (see Table 4-2)

1. The availability and receptor binding of specific neu-
    rotransmitters is a basic **determinant of mental health.**
2. The **associations among neurotransmitters** are highly
    complex. Evidence for these associations is based on me-
    tabolite levels in body fluids, as well as the observed re-
    sponse to pharmacologic agonists and antagonists.
    Example: Low levels of GABA may lead to increased glu-
    tamate release.

III. Neuroendocrinology

A. The **endocrine system** strongly influences **mood** and symptoms of **anxiety.**

B. **Changes in production and availability of thyroid
hormone** can lead to symptoms of increased anxiety, poor
concentration, emotional lability, memory impairment, depression, and psychosis.
1. Levels of thyroid-stimulating hormone **(TSH)**, thyroxine
    (T_4), and free triiodothyronine (T_3) should be obtained as
    part of a screening evaluation for psychiatric disorders
    (see Chapter 9).
2. **Lithium therapy** may lead to **hypothyroidism** in about
    10% of treated patients.

C. **Dysfunction of the hypothalamic-pituitary-adrenal axis**
(HPA) can lead to mood and anxiety disorders.
1. **Cushing's syndrome**, which results in **hypercortisolism**
    (high levels of cortisol), is associated with psychiatric
    symptoms such as delirium, mood and personality
    changes, and symptoms of anxiety.
2. **Hypocortisolism** (low levels of cortisol) may lead to
    paranoia and mood disorders.
3. **Failure of the negative feedback loop** and **hypersecre-
    tion of cortisol** may occur secondary to hypersecre-
    tion of corticotropin-releasing factor **(CRF)**, despite ele-
    vated levels of cortisol in the bloodstream.
    • This response is demonstrated in the **dexamethasone
      suppression test** by the patient's inability to suppress
      cortisol release upon administration of dexamethasone.
4. CRF initiates the main initial stress response (see Figure
    3-1); thus, **hypersecretion of CRF** is implicated in
    some **anxiety disorders.**

D. **Hypoparathyroidism and hyperparathyroidism** may lead
to personality changes and delirium.

IV. Behavioral Genetics

A. The manifestation of behavioral traits and psychiatric disorders in any individual is a result of the action of **biological, psychosocial,** and **environmental factors** on genetics.

B. **Types of genetic studies**
• Several types of studies provide evidence of the involvement
  of genetic factors in the development of many psychiatric
  disorders (Table 4-3).

Psychiatric disorders
may occur when
psychosocial and
environmental influ-
ences act on ge-
netically vulnerable
individuals.

TABLE 4-2 Neurotransmitters and Associated Psychiatric Conditions

Class/Neurotransmitter	Distribution	Receptor Type	Psychiatric Condition and Impact
Biogenic Amines			
Dopamine (DA) Type: Catecholamine Precursor: Tyrosine Metabolite: Homovanillic acid (HVA)	Nigrostriatal tract: regulates muscle tone and movement Tuberoinfundibular tract: regulates prolactin secretion from pituitary Mesolimbic and mesocortical tracts: modulate mood and reality-based thought and behavior	D_1–D_5 D_2 has most important behavioral associations	↑ DA activity: schizophrenia and other psychoses ↓ DA activity: Parkinson's disease and depression DA activity is implicated in the brain's reward system and in addiction
Norepinephrine (NE) Type: Catecholamine Precursor: Tyrosine→dopamine→NE Metabolite: 3-methoxy-4-hydroxyphenglycol (MHPG)	Neurons originate in locus ceruleus, with projections to forebrain (including amygdala and hypothalamus), cerebellum, and spinal cord	α_1, α_2, β_1, β_2	↑ NE activity: anxiety ↓ NE activity: depression
Serotonin (5-HT) Type: Indoleamine Precursor: Tryptophan Metabolite: 5-hydroxyindoleacetic acid (5-HIAA)	Neurons originate in raphe nucleus and are widely distributed to basal ganglia, limbic system, and cerebral cortex	More than 14 receptors identified; 5-HT$_1$, 5-HT$_2$, and 5-HT$_3$ most often associated with behavioral and pharmacologic effects	↑ 5-HT: psychosis ↓ 5-HT: depression and anxiety Low levels of 5-HIAA: found in body fluids of individuals displaying aggressive and suicidal behaviors
Acetylcholine Type: Quaternary amine Precursor: Acetyl coenzyme A and choline Metabolites: Choline and acetic acid (by acetylcholinesterase)	Projection from nucleus basalis of Meynert to cerebral cortex and limbic system Also found in reticular activating system and thalamus	Muscarinic and nicotinic	Memory deficits and dementia (e.g., Alzheimer's dementia)
Histamine (H) Type: Ethylamine	Neurons in hypothalamus projecting to cerebral cortex, limbic system, and thalamus	H_1–H_3	Histaminic side effects (e.g., weight gain and drowsiness) of many psychopharmacologic agents
Amino Acids			
γ-Aminobutyric acid (GABA) Metabolite: Glutamic acid	Widely distributed throughout brain as primary inhibitory neurotransmitter, with receptors on many types of neurons	GABA$_A$ and GABA$_C$ act directly on Cl$^-$ channels, facilitating influx and hyperpolarization GABA$_B$ sites are G protein–associated, acting via second messengers	Underactivity: anxiety disorders, withdrawal syndromes (e.g., alcohol withdrawal), and onset of seizure activity

Neurotransmitter	Receptor/Mechanism	Distribution	Significance
Glutamate Precursors: Glucose and glutamine Metabolite: Glutamic acid	N-methyl-D-aspartate (NMDA) and non-NMDA Receptors work in concert with depolarization, binding of glutamate and glycine, and expulsion of Mg^{2+} at receptor to allow influx of Na^+ and Ca^{2+}	Diffusely distributed as principal excitatory neurotransmitter of central nervous system	Excessive glutamate receptor stimulation: may cause neurotoxicity as a result of increased concentrations of Ca^{2+} and nitrous oxide ↓ NMDA receptor activity, seen with use of PCP (phencyclidine hydrochloride): may cause psychosis ↑ Glutamate: withdrawal syndromes and seizure activity Antagonists cause convulsions
Glycine	Cl^- channels May act together with glutamate as excitatory neurotransmitter on NMDA receptor, or alone as inhibitory neurotransmitter	Widely distributed, with highest concentration in spinal cord	
Neuropeptides			
Enkephalins, endorphins, dynorphins Type: Endogenous opioids	δ, μ, κ	Nerve cell bodies in medial hypothalamus, diencephalon, pons, hippocampus, and midbrain, with diffuse projection of axons	Endogenous analgesia Associated with reward system in addiction May play a role in anxiety and depression
Substance P	—		Identified primarily in neurotransmission of pain perception but also implicated in depressive states, Alzheimer's dementia, and Huntington's disease
Cholecystokinin	—		Implicated in schizophrenia, eating disorders, and movement disorders Triggers panic attacks in individuals with panic disorder
Neurotensin	—	Coexists with DA in some axons	Implicated in pathophysiology of schizophrenia
Vasopressin and oxytocin	—	Synthesized in hypothalamus, with release in the posterior pituitary	May be involved in regulation of mood

—, not known or certain.

TABLE 4-3 Psychiatric Disorders and Associated Familial Risk

Psychiatric Disorder	Lifetime Prevalence	Risk in First-degree Relatives	Risk in Monozygotic Twins	Other Disorders With Higher Risk in Relatives
Schizophrenia	1%	10%	50%	Schizoid and schizotypal personality disorders Bipolar disorder Major depressive disorder
Bipolar type I	1%	25%	75%	Major depressive disorder Schizophrenia
Major depressive disorder	15%	15–20%	50%	Bipolar disorder Schizophrenia
Alcohol dependence	16%	30%	60%	Mood and anxiety disorders Antisocial personality disorder
Anxiety disorders Obsessive-compulsive disorder	3%	35%	25–30%	Tourette's disorder
Panic disorder	1–2%	8–20%	33–43%	Agoraphobia, social phobia, generalized anxiety disorder
Generalized anxiety disorder	5%	20%	22%	Panic disorder, agoraphobia, social phobia, major depressive disorder
Social phobia	3–13%	5%	24%	Panic disorder

1. **Family studies**
    * These studies are initiated by creating a **genogram** of the affected individual (the **proband**) and any of the immediate and ancestral family members who may have displayed the illness.
    a. **First-degree relatives** (e.g., parents, siblings, and children) share 50% of the proband's genetic information, or 100% in the case of monozygotic twins (who develop from the same ovum).
    b. **Second-degree relatives** (e.g., grandparents, grandchildren, nieces, nephews, aunts, and uncles) share 25% of genetic information with the affected individual, or 50% in the case of an aunt or uncle who is a monozygotic twin of a parent.
    c. **Penetrance** describes the proportion of family members who will display symptoms of the illness.
        * In **complete penetrance**, all members with the genotype for the disorder will display the symptoms.
    d. **Heritability** refers to the extent to which genetic factors determine phenotype.
        * In some genetic illnesses, affected individuals may vary in the degree to which the phenotype (i.e., symptomatology) is manifested, referred to as **expression**.

Schizophrenia and bipolar disorder are strongly linked to familial inheritance.

      e. If the relatives of probands are significantly more likely to have the psychiatric condition than relatives of controls, the illness has a **familial inheritance.** **Example: Obsessive-compulsive disorder** has a lifetime prevalence of 2–3% in the general population but a 30% prevalence in monozygotic twins.

      f. Family members may also display other psychiatric disorders with more frequency. **Example: Major depression** is more likely to occur in family members of persons with **bipolar disorder.**

2. **Twin studies**
   - These studies compare the rates at which monozygotic and dizygotic twins share the same illness.

         a. If the illness is manifested in both twins, the individuals are said to be **concordant.**

         b. Because environmental factors may vary, even for twins who are raised together, twin studies highly **suggest** (but do not prove) **genetic inheritance** of any particular condition.

3. **Adoption studies**
   - These studies compare genetic and environmental influences by studying the **prevalence** of an illness in **biological versus adoptive relatives.**

4. **Molecular genetic studies**
   - These studies evaluate genetic material obtained from **control** and **affected individuals** in the **same family.**

         a. **Restriction fragment length polymorphism (RFLP) studies** proceed through the genome, searching for genetic markers that are linked to the phenotype in question.

         b. A few neuropsychiatric illnesses have specific genetic associations with one gene or a short network of genes; however, **most psychiatric illnesses** appear to be **multifactorial,** with few clear-cut markers and great variation in expression of the phenotype.

5

Psychosocial Theories of Behavior

Target Topics

▸ Psychosocial theorists
▸ Learning theory; classical and operant conditioning
▸ Cognitive and social cognitive theories
▸ Psychoanalytic theory; defense mechanisms
▸ Family systems theory

I. Biopsychosocial Model
- This model, developed by **George Engel**, is the most widely accepted approach used to evaluate and treat patients with psychiatric and medical disorders.
  A. It emphasizes the importance of **biological, psychological, and social factors** in the etiology and treatment of illness.
  B. The comprehensive approach to the **assessment of a patient** results in more effective treatment and improved outcomes.

II. Learning Theory
  A. Overview
  1. **Learning** is defined as a **long-term change in behavior** that results from practice or previous experience.
  2. Learning theory applies principles of learning to the **development** and **modification** of **patterns of behavior**.
  3. This theory is the **basis for behavioral therapies**, which utilize learning concepts to strengthen adaptive behaviors and reduce unwanted behaviors (see Chapter 11).
  B. Classical conditioning
  1. Classical, or respondent, conditioning involves **learning**

Classical conditioning involves learning an association between a neutral stimulus and a stimulus that elicits a physiologic reflex.

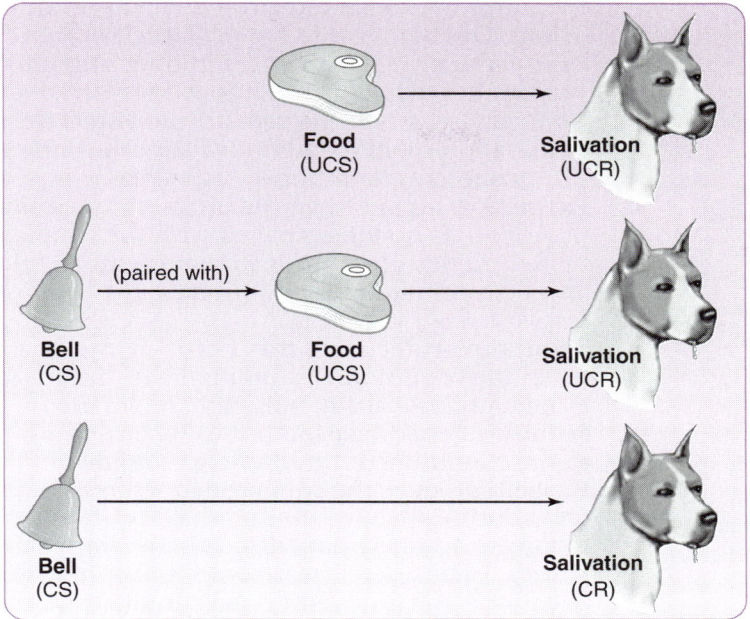

Figure 5-1   An unconditioned stimulus (UCS) naturally elicits an unconditioned response (UCR). A conditioned stimulus (CS) is a new stimulus delivered simultaneously with the UCS until it elicits the same response, which is then called a conditioned response (CR).

an association between a stimulus that evokes a physiologic reflex and a new stimulus.

2. **Ivan Pavlov's** experiments on the gastric secretions of dogs led him to develop the principles of classical conditioning (Figure 5-1).
   - Pavlov observed that the dogs would begin salivating at the sight or sound of other stimuli that had occurred repeatedly at the time of feeding (e.g., at the sight of the experimenter).
   a. The **unconditioned stimulus** is the stimulus that naturally elicits the reflexive response.
      - In the case of Pavlov's dogs, **food** is the unconditioned stimulus.
   b. The **unconditioned response** is the reflexive response.
      - In the case of Pavlov's dogs, **salivation** is the unconditioned response.
   c. The **conditioned stimulus** is any neutral stimulus that is repeatedly paired with the unconditioned stimulus until it elicits the same response, the **conditioned response**.
      - Pavlov **rang a bell** each time the dogs were fed, and eventually the dogs **salivated** (conditioned response) at the **sound of the bell** (conditioned stimulus).

- **Example:** A 3-year-old girl has recurrent ear infections. On each visit to her pediatrician, pain from the ear examination (unconditioned stimulus) causes her to cry (unconditioned response). On the fourth visit, when the pediatrician enters the examination room (conditioned stimulus), the girl begins to cry (conditioned response).

    d. **Extinction** occurs when the unconditioned stimulus (e.g., food) is no longer paired with the conditioned stimulus (e.g., bell) so that eventually the conditioned stimulus ceases to produce the conditioned response (e.g., salivation).

    e. **Spontaneous recovery** may occur after extinction when the conditioned stimulus elicits the conditioned response again, but only temporarily.

    f. **Stimulus generalization** occurs when stimuli similar to the conditioned stimulus (e.g., sounds similar to the bell) produce the conditioned response (e.g., salivation).
    Example: In many patients, chemotherapy produces nausea. After several treatment sessions in which chemotherapy (unconditioned stimulus) and nausea (unconditioned response) repeatedly are paired, the patient may experience nausea (conditioned response) when exposed to stimuli associated with the treatment environment (e.g., the waiting room, the hospital parking lot).

    g. **Discrimination** is the process by which the differences between similar stimuli are learned.
    - In the case of Pavlov's dogs, after a conditioned response develops to the sound of a bell, salivation may occur after hearing other sounds (e.g., a buzzer). However, if food is presented only with the sound of a bell, but not with a buzzer, eventually the conditioned response will be elicited only with the sound of the bell.

    h. **Aversive conditioning** occurs when an unpleasant stimulus is paired repeatedly with an unconditioned stimulus, resulting in the reduction of the original response.

    3. **Emotional responses**, especially **fear** and **anxiety**, can be developed through the process of classical conditioning.
    Example: Patients with posttraumatic stress disorder exhibit a strong fear response in new situations that are similar to the traumatic event. The principles of classical conditioning help to explain the case of a combat veteran who experiences a high level of anxiety at the sound of a helicopter or when viewing war scenes in a movie.

C. **Operant conditioning**

    1. **Operant conditioning** involves **voluntary responses**

Operant conditioning involves learning an association between a response and its consequence.

and is based on the principle that **behavior is a function of its consequences.**

    a. Responses followed by **positive consequences** will **increase** in frequency.

    b. Responses followed by **adverse consequences** or no **consequences** will **decrease** in frequency.

  2. **B.F. Skinner** developed the principles of operant conditioning through research examining the behavior of animals as they learned to obtain food under different patterns of reinforcement.

    a. Positive consequences are referred to as rewards or **positive reinforcement.**

    b. **Punishment** involves the presentation of adverse consequences or the removal of positive consequences.

    c. **Negative reinforcement** involves the removal of an adverse stimulus, which strengthens the behavior that caused the adverse stimulus to cease.
     Example: A child is throwing a tantrum because he wants a toy, and his parents agree to buy it so that he will stop crying. The parents' response of giving in to the child's demands now has been negatively reinforced. The next time the child throws a tantrum, the parents will be more likely to give in because the aversive event (i.e., crying) ceased with this behavior.

    d. The **schedule of reinforcement,** or pattern of reinforcement, affects the resulting pattern of behavior (Table 5-1).
      • **Behaviors** that have been **reinforced** on an **intermittent** basis are **more resistant to extinction** than behaviors that are reinforced on a continuous basis.

    e. **Extinction** occurs when reinforcement is discontinued, resulting in a cessation of the previous response.
     Example: The parents of an 18-month-old girl pick her up each time she cries at night and rock her back to sleep. They seek advice on how to reduce nighttime crying and are instructed by their pediatrician to briefly comfort their daughter when she cries but not remove her from her crib. After several nights of this routine, the child stops crying during the night.

    f. An **extinction burst** describes an increase in behavior that may occur as the initial response to extinction. Using the previous example, the girl might cry more than usual during the first few nights with this new routine before her bouts of crying eventually decrease and stop.

    g. **Shaping** is the process of reinforcing behaviors that increasingly approximate a desired behavior (Box 5-1).

TABLE 5-1   Schedules of Reinforcement

Type of Schedule	Definition	Example	Impact on Behavior
Continuous reinforcement	Reinforcement occurs after each response	A young girl receives a sticker on a chart for each morning she gets ready for school on time.	Helps establish new behavior Extinguishes quickly; to maintain behaviors established by continuous reinforcement, the frequency of reinforcement gradually is decreased
Fixed ratio	Reinforcement occurs after a specific number of responses	A typist receives a certain amount of money for each page typed.	Produces a high response rate
Variable ratio	Reinforcement occurs on a specified average number of responses	Slot machines are set to pay off on an average of a certain number of plays.	Produces a high response rate Resistant to extinction, because it is difficult to determine if reinforcement actually has stopped
Fixed interval	Reinforcement occurs after a fixed interval of time	A mother tells her son that she will check on him every 15 minutes to see if he is doing his homework. If he is working, he receives a star on a chart, which can be accumulated and exchanged for a reward.	Responses increase immediately before the reinforcement When graphed, the frequency of responding produces a scalloped pattern
Variable interval	Reinforcement occurs at variable time intervals	A mother tells her son that she will check on him at undetermined time intervals to see if he is working on his homework.	Produces a slow, steady response rate

III. **Cognitive Theory**
   A. **Overview**
      1. **Cognitive theory** focuses on the important effect of **cognitions** (e.g., thoughts, beliefs, expectations, perceptions, and interpretations) on **feelings** and **behavior**.

Cognitive theory focuses on the importance of thoughts, beliefs, and perceptions in influencing mood and behavior.

      2. **Cognitive therapy**, pioneered by **Aaron Beck** and **Albert Ellis**, involves the identification and modification of distorted thoughts in the treatment of mental health disorders (see Chapter 11).
   B. **The ABC model**
      • The ABC model postulates that a person's **interpretation of events**, rather than the events themselves, influences changes in moods and behaviors.
      1. "A" represents **antecedent events** (e.g., receiving a failing grade on an examination).
      2. "B" represents the individual's **beliefs** or interpretation of the event (e.g., "I'm not smart enough to succeed in medical school"; "I need to spend more time studying").

BOX 5-1	**The Patient Whose Health Behavior Is Modified Through Shaping**

A 52-year-old man with a family history of cardiovascular disease has developed moderate hypertension. His physician makes several treatment recommendations, including dietary modifications that reduce sodium intake. At the first and second follow-up visits, knowing that the patient has been accustomed to having high levels of sodium in his diet, the physician praises the patient for reducing his sodium intake and encourages him to continue the reduction process until he meets the recommended goal. By the third visit, the patient is maintaining his sodium intake within the recommended limit.

3. "C" represents the affective and behavioral **consequences** (e.g., depressed mood; spending more time studying).
C. **Social cognitive theory**
  1. **Overview**
     a. Social cognitive theory (also known as social learning theory) was developed by **Albert Bandura** and is based on the idea that human behavior is caused by the **reciprocal interactions** of **cognitive factors**, **behavior**, and the **environment**.
     b. Like cognitive theory, the focus is on cognitive factors such as expectations. However, social cognitive theory also emphasizes **bidirectional influences** and **learning by observation of others**.
  2. A fundamental concept is that observational learning, or **modeling**, plays a major role in influencing behavior or acquiring new behaviors.
     a. Modeling is a significant **influence** in the development of **aggressive behavior** and **emotional responses**.
     b. **Modeling approaches** have been used in the treatment of **anxiety responses**, including medical and dental phobias.
        Example: Children who are scheduled for surgery are shown a videotape of a child who models methods of coping with hospitalization and surgery. The children who view the videotape experience less anxiety because they have learned ways of managing their fear by watching the child in the videotape.
  3. **Self-efficacy**, or a person's confidence in his or her ability to carry out a behavior, is another central concept.
     • Self-efficacy is an important factor in changing health-risk behaviors, increasing adherence to medical advice, and coping with chronic pain (see Chapter 3).

> Social cognitive theory addresses learning by observation of others.

IV. **Psychoanalytic Theory**
   A. **Overview**

Psychoanalytic theory emphasizes the importance of unconscious processes in human behavior.

   1. Psychoanalytic theory, developed by **Sigmund Freud**, is based on the notion that **behavior** is deeply **influenced by early experiences** in important relationships, and that these influences usually are **unconscious** (outside of awareness).
   2. **Psychoanalysis** is a therapeutic approach based on this theory (see Chapter 11).
   3. Later theorists adapted and modified Freud's concepts to develop theories that are collectively referred to as **psychodynamic theory**. Therapies based on psychodynamic theory include psychoanalytic psychotherapy, psychodynamic psychotherapy, and brief dynamic psychotherapy (see Chapter 11).
   B. **Freud's theories of the mind**
   1. Freud initially described the **topographic theory of the mind**, which identifies three levels of awareness.
      a. The **conscious mind** contains thoughts of which an individual is aware. It utilizes **secondary process thinking**, which is logical and rational in nature.
      b. The **preconscious mind** contains thoughts of which an individual is *not immediately* aware; however, these thoughts can be accessed by focusing attention on them (e.g., a patient may not be thinking about her psychiatric treatment history but can recall and describe it when asked).
      c. The **unconscious mind** contains thoughts that are kept out of awareness by repression and other defense mechanisms.
         (1) Mental activity in the unconscious mind is characterized by **primary process thinking**, a primitive, illogical form of thinking that centers on **wish fulfillment.**
         (2) Freud believed that **dreams** are symbolic representations of wish fulfillment.
         (3) Unconscious thoughts can be revealed through **dreams** and **free associations** (the verbalization of uncensored thoughts that is encouraged in psychoanalysis).
   2. Freud later developed the **structural model of the mind**, which identifies three parts of the mind: the id, the ego, and the superego.
      a. The **id** is part of the **unconscious** mind. It involves **instinctual drives** and operates under the **pleasure principle**—pursuing pleasure and avoiding pain without consideration of consequences.
      b. The ego operates under the **reality principle**—perceiving the external world and solving problems in a realistic way.

      (1) The ego **moderates the drives of the id** so that its expression is appropriate for external circumstances.

      (2) The **functions of the ego** are carried out primarily in the **conscious** and **preconscious** mind and include **cognitive functions** (e.g., memory, language, learning, attention). **Unconscious** aspects of the ego are involved in **defense mechanisms.**

    c. The **superego** represents the individual's **moral values** and **standards of behavior** against which the individual's specific behavior is evaluated. These activities primarily occur unconsciously.

      (1) The **conscience** is the part of the superego that **prohibits** behaviors that are wrong and **punishes** the individual for transgressions through **guilt.**

      (2) The **ego ideal** prescribes behaviors that the individual aspires to or expects to achieve. Consequently, an individual whose behavior falls short of his or her moral ideal experiences **shame.**

C. **Defense mechanisms** (Table 5-2)

    1. Unacceptable impulses or painful feelings that threaten to break into the conscious mind can cause intrapsychic conflict (i.e., conflict between the demands of the id, ego, and superego), resulting in anxiety. The **ego** uses **defense mechanisms** in response to the signal of **anxiety.**

    2. **Repression** is the **primary defense mechanism** and involves blocking unacceptable impulses and painful feelings from conscious awareness.

> Defense mechanisms prevent unacceptable impulses or painful feelings from entering conscious awareness.

V.   Family Systems Theory

A. Overview

    1. Family systems theory is based on the assumption that an **individual** can be **understood best** in the **context of** his or her **family.**

    2. In **family therapy,** which has developed from family systems theory, the family is considered to be the patient.

    3. **Psychological symptoms** of individual family members are thought to indicate **disturbances in the family system** (see Chapter 11). These symptoms may serve to **maintain homeostasis,** or stability of the family system.

> Family systems theory emphasizes the importance of the family as a context for understanding each individual member.

B. Family structure and function

    1. **Structure** refers to how the family is **organized.**

      a. The **power hierarchy,** or how authority is distributed within the family, is an aspect of family structure. In healthy families, the hierarchy is clear and flexible, and authority lies with the **most competent members.**

      b. **Boundaries** determine how subsystems of the family

TABLE 5-2 Defense Mechanisms

Defense Mechanism	Description	Example
Acting out	Expressing an unacceptable feeling through actions	A woman who is angry at her mother throws a glass vase on the floor.
Altruism	Engaging in service to others to help deal with painful feelings	A man who lost a leg in an accident volunteers at camps for children with physical disabilities.
Denial	Refusing to acknowledge anxiety-provoking events	A 50-year-old woman with a family history of breast cancer finds a lump in her breast but waits 2 months before seeing her physician.
Displacement	Redirecting feelings from an original source to a more acceptable substitute	A resident feels humiliated by her attending physician and then is overly critical of the medical student under her supervision.
Humor	Finding amusing aspects of a stressful situation	A man who is in the hospital recovering from bypass surgery jokes frequently with medical staff.
Identification	Imitating the behavior of a more powerful person	A young boy who has witnessed his father hitting his mother on several occasions becomes physically aggressive with other children.
Intellectualization	Excessive focus on intellectual aspects of difficult situations to avoid painful feelings	A physician tells a married couple that the woman has lung cancer. When the couple returns home, the husband sits at the computer for several hours, reading about treatments for lung cancer.
Isolation	Separating painful feelings from stressful situations	A patient describes her history of childhood sexual abuse in an objective, unemotional manner.
Projection	Attributing unacceptable thoughts or feelings to others	A married man who is attracted to a female friend suspects that his wife may be having an affair.
Rationalization	Justifying unreasonable feelings or behavior with logical explanations	A mother who dipped her son in scalding water for punishment says that the boy needs to learn to respect authority.
Reaction formation	Adopting behaviors that are the opposite of one's unacceptable impulses	A woman who has strong unconscious feelings of anger and aggression is always nice to everyone and never loses her temper.
Regression	Returning to earlier patterns of behavior in response to stress	A hospitalized 5-year-old boy returns to sucking his thumb and wetting the bed.
Repression	Blocking unacceptable impulses and painful feelings from conscious awareness	A young girl witnesses a playmate being struck and killed by a car. As an adult, she has no memory of the event.
Splitting	Feelings about people and situations are either all positive or all negative	A patient is extremely satisfied with her physician. One day he advises her to lose weight because of her hypertension. She becomes very angry and says he is the worst doctor she has ever known.
Sublimation	Channeling unacceptable drives and impulses into socially acceptable activities	A rape victim who initially fantasized about revenge works to improve services for other rape victims.
Suppression	Voluntarily postponing attention to unwanted thoughts or feelings	A physician feels sexually attracted to a patient but consciously directs his attention back to the medical interview.

interact with one another and how the family inter-acts with the outside world.

    (1) Members of **disengaged families** are **isolated** from one another. The boundaries between family members are too rigid, and the bound-aries between the family and the outside world are too diffuse.

    (2) Members of **enmeshed families** are **overly in-volved** with each other. The boundaries between family members are too diffuse, and the boundaries between the family and the outside world are too rigid.

  c. Families have implicit and explicit **rules to maintain their structure.** Healthy families have clearly iden-tified, fair, and consistent rules that can be adapted to changing circumstances.

2. **Function** refers to how well a family **meets the needs of its members.**

  a. **Family cohesion** is the degree to which there is a balance between the functions of providing **support** to family members and establishing the **autonomy** of each member.

  b. **Family adaptability** is the degree to which there is a balance between the functions of maintaining sta-bility and adjusting to change.

Human Development and the Life Cycle

6

Pregnancy Through Adolescence

Target Topics

▷ Psychosocial concerns in pregnancy, childbirth, and the postpartum period
▷ Major theories of development: Freud, Piaget, Erikson
▷ Normal development in infancy through adolescence
▷ Developmental issues affecting care of infants, children, and adolescents
▷ Responses to hospitalization based on developmental stage
▷ Tanner stages of secondary sex characteristics

I. **Overview of Normal Human Development**
  A. **Knowledge of normal human development** helps the physician to:
    1. **Recognize developmental problems** and ensure appropriate treatment
    2. **Offer anticipatory guidance** to patients to facilitate developmental changes
    3. **Help patients adjust to adverse medical events**
  B. **Stages of development and expected ages of accomplishing milestones** are approximate. Development may be affected by the following factors:
    1. **Genetics**
    Example: Down syndrome, a common form of mental retardation, is caused by a chromosomal abnormality.

2. **Gender**
   Example: Girls begin puberty earlier than boys, but puberty tends to last longer in boys.
3. **Chronic illness**
   Example: Chronic illness may delay the onset of puberty in adolescents.
4. **Culture**
   Example: The cultural group to which a child belongs may influence the age at which he or she is expected to be self-sufficient.
5. **Social environment**
   Example: An impoverished environment with little stimulation may slow cognitive development.

II. **Pregnancy, Childbirth, and the Postpartum Period**
   A. **Adaptation to pregnancy**
      1. **Factors affecting a woman's emotional response to pregnancy**
         a. Whether the pregnancy was planned and the infant is wanted
         b. Relationship with the infant's father
         c. Her psychological well-being
         d. Confidence that she will be a good mother
      2. The **emotional bond** between mother and child begins during pregnancy.
      3. Both parents develop hopes and fears for their future child.
      4. A **miscarriage**, or intrauterine death, is emotionally very difficult for expectant parents, who grieve the loss.
   B. **Pregnancy and the marital relationship**
      1. Throughout pregnancy, expectant **parents prepare for their new roles** and responsibilities.
      2. **Sexual activity may decrease** because of a reduction in the woman's sexual desire, a decrease in the man's interest due to the pregnancy, or concern about harming the infant.
      3. The risk of **intimate partner abuse** is **increased** during pregnancy.
   C. **Factors affecting prenatal development**
      1. **Genetics:** Genetically transmitted diseases, such as Tay-Sachs disease or Turner syndrome, may affect fetal development.
      2. **Maternal health and lifestyle**
         a. **Medical conditions:** Diabetes, hypertension, and malnutrition are associated with prematurity and intrauterine growth retardation.
         b. **Infections:** Rubella, herpes, and syphilis are associated with fetal malformations.
         c. **Alcohol, drug, and tobacco use**
            (1) **Moderate to heavy alcohol consumption** during pregnancy may cause **fetal alcohol syndrome**, characterized by intrauterine growth

TABLE 6-1 Apgar Evaluation of Newborn Infants

Category	0	1	2
Appearance (color)	Blue, pale	Blue extremities, pink trunk	Pink
Pulse	Absent	< 100	> 100
Grimace (response to catheter in nostril)	No response	Grimace	Cough or sneeze
Activity (muscle tone)	Limp	Some movement	Active
Respiration	Absent	Irregular, slow	Regular, crying

retardation, facial abnormalities, below-normal intelligence, attention-deficit/hyperactivity disorder, and learning disorders. (The amount of alcohol that presents a risk to the fetus has not been determined; however, the potential for harm is greater with higher amounts of alcohol consumption.)

(2) Infants born to mothers who are dependent on **narcotics** go through **withdrawal at birth** and are at increased risk of developing **behavioral problems.**

(3) Maternal **cigarette smoking** is associated with **low birth weight.**

    d. **Prescription drug use:** Fetal abnormalities may result from prenatal exposure to many drugs, including tetracycline, lithium, and antiseizure medications.

    e. **Emotional state:** Maternal stress and anxiety are associated with miscarriage, premature birth, and low birth weight.

  3. **Lack of prenatal care** is associated with **increased infant morbidity** and **mortality rates** and is more likely to occur among adolescents and women of low socioeconomic status.

D. **Low birth weight** caused by premature birth (**< 37 weeks' gestation**) or intrauterine growth retardation (**birth weight < 2500 g**) increases the risk of **developmental, medical, behavioral, and learning problems** and is associated with mothers who are teenagers or of low socioeconomic status.

E. **Childbirth preparation** and emotional support during labor and delivery are associated with **improved outcomes** for newborn infants and mothers.

F. **Apgar score**
  1. The Apgar score is a method of assessing the condition of newborn infants immediately after birth.
  2. **Scores of 0–2** are given in each of five categories (Table 6-1).

Apgar score:
Appearance
Pulse
Grimace
Activity
Respiration

G. **Postpartum mood disturbances** (see Chapter 13)
   1. **Postpartum blues or "baby blues"**
      a. Seen in up to **70%** of postpartum women
      b. Onset is **within 2–3 days after delivery**; may last up to 2 weeks
      c. **Symptoms are mild** and include mood lability, sadness, tearfulness, and anxiety.
      d. Dramatic **changes in hormonal levels** after birth likely play a key role in the development of postpartum blues.

Postpartum blues occur in up to 70% of postpartum women.

   2. **Postpartum depression** (major depressive disorder with postpartum onset)
      a. Occurs in **5–10%** of postpartum women
      b. Symptoms of a **major depressive episode** begin within **4 weeks after delivery.**
      c. **Risk factors** include a personal or family history of mood disorders, high levels of stress, and lack of social support.
      d. Mothers experiencing postpartum depression may have difficulty providing infant care.

Postpartum depression occurs in 5–10% of postpartum women.

   3. **Postpartum psychosis** (brief psychotic disorder with postpartum onset)
      a. Symptoms include **severe depression,** hallucinations, delusions, and **thoughts of infanticide or suicide.**
      b. **Inpatient treatment is indicated** because of the risk of harm to infant and mother.

III. **Major Theories of Development** (Table 6-2)
   A. **Sigmund Freud: Psychosexual development**
      1. Freud's model describes **five stages** of psychosexual development during childhood, corresponding with the areas of the body where pleasurable sensations primarily occur.
      2. The **successful resolution** of each stage leads to **effective adult functioning.**
      3. **Difficulties** experienced during a stage lead to predictable patterns of **problematic behavior in adulthood.**
   B. **Erik Erikson: Psychosocial development**
      1. Erikson identified **eight stages** of psychosocial development across the lifespan, with each stage having a specific task to be accomplished during that stage.
      2. The degree to which each task is achieved affects the outcome of the following stages.
      3. The ultimate **goal** is attainment of a **sense of personal identity.**
   C. **Jean Piaget: Cognitive development**
      1. Piaget identified **four stages** that describe how children understand the world.
         a. **Sensorimotor:** infants learn through interacting with the environment.

TABLE 6-2   Stages of Development According to Freud, Erikson, and Piaget

Developmental Stage	Freud	Erikson	Piaget
Infancy	Oral (birth–1 year)	Trust vs. mistrust (birth–1 year)	Sensorimotor (birth–2 years)
Toddler	Anal (1–3 years)	Autonomy vs. shame and doubt (1–3 years)	Preoperational (2–7 years)
Early childhood	Phallic or oedipal (3–6 years)	Initiative vs. guilt (3–6 years)	(Preoperational)
Middle childhood	Latency (6–12 years)	Industry vs. inferiority (6–12 years)	Concrete operational (7–11 years)
Adolescence	Genital (12 years–adulthood)	Identity vs. role confusion (12–18 years)	Formal operational (11 years–end of adolescence)
Young adulthood	—	Intimacy vs. isolation (early adulthood)	—
Middle adulthood	—	Generativity vs. self-absorption (middle adulthood)	—
Older adulthood	—	Ego integrity vs. despair (older adulthood)	—

      b. **Preoperational:** children begin to use language and symbols.

      c. **Concrete operational:** children acquire the ability to reason, classify, and order (logical thought), and to understand cause and effect.

      d. **Formal operational:** children develop the capacity for abstract thinking.

  2. Knowledge of these stages helps ensure developmentally appropriate patient education for children and adolescents.

IV. Infancy: Birth to 18 Months

  A. **Reflex behaviors**

    1. Are **present at birth**, then **disappear** during the **first year of life** (Table 6-3)

    2. Absence or persistence is an indicator of central nervous system (CNS) dysfunction.

  B. **Attachment**

    1. Attachment is the enduring emotional **bond** that develops over time between an **infant and its caregiver(s).**

    2. The quality of attachment is affected by the responsiveness of both the caregiver and the infant.

    3. **Risk factors for poor attachment**

      a. **Decreased sensitivity of caregiver to infant's needs** (e.g., because of depression, substance abuse)

Suspect CNS dysfunction in children with absent or persistent infant reflexes.

The quality of attachment in infancy has profound influences on a child's development.

TABLE 6-3   Reflex Behaviors in Newborn Infants

Reflex	Description	Age at Which Reflex Disappears
Stepping	When held upright, makes walking movements	2–3 months
Rooting	When cheek is stroked, turns head in same direction and opens mouth	3–4 months
Moro or startle	When startled or in response to falling, throws out arms symmetrically	3–6 months
Tonic neck	When head is turned to one side while supine, the arm on the same side of the head extends while the other arm flexes (known as "fencer's position")	4–9 months
Grasp or palmar	Grasps objects placed in palm of hand	5–6 months
Babinski or plantar	When sole of foot is stroked, extends big toe and fans other toes	12–14 months

        b. **Decreased responsiveness of infant** (e.g., because of disability)

        c. **Infant characteristics** that make caregiving challenging (e.g., physical handicaps, difficult temperament)

        d. **Prolonged separation** between caregiver and infant (e.g., long-term hospitalization)

           • **Rene Spitz** observed that infants who experience **long-term deprivation of responsive caregiving** (e.g., they live in an understaffed institution) exhibit symptoms of **anaclitic depression**, becoming withdrawn, unresponsive, delayed in development, and susceptible to illness.

    4. **Effects of poor attachment**

        a. **Immediate consequence: failure to thrive** (reduced growth and delayed development)

        b. **Long-term consequences:** lack of trust, depression, substance abuse, and aggressive behavior

  C. **Temperament**

    1. **Chess and Thomas** described temperament as stable or relatively stable individual differences in behavioral style that influence development and are evident early in life.

    2. Dimensions that are used to describe temperament include **activity** level, **adaptability**, and quality of **mood.**

    3. The "**goodness of fit**" between a child's temperament and the parents' responses is a key factor in the child's development.

D. Developmental milestones
1. Motor, language, cognitive, and social developmental milestones in infancy are summarized in Table 6-4.
2. **Developmental screening**
   a. The **Denver II Developmental Screening Test** is used to assess motor, language, and social development of infants and children up to 6 years of age.
   b. Additional developmental evaluation is warranted if a developmental delay or abnormality is suspected.
E. Common developmental issues
1. **Prolonged crying (colic)**
   a. Colic usually occurs in a **healthy, well-fed infant**, commonly in the late afternoon or evening, and may persist for several hours at a time.
   b. If the physical examination is negative, parents should be informed that crying in normal infants peaks at 2–3 hours per day at the age of 6 weeks, and then decreases to about 1 hour per day by the age of 3 months.
   c. **Soothing techniques** include cuddling, repetitive motion (e.g., rocking), use of a pacifier, and sound (e.g., soft music).
2. **Anxiety reactions**
   a. **Stranger anxiety**
      (1) Develops at about **8 months** of age
      (2) Is characterized by **crying** and **clinging** when a stranger approaches
      (3) Is likely to be stronger in infants who have one primary caregiver
   b. **Separation anxiety**
      (1) First appears between **10 and 18 months** of age
      (2) Involves **crying** and **fearfulness** when the infant is separated from an attachment figure
F. Responses to hospitalization
1. Separation from parents during hospitalization can be emotionally traumatic for infants **after 6 months** of age.
2. Parents should be encouraged to be present and to provide as much of the infant's care as possible.

The leading cause of infant deaths is congenital malformations.

G. Leading causes of death in infancy
1. Congenital malformations
2. Disorders related to short gestation and low birth weight
3. Sudden infant death syndrome (SIDS)

V. Toddler: 18 Months to 3 Years
A. Developmental milestones (see Table 6-4)
B. Common developmental issues
1. **Toilet training**
   a. The majority of children are usually toilet trained by 2½ **years** of age.
   b. Training should incorporate positive consequences for using the toilet. **Punishment should *not* be used.**

TABLE 6-4   Normal Development: Infancy Through Age 6 Years

Approximate Age	Gross Motor and Fine Motor Skills	Cognitive and Language Skills	Social Skills
2–3 months	Holds head up briefly	Makes some vowel sounds; coos and gurgles	Smiles responsively ("social smile")
4–5 months	Rolls over front to back Reaches for objects Brings hand and objects to mouth	Babbles one-syllable sounds Stares at own hand	Laughs Becomes excited at sight of food
7–10 months	Sits without support Crawls or creep-crawls Transfers objects hand to hand Pulls self to standing position Points with index finger Walks holding furniture ("cruises") Uses pincer grasp (thumb and index finger)	Bangs two cubes Shakes rattle Uncovers objects hidden beneath a cloth Babbles with multiple-syllable sounds	Shows stranger anxiety Enjoys showing things to parents Plays social games (e.g., "peek-a-boo") Waves "bye-bye" Starts to imitate actions and sounds
12–13 months	Walks with one hand held or alone Turns pages of a book	Speaks a first word Responds to simple statements (e.g., "give me") Speaks a few words	Cooperates when being dressed Engages in pretend play with self (e.g., pretends to drink from a cup)
15 months	Builds tower of two cubes Walks alone Creeps up stairs		Shows separation anxiety Indicates desires by pointing
18 months	Runs Throws a ball Feeds self, but makes a mess	Names pictures Scribbles Uses 10–20 words Understands up to 150 words	Becomes more clingy with parents ("rapprochement") May use transitional object (e.g., blanket, doll) Engages in pretend play with dolls Says "no" often
2 years	Kicks a large ball Walks up and down stairs Opens doors Jumps	Uses two to three words together Knows full name	Engages in parallel play (plays side by side with other children without direct interaction)
3 years	Rides a tricycle Copies a circle Cuts paper with scissors Unbuttons buttons Feeds self well	Gender identity (perception of being male or female) has been established Uses complete sentences Knows age	Understands taking turns Has usually achieved urinary and bowel control
4 years	Brushes own teeth Copies a cross Hops on one foot	Tells a story	Plays cooperatively with other children
5 years	Skips Copies a square Draws a person Dresses and undresses independently	Understands concepts of past and future	Can participate in group games or projects
6 years	Ties shoelaces Copies a triangle Prints letters Rides a bicycle	Begins to develop a conscience Begins to read	Begins to develop empathy

2. **Autonomy**
   a. Toddlers have a strong **need for autonomy**, which is often expressed as **negativity** and **tantrums.**
   b. Constructive responses to a child's misbehavior at this stage include use of distraction and brief periods of "time out."
3. **Feeding problems**
   a. Often result from a **decreased appetite** associated with decreased growth rate and increased interest in activities
   b. Parents should be cautioned to **avoid forced feeding.**
4. **Thumb sucking and use of transitional objects** (e.g., a special blanket, stuffed animal)
   a. These behaviors may increase at approximately **16–24 months** of age.
   b. Orthodontic problems will arise only if thumb sucking continues on a frequent basis after age 6.

C. **Responses to hospitalization**
   1. Separation from parents during hospitalization is the most difficult issue for toddlers.
   2. The presence of parents and transitional objects is helpful.

D. **Adoptive families**
   1. **Children** in adoptive families **should hear** the words "adopted" and "adoption" used comfortably in conversation by their parents during the toddler years, even before the meaning of these words is fully understood.
   2. **Ongoing discussion of adoption** should occur during conversations about family, according to the child's desire to know more, rather than having a one-time discussion in which the child is told that he or she is adopted.

E. **Leading causes of death of toddlers**
   1. Unintentional injury: most commonly motor vehicle crashes or drowning
   2. Congenital malformations
   3. Malignant neoplasms: most common types are leukemia and brain or CNS tumors

The leading cause of death of children aged 18 months to 11 years is unintentional injury (motor vehicle accidents, drowning).

VI. **Early Childhood: 3–6 Years**
   A. **Developmental milestones** (see Table 6-4)
   B. **Common developmental issues**
      1. Common **fears** include the **dark, animals, monsters, or ghosts.**
      2. **Interest in their bodies** and in **physical differences** lead children in this age group to explore their own genitalia and play "doctor."
      3. **Imaginary friends** are common among children aged 3–10 years.
   C. **Responses to illness, hospitalization, and death**
      1. Anxiety about physical injury is common.

Minimize separation from parents during hospitalization, especially for children ≤ 6 years.

2. Children may interpret **illness as a punishment** for misbehavior.
3. Role-playing or practicing medical procedures with the child is more effective than verbal descriptions in preparing a young child for hospitalization and medical care.
4. Separation from parents during hospitalization remains difficult.
5. **Regression to earlier behaviors** (e.g., thumb sucking, wetting accidents) may occur during hospitalization or other stressful events.
6. Children in this age group *do not* understand the finality of death.

> Regression to earlier behaviors is common in young children during hospitalization.

VII. **Middle Childhood: 6–11 Years**
  A. **Motor and cognitive development**
    1. **Gross motor and fine motor skills:** dramatic improvement in these skills occurs, enabling the child to participate in sports and to write and draw well.
    2. **Cognitive abilities: thinking** becomes organized and **logical,** and the ability to solve problems and **delay gratification** improves.
  B. **Social development**
    1. **Same-gender friendships,** participation in clubs and organizations, and an emphasis on acceptance by peers
    2. The ability to **distinguish right from wrong** and follow rules
    3. Collecting objects of interest (e.g., dolls, cards, rocks)
  C. **Common developmental issues**
    1. Success in **school, social interactions,** and other arenas is an important aspect of development for children in this age group (for whom Erikson identifies "industry" as the primary psychosocial task).
    2. **Self-esteem** is a key issue because of the child's newly developed ability to evaluate himself or herself and to perceive others' evaluations.

> A sense of achievement is very important to children during middle childhood.

  D. **Responses to illness, hospitalization, and death**
    1. Children in this age group **cope well** with illness and hospitalization, especially if they are well-supported by their parents.
    2. **Understanding of death becomes more realistic.**
    3. **Fear of being abandoned** through the death of their parents may be present.
  E. **Adoptive families**
    1. Children's **questions** about their birth and adoption become **more specific** during this period.
    2. Parents should provide information in a direct and positive manner, **emphasizing the permanence** of the adoptive parents in the child's life.
  F. **Leading causes of death in early to middle childhood**
    1. Unintentional injury: most commonly motor vehicle crashes or drowning

TABLE 6-5   Tanner Stages of Development of Secondary Sex Characteristics

Stage	Breast Development in Girls	Genital Development in Boys
1	Appearance typical of preadolescent	Appearance typical of preadolescent
2	Breast bud stage Breasts and papillae are elevated, forming small mounds Areolar diameter increases	Scrotum and testes increase in size Skin of scrotum reddens
3	Breasts and areolae increase in size, with no separation in their contours	Penis begins to lengthen Testes and scrotum continue to increase in size
4	Areolae and papillae form secondary mounds projecting above the breast	Penis continues to enlarge in both length and diameter Glans penis develops Testes and scrotum enlarge further Skin of scrotum darkens
5	Adult appearance; areola is part of the general breast contour	Adult appearance

    2. Malignant neoplasms: most common types are leukemia and brain or CNS tumors

    3. Homicide

VIII. Adolescence: 11–21 Years

  A. Stages

    1. **Early** adolescence: **11–14** years

    2. **Middle** adolescence: **15–17** years

    3. **Late** adolescence: **18–21** years

  B. Physical development

    1. Puberty

      a. Puberty is marked by the **secretion of sex hormones** that create the bodily changes necessary for reproduction as well as secondary sex characteristics (e.g., growth of pubic hair).

      b. **Average age of onset:** girls, 11 years; boys, 13 years

        (1) **Menarche** (the first menstruation in girls) begins at an average age of 12½ years.

        (2) The **first ejaculation** in males occurs at an average age of 14.

      c. **Tanner stages** classify the development of secondary sex characteristics for boys and girls across five stages (Table 6-5).

      d. **Early pubertal development** tends to be a positive phenomenon for boys, but often it is a negative experience for girls.

    2. Other physical changes

      a. Rapid skeletal growth

      b. Deepening of the voice in boys

TABLE 6-6   Cognitive and Social Development in Adolescence

Period	Developmental Characteristics
Early adolescence (11–14 years)	Adjusts to physical changes of puberty: "Am I normal?" Sensitivity to physical appearance increases Peer group involvement increases; family involvement decreases Sexual curiosity and masturbation are common Peer group is same gender Privacy needs increase Crushes on adults are common
Middle adolescence (15–17 years)	Conflict with parents increases; testing of rules and questioning of authority occurs Experimentation with sex and drugs is common, including homosexual experiences Experiments with different images or appearances to develop a sense of identity Peer group is composed of males and females Ability for abstract thinking and planning for the future increases Feelings of invincibility; risk-taking behavior is common Forms own value system as distinct from value system of parents
Late adolescence (18–21 years)	Individual relationships are more important than peer group Family relationships improve Abstract thinking is further developed, characterized by an increased capacity to see other points of view, appreciate long-term consequences of behavior, and appreciate multiple causes and interrelationships Self-sufficiency, career planning, and social roles are major concerns High-risk behaviors are common Sexuality begins to be an expression of caring and intimacy Idealism and an increased concern for others is common Sense of morality and personal ethics are developed

     c. Increased muscle mass in boys

     d. Increased proportion of body fat to body weight in girls

C. **Cognitive and social development** (Table 6-6)

D. **Common health problems**

    • Health problems in adolescents generally are related to health-risk behaviors.

    1. Teenage pregnancy

      a. Statistics

        (1) The rate of adolescent pregnancy in the **United States** is the **highest among developed countries.**

        (2) Of all teen pregnancies, **80% are unintended** and approximately 25% end in abortion (both rates have declined in recent years).

        (3) Pregnancy rates are **more than twice as high** among **black and Hispanic** teenagers as among white teenagers.

Common health problems among adolescents include unintended pregnancy, sexually transmitted diseases, and substance use.

Among developed countries, the US has the highest rate of teenage pregnancy.

BOX 6-1	The Adolescent Patient Who Is Nonadherent with Medical Treatment

A 15-year-old girl seeks treatment for an exacerbation of asthma symptoms. The girl, who is accompanied by her mother, says that for the past month she has been performing the recommended breathing treatments only 4–5 times a week instead of twice a day. The physician acknowledges that it is difficult to complete two breathing treatments every day, but he points out that the treatments increase the likelihood that the teenager will not miss favorite activities because of illness. He asks the girl about the recent difficulties in carrying out treatments, as well as strategies she thinks will help her adhere to the recommended schedule more closely. He also mentions that several of his teenage patients find it easier to complete their daily treatments if friends encourage them or keep them company during the treatments. At the conclusion of the office visit, the physician gives the girl and her mother educational materials designed for adolescents with asthma and their parents.

Teenage pregnancy is associated with negative outcomes for both mothers and infants.

The leading causes of adolescent deaths are unintentional injury, homicide, and suicide.

    b. Maternal and infant outcomes
        (1) Maternal complications during pregnancy occur at an increased rate in teenagers because of physical immaturity and lack of prenatal care.
        (2) Teenage mothers are less likely to complete schooling or pursue advanced educational achievement and are more likely to require public assistance.
        (3) Infants of teenage mothers are more likely to experience poor health outcomes, child abuse and neglect, and behavioral and educational problems.
  2. Sexually transmitted diseases (STDs)
    • Approximately **50%** of all students in grades 9–12 have had **sexual intercourse**, and about 40% did not use a condom during their last intercourse, placing them at risk of contracting STDs.
  3. Alcohol, drug, and tobacco use
    • Approximately **50%** of high school students have **drunk alcohol** within the past month, 35% have smoked cigarettes, and 25% have smoked marijuana.
E. Common developmental issues in the medical care of adolescents
  1. Because the capacity for abstract thought (Piaget's formal operational stage) does not develop fully until late adolescence or beyond, **patient education about health risk behaviors** should focus on short-term positive consequences rather than on long-term consequences.
  2. Nonadherence to medical recommendations is common

during adolescence and can be especially serious for patients with chronic illnesses (Box 6-1).

    a. **Adolescents with chronic illnesses** or **physical handicaps** often are especially sensitive to physical differences from peers and any restrictions on independent activities.

    b. **Strategies to maximize adherence** include:

        (1) **Involving** the adolescent **in management plans**

        (2) **Giving** the adolescent as much **responsibility** as possible for his or her **own care**

        (3) **Involving friends** and **other teens** with similar medical problems for support

  3. **The loss of autonomy and privacy** are difficult aspects of hospitalization for teens.

F. **Adoptive families**

  1. Adolescents in adoptive families often **want to contact their birth parents.**

  2. Adoptive parents should be reassured that this interest is *not* an indication of dissatisfaction with the adoptive parents and usually results in a **strengthened relationship** with the child.

G. **Leading causes of death in adolescence**

  1. Unintentional injury: most involve motor vehicle crashes

  2. Homicide

  3. Suicide

7

Adulthood, Aging, Death, and Bereavement

I. Overview of Adult Development

A. **Stages of adult development** are associated with **major tasks and needs**, although these stages are *not* related as closely to age or unfolding biological events as are stages of child development.

B. Three **changes in the 20th century** profoundly influenced the nature and timing of adult development:

    1. An **increase** in the percentage of **high school graduates attending college** has delayed the time at which many young people enter the adult world (e.g., when they begin their occupational careers, marry, and become parents).

    2. **Greater availability of effective contraceptives** has influenced decisions about sexual activity, marriage, parenthood, and work.

    3. An **increase in life expectancy at birth** (from 47 years in 1900 to 77 years in 2000) has increased the upper boundary of midlife by about 20 years and resulted in many more people living into late adulthood.

II.   Young Adulthood: 22–44 Years
A.   Transition to adulthood
1. The transition to adulthood may begin during the **late teens** and persist until the **mid-20s.**
2. By their late 20s or early 30s, most individuals view themselves as having reached adulthood.
B.   Psychosocial issues in young adulthood
1. Young adults become **self-sufficient** and **autonomous** by developing an identity separate from that of their parents or birth family.
2. An important task during this period is learning how to **form intimate relationships** with others.
C.   Leading causes of death in young adulthood
1. Unintentional injury
2. Malignant neoplasms
3. Heart disease

III.   Middle Adulthood: 45–64 Years
A.   Midlife transition
1. No universal event marks the transition to middle adult-hood or the realization that an individual is now middle-aged.
2. Most people experience a "**midlife transition**," a time when they realize that they are no longer young; for some individuals, the transition can be so distressing that it may be viewed as a "**midlife crisis.**"

> For some people, the transition to midlife may cause a "midlife crisis."

3. Midlife can be a time for individuals to **reassess life values** and **goals** and to demonstrate increased **generativity** (reorienting themselves toward helping younger people to thrive).
B.   Menopause
1. **Physiologic changes**
   a. Menopause (the permanent cessation of menses) is the **most pronounced biological change** in women in middle adulthood.
   b. It is one aspect of the **climacteric**, a period of several years' duration during which women experience endocrine, somatic, and psychological changes.

> Most women accept menopause as a normal life cycle event.

   c. About 40% of menopausal women seek treatment for symptoms related to estrogen deficiency, such as **hot flashes** or vasomotor flushes and **sleep disturbances.**
2. **Median age of onset: 51 years,** but it may occur as early as age 40 or into the late 50s.
3. Most women accept menopause as a normal life cycle event; 70% of menopausal women express relief or have neutral feelings about the cessation of menses.
4. Menopause is *not* specifically associated with an increased rate of psychiatric disorders.

C. **Health issues during middle adulthood**
1. Most **mental functions peak** during middle adulthood.
2. The gradual decline in some mental and physical functions that begins during this period has minimal impact on daily life because of reserve capacities, adaptation, and compensation.

D. **Leading causes of death in middle adulthood**
1. Malignant neoplasms
2. Heart disease
3. Unintentional injury

IV. **Older Adulthood: 65 Years and Older**
A. **Demographics**
1. In **2000, life expectancy** for the United States general population was **76.9 years.** Males had a life expectancy of 74.1 years and females, 79.5 years.
2. **Adults 65 years of age and older** currently constitute about **12%** of the population; by 2030, this figure is expected to increase to about 20%.
3. In 2000, the percentage of **minority elders** in the 65-and-older population was **16.4%;** by 2030, it is expected to be 25.4%.
4. The fastest growing group of elders is **85 years** of age **and older,** and this group has the **greatest number of health problems** and the **greatest need** for **long-term care.**

B. **Physiologic changes of normal aging**
1. Aging **begins in early adulthood** and is a gradual and variable process.
2. **Chronological age** may not match **physical age;** organ systems in the same individual may age at different rates.
3. **Normal changes in body systems** are contrasted with age-related pathologies in Table 7-1. Most older adults experience the following changes:
   a. Greater difficulty maintaining homeostasis
   b. Decreased reserve capacities in body systems
   c. Impaired immune responses
   d. Longer recovery period from disease or injury and often an incomplete recovery
4. **Physicians** should carefully evaluate all signs and symptoms in older adults to determine whether they are a result of normal aging, disease, or disuse and should **avoid the tendency to automatically attribute these changes to "old age."**

C. **Leading causes of death in older adulthood**
1. Heart disease
2. Malignant neoplasms
3. Stroke

D. **Changes in functional status** (Box 7-1)
1. Functional status is often equated with health by elders and **determines** their **independence.**
2. **Significant losses in function** commonly occur in the

The fastest-growing group of elders is aged 85 years and older.

The leading cause of death in older adults is heart disease.

Optimizing functional status is an important objective in the care of older adults.

TABLE 7-1   Comparison of Normal Changes and Age-related Pathologies

System	Normal Changes	Age-related Pathologies
Skin	Thinner, drier, less elastic skin Fewer and less efficient sweat glands	Malignant melanoma
Cardiovascular	Increase in blood pressure Diminished cardiac reserve Decline in maximum heart rate	Hypertension Atherosclerotic heart disease Congestive heart failure
Pulmonary	Decreased pulmonary function reserves Less forceful cough Stiffening of chest wall	Emphysema Lung cancer
Urinary	Decline in glomerular filtration rate Impairment of renal concentrating and diluting abilities Prostatic hypertrophy	Urinary incontinence
Gastrointestinal	Slowing of peristalsis	Diverticulosis
Musculoskeletal	Decrease in muscle mass, muscle strength, endurance, lean body mass, and bone density	Osteoporosis Osteoarthritis
Central nervous system	Decrease in brain weight and in cerebral blood flow Enlargement of sulci and ventricles	Alzheimer's disease
Sensory Vision	Gradual loss of lens elasticity (presbyopia) Slower adaptation to the dark Decline in contrast and color sensitivities Increased susceptibility to glare	Cataracts Macular degeneration Glaucoma
Hearing	Loss of high- then low-frequency sounds (presbycusis)	Cerumen impaction Noise-exposure deafness Inner and middle ear diseases
Reproductive Women	Decrease in estrogen level, associated with increased vaginal dryness and thinning of vaginal lining	Breast cancer
Men	Decreased testosterone level, associated with longer time to achieve erection and longer refractory period	Impotence Prostate cancer

urinary, musculoskeletal, and central nervous systems, and in hearing and vision.

3. In addition to normal age-related changes, most people aged 65 and older have at least one chronic condition and many have multiple **chronic conditions,** such as arthritis, hypertension, hearing loss, heart disease, and cataracts.

4. A common way to determine functional status is to **assess activities of daily living** (ADLs) and **instrumental activities of daily living** (IADLs).

   a. ADLs consist of **basic activities** such as dressing, bathing, eating, and toileting.

| BOX 7-1 | **The Patient With Impaired Functional Status** |

An 80-year-old man whose wife died 5 months ago comes to the physician's office with symptoms of an upper respiratory infection. The physician prescribes an antibiotic to treat the infection, but she notices that the patient has lost weight since she last saw him 3 months ago. When the physician mentions this, he tells her that he has not been eating well lately. He says it is painful for him to prepare a meal because the arthritis in his hands has worsened, and he is afraid he might drop the hot pots while cooking. As a result, he has been eating mostly cereal and sandwiches. He says he has not mentioned this before "because it's just due to old age and there's nothing you can do to help with that." The physician assures him that there are treatments for arthritis and assistive devices that may help him gain more functional use of his hands. She also gives him information about Meals-on-Wheels and the telephone number of the local senior center, where he can go to have a hot meal and socialize with other seniors on weekdays.

    b. IADLs are more **complex activities** that are essential for independent living such as going shopping, preparing a meal, handling finances, and taking medication.

  E. **Psychological aspects of aging**

    1. **Cognitive changes associated with aging**

      a. Decline in motor speed, reaction time, and cognitive processing

      b. Decline in the ability to solve new problems

      c. Some **short-term memory loss**, which does not cause problems with daily functioning

    2. Accumulated knowledge and experience and the ability to access this information remain the same or improve until very late in life

    3. **Personality** tends to remain **stable over a lifetime.**

    4. **Sexuality and sexual functioning**

      a. Most older adults remain interested in **sexual activity.**

      b. **Factors associated with sexual activity after age 65**

        (1) Previous sexual activity

        (2) Good health

        (3) Availability of a capable and interested partner

    5. **Mental health problems**

      a. **Depression**

        (1) Between **5% and 20% of elders** 65 years of age and older are affected by **major depression** and **related disorders**, making depression the most common mental health disorder in later life.

        (2) The prevalence is higher for elders in hospitals and nursing homes.

        (3) The risk of **suicide** is highest among people aged 65 years and older, especially among **white men.**

Depression is the most common mental health disorder among older adults.

The risk of suicide is highest among older adults, especially white men.

    b. **Dementia:** prevalence increases with age (see Chapter 20).

    c. **Substance abuse**

        (1) Older adults may become dependent on **alcohol** or **prescription medications.**

        (2) About **10%** of older adults are **alcoholics,** with a 5:1 male-to-female ratio.

        (3) Of older adults who are alcoholics, 30–50% begin drinking late in life, often in **response** to a **stressful life event.**

    d. **Anxiety disorders:** most common are generalized anxiety disorder, phobias, and anxiety disorder due to a general medical condition.

    e. **Diagnosis and treatment of mental health problems**

        (1) Mental health problems in the elderly are often **underdiagnosed** and **undertreated,** with most problems being brought to the attention of a primary care physician rather than a mental health practitioner, most often as physical problems.

        (2) **Diagnosis** of a mental health problem may be **confounded** with **physical health problems** and their associated treatments.

        (3) Many mental health problems are **treatable** using modalities such as individual and group therapy and pharmacotherapy.

F. **Social aspects of aging**

  1. Later life is a time of adapting to many changes and losses.

  2. The **transition to retirement** can have both **positive** and **negative** aspects, influenced by the following factors:

    a. Commitment to work

    b. Financial situation

    c. Health status

    d. Support network

    e. Non–work-related interests

  3. **Financial status:** Among elders 65 years of age and older, median income declines and the percentage of people living in poverty rises.

  4. **Living arrangements**

    a. **Most** elders are community-based and **live with a spouse** until the spouse's death or placement in an institution.

    b. About **30%** of noninstitutionalized elders **live alone,** with the greater proportion of these being older women.

    c. About **5%** of elders 65 years of age and older **live in institutions** (e.g., nursing homes, veteran's administration facilities). The percentage increases with age (18% for those 85 years of age and older).

> Approximately 10% of those aged 65 and older live in poverty.

> About 5% of people aged 65 and older live in institutions.

TABLE 7-2 Changes in Death and Dying in the United States, 1900–2000

Characteristic	1900	2000
Life expectancy	47 years	77 years
Timing of death	Death occurs at all ages, with high childhood mortality	Death occurs mostly at older ages
Causes of death	Infectious diseases and accidents; death occurs quickly	Chronic diseases: cardiac, cancer, stroke; dying is prolonged
Place of death	Home: familiar to patient; little technology	Institutions: strange environment; often frightening technology
Focus of medicine	Palliative: caring, comfort	Curative: prolonging living with chronic illness
Caregivers	Family	Institutional staff; minimal family involvement
Perception of death	Familiar, natural, accepted part of life	Unfamiliar, to be avoided at all costs, unacceptable part of life
Expense	Minimal	Very costly for an extended period of time
Financing	Primarily from family	Most from Medicare and Medicaid

   5. Social support
      a. **Family** is the most important source of social support for elders.
      b. Older men are more likely to be married than older women, and more older women are widowed than older men.
      c. **Family members** (usually women) **provide 70–80%** of the **care** to sick elders.
      d. **Demographic changes** (e.g., smaller families, an increase in the number of working women, and an increase in geographic mobility) are affecting family **caregiver availability**, particularly that of adult children.
      e. **Social isolation** is a **risk factor for elder abuse** (see Chapter 21).

V. End-of-Life Issues
   A. Perspectives on death and dying
      1. Death and dying are influenced by the social, historical, and cultural environment as well as by biological and psychological factors.
      2. **Contemporary United States society** has been called a **"death-denying" society**—one in which independence, youth, and productivity are valued and caring for one another, age, and family are devalued.
      3. The **experience of death and dying** has **changed** greatly **since the early 1900s** (Table 7-2).
      4. Less than 10% of the population will die suddenly; more than 90% will die after a prolonged illness.

TABLE 7-3 Leading Causes of Death for the General Population in the United States in 2000

Cause of Death	Death Rate per 100,000 Population
Heart disease	258.2
Malignant neoplasms	200.9
Cerebrovascular diseases	60.9
Chronic lower respiratory diseases	44.3
Accidents (unintentional injuries)	35.6
Diabetes mellitus	25.2
Influenza and pneumonia	23.7

Source: Anderson RN. Deaths: Leading causes for 2000. *National Vital Statistics Reports.* Vol 50, No 16. Hyattsville, Md: National Center for Health Statistics; 2002.

5. Most people **want to die at home,** although only about 20% actually do.
6. **Leading causes of death** vary by age, sex, and race or ethnic group. Statistics for the population as a whole are summarized in Table 7-3.

B. **Elisabeth Kübler-Ross: Stages of dying**
1. Patients do *not* necessarily go through all stages or go through stages in the specified order, and they may experience more than one stage simultaneously.
    a. **Denial:** the patient refuses to believe that the diagnosis and prognosis are true.
    b. **Anger:** the patient asks: "Why me?" Physicians and family members are prime targets for the anger.
    c. **Bargaining:** the patient usually bargains with a higher power or fate and wants to trade good behavior for good health or at least a postponement of death.
    d. **Depression:** the patient faces the reality of the situation, experiences sadness and distress, and stops fighting to survive.
        • **Anticipatory grief** may occur, in which the patient grieves the prospect of his or her own death.
    e. **Acceptance:** the patient is calm and more peaceful and may take care of unfinished business.
2. This theory does *not* fully acknowledge the importance of anxiety in the dying patient.

C. **Bereavement, grief, and mourning**
1. **Bereavement**
    a. Begins with the **death of a loved one** and with most **other significant losses** (e.g., spinal cord injury, divorce)
    b. Bereaved people have **higher morbidity** and **mortality rates** for at least the first **6 months after the loss.**
    c. **Social** and **emotional support** are extremely helpful for bereaved people.

More than 90% of the general population will die after a prolonged illness.

Kübler-Ross's five stages of dying: denial, anger, bargaining, depression, acceptance

TABLE 7-4   Comparison of Normal Grief and Clinical Depression

Normal Grief	Clinical Depression
Exhibits feelings of sadness; cries	Feels hopeless and worthless
Has a reduced ability to enjoy activities	Has a significantly diminished ability to enjoy usual activities
Relates depressed feelings to the loss	Does not relate depressed feelings to any specific event
Expresses guilt over some aspect of the loss	Feels excessive or inappropriate guilt
Experiences a lack of or a temporary loss of self-esteem	Experiences a loss of self-esteem over an extended period of time
Has thoughts of being better off dead or that he or she should have died with the deceased	May have suicidal thoughts
Hears the voice or briefly sees the image of the deceased	May have hallucinations or delusions

2. **Normal grief** shares some of the features of **clinical depression** (Table 7-4; see also Chapter 13). **Characteristics of normal grief** include the following **responses:**
   a. **Physical:** Chest tightness, heart palpitations, decreased energy, weight loss or gain, sleep disturbances
   b. **Psychological:** Emotional numbness, sadness, anger, guilt, anxiety
   c. **Cognitive:** Disbelief, confusion, inability to concentrate, low self-esteem, preoccupation with or hallucinations or dreams about the deceased
3. **Normal grief reactions** may resurface on anniversaries ("**anniversary reaction**") such as the deceased's birthday or date of death, or in special places such as a favorite restaurant of the survivor or the deceased or the park they used to walk in.
4. **Complicated grief**
   a. Is greatly **prolonged**, very **intense, postponed**, or **suppressed**
   b. Interferes with health or ability to function
5. **Mourning** involves the following tasks:
   a. **Accepting** the reality of the loss
   b. **Working through** the pain of the grief
   c. **Adjusting** to living without the deceased
6. Most people go through the grief and mourning process without need for medical treatment.
7. The **physician** should be **supportive** and **empathic** with the survivor and **evaluate the survivor for complicated grief reactions** during office visits after the loss.

8

Clinical Assessment

Target Topics

▸ Psychiatric evaluation, clinical interview, and mental status examination

▸ Frequently used psychological tests

▸ DSM-IV-TR multiaxial classification

I. General Considerations

- Patients with medical illnesses often have **comorbid psychiatric disorders** as well as psychosocial factors, such as stressful life events and lack of social support, that can significantly affect functioning.

> Common responses to illness include fear, anxiety, anger, denial, depression, and regression.

A. Primary care setting

1. More patients are treated for psychiatric disorders by primary care physicians than by mental health professionals.

2. The most common psychiatric problems in the outpatient setting are the following disorders: **mood, anxiety, substance use**, and **somatoform**.

> Significant psychosocial problems may be present in 50–70% of patients who visit primary care physicians.

B. Hospital setting

1. **Psychological disturbances** may emerge in hospitalized patients with or without a history of psychiatric illness.

2. The most common psychiatric problems are those associated with **cognitive impairment** (e.g., delirium), **depression**, and **substance abuse**.

3. Patients who are **postoperative**, undergoing **renal dialysis**, or admitted to an intensive care unit (**ICU**) or a critical care unit (**CCU**) are at higher risk for emotional problems.

> Approximately 40–50% of hospitalized patients with a general medical condition have a diagnosable psychiatric disorder.

BOX 8-1	Components of the Clinical Interview

A. **Identifying information:** patient's name, age, sex, marital status, ethnicity, educational level, occupation
B. **Chief complaint:** description of the problem using patient's own words (if patient is unable to offer a chief complaint clearly or lacks awareness of the problem, may also include physician's assessment of patient's problem)
C. **History of present illness:** onset; symptoms; impact on patient's social, family, and work functioning; recent life stressors; coping strategies; support system
D. **Psychiatric history:** history of psychiatric illness or chemical dependency; inpatient or outpatient treatments; medications taken and result; history of suicide attempts, psychotic symptoms, obsessions, fears, problems with anxiety or depression
E. **Medical history:** allergies, recent or ongoing health problems, past surgery, current medications, risk factors (e.g., smoking or hypercholesterolemia), recent findings from physical examination or laboratory evaluation
F. **Family history:** disease history in patient's immediate family and family of origin; construct a genogram of serious familial disorders, as pertinent (e.g., in the case of a depressed patient, determine whether there is a family history of mental illness, substance abuse, or suicide)
G. **Social history:** current and past family and marital relationships; history of emotional, physical, or sexual abuse or trauma; sexual preference and history; current sexual functioning; legal or financial problems; cultural and religious background; hobbies, interests, and leisure activities; educational and work history, including experiences in the armed services; use of alcohol or drugs
H. **Review of systems:** always perform a thorough review of systems

II. The Psychiatric Evaluation

A. The psychiatric evaluation applies the same principles used to assess patients with physical disorders, paying particular attention to **behavioral** and **psychological symptoms.**
   1. Follows the general format of the medical history and uses a biopsychosocial approach
   2. Information can be pursued and expanded on by the physician to clarify the diagnosis, as indicated by the patient's chief complaint or positive responses to psychiatric screening questions.
B. **Clinical interview** (Box 8-1)
   1. When conducting the clinical interview, the **patient should be encouraged to speak freely.**
   2. The physician should screen for the presence of **substance abuse, suicidal** or **homicidal ideation,** and **mood** and **anxiety disorders.**
C. **Mental status examination**
   1. This examination is an essential part of the psychiatric

Always assess for and record suicidal or homicidal ideation.

evaluation and provides information about a patient's current cognitive and affective state (Table 8-1).

2. A patient's mental status may change and should be **observed and documented with each patient encounter** to monitor these changes.

3. **Abnormal findings**, particularly signs of **cognitive impairment**, should prompt **further screening** with the Mini-Mental State Examination (MMSE) or another commonly used screening test (Table 8-2).

Evaluate and document mental status with each patient encounter.

III. **Psychological Tests**
   A. **Uses**
      1. Psychological tests are **standardized tests** used in a variety of settings, including health care, education, industry, and criminal justice.
      2. In the health care setting, psychological testing is an **extension of the clinical interview** and is intended to supplement the interview but not replace it.
   B. **Screening tests and batteries**
      1. A **screening test** is designed to identify specific symptoms and syndromes (e.g., depression, dementia) (Box 8-2; see Table 8-2).
         a. **Identifies** the likely **presence of a diagnosable disorder** and the need for comprehensive clinical evaluation
         b. *Not used independently* to diagnose a mental health disorder
         c. Some tests can be used repeatedly and are **useful as measures of change** and to **evaluate treatment outcomes.**
      2. **Batteries** are groups of standardized tests used to assess a **specific mental problem.**
         • These tests are usually **individualized for each patient** (i.e., the psychologist chooses a group of tests that directly address the suspected patient problem).
   C. **Frequently used psychological tests** (Tables 8-3 and 8-4)
      1. **Personality tests** measure patterns of perceiving, responding to, and thinking about the world.
         a. **Objective tests** are highly structured, consist of questions with a limited number of possible answers, and yield **statistically based descriptions of specific aspects of personality.**
         b. **Projective tests** are **qualitative** tools in which patients are asked to create imaginative responses to ambiguous stimuli. These tests yield **theory-based descriptions of various aspects of personality.**
      2. **Intelligence tests** measure perceptual, integrative, memory, and motor skills that are highly related to educational success.
         a. **Performance** on these tests is influenced by patient motivation, emotional state, and cultural factors.

TABLE 8-1   Mental Status Examination

Case Description: A 22-year-old woman is brought to the physician by her mother, who has noticed that her daughter has not been eating and has withdrawn from her usual activities. The mother is concerned that her daughter may be anemic.

Category	Components	Observations
Appearance, attitude, and behavior	Grooming, hygiene, dress	The patient is a disheveled young woman, who has poor eye contact and responds to questions in a terse, hostile manner.
	Psychomotor activity	She is slumped in her chair and biting her nails.
Orientation and sensorium	Level of consciousness	She is alert.
	Orientation to person, place, and time	She knows her name, her current location (e.g., town, state), and the day and date.
Mood and affect	Description of emotional state (e.g., dysphoric, euphoric, expansive, irritable)	She describes feeling sad and hopeless.
	Range of affect (e.g., blunted, flat, restricted, labile, inappropriate)	Her affect is flat, and she shows little emotional expression.
	Congruence of affect with mood	She begins to cry when describing her feelings of worthlessness and helplessness.
Speech	Rate, quality, quantity, prosody	Her speech is of normal rate, but she stutters occasionally. She speaks softly and in a monotonous tone of voice.
Thought and language	Thought content	The content of her thought includes some passive suicidal ideation. She wishes to die of natural causes and has no active intent to harm herself. There are no signs of paranoia, delusions, ideas of reference, obsessions, or homicidal ideation.
	Thought process	Her thought process is organized and logical, without signs of flight of ideas or thought blocking.
	Perception	She denies auditory or visual hallucinations, or illusions (i.e., misinterpretation of sensory stimuli).
Memory and cognition	Immediate recall and short-term memory	She can repeat three words but is unable to name them after a 5-minute delay.
	Recent memory	She is unable to remember what she ate for breakfast or dinner yesterday and reports lapses in her memory across the day.
	Long-term memory	Her memory for life events and personal information, such as her birthday, is intact. She can name the past three presidents.
	Calculation, reading, construction	She can read a simple paragraph, do single digit addition, and copy intersecting pentagrams.
Concentration	Attentional ability	When asked to subtract "7 from 100" and to keep subtracting "7's" until told to stop, she makes four errors out of five responses.
Intelligence	Estimate of below-average, average, or above-average intelligence	Her responses indicate below-average IQ, based on her fund of knowledge and vocabulary.
Insight	Awareness of being ill or having a problem	She shows poor insight, because she does not feel she has a problem or needs help.
Judgment	Capacity to judge social and other situations	Formal testing with proverbs and problem-solving scenarios indicates poor abstract reasoning and judgment.

TABLE 8-2   Frequently Used Screening Tests

Screening Test	Description
Beck Anxiety Inventory (BAI)	Differentiates between anxious and nonanxious patients Appropriate for ages 17–80 years
Beck Depression Inventory–II (BDI-II)	Measures symptoms of depression Used for initial screening and to assess changes in the patient's symptoms Appropriate for ages 13–80 years
Dementia Rating Scale–2 (DRS-2)	Measures cognitive status in older adults Used for initial assessment and to follow changes in the patient's status Appropriate for ages 55–89 years
Mini-Mental State Examination (MMSE)	Measures cognitive status Used for initial screening and to follow cognitive changes over time Appropriate for adults

BOX 8-2	The Patient Who Is Undergoing Psychiatric Evaluation and Screening

A 72-year-old married woman tells her physician that she is forgetful and lacks interest in her usual activities. During the interview, she is confused about the date and cannot remember where she is, other than that she is at the physician's office. The physician administers a Mini-Mental State Examination (MMSE) and the Beck Depression Inventory–II (BDI-II) to aid in differential diagnosis. Results of the MMSE indicate significant cognitive impairment consistent with that seen in dementia. The BDI-II reflects the presence of only a mild mood disturbance. Based on interviews with the patient and her husband and the results of her initial cognitive screening, the physician decides to pursue a diagnostic workup for dementia.

TABLE 8-3   Frequently Used Personality Tests

Test	Description
Objective	
Minnesota Multiphasic Personality Inventory (MMPI)	True/false items measure test-taking attitudes, bodily concerns, depression, naivete and defensiveness, anger, gender-related interests, paranoia, anxiety, unconventional thinking, energy, and social introversion Appropriate for adults
Personality Assessment Inventory (PAI)	Measures syndromes, such as depression, anxiety, mania, paranoia, and schizophrenia Appropriate for adults
Projective	
Rorschach Technique	Patient responds to 10 inkblot designs Appropriate for children, adolescents, and adults ($\geq$ 5 years)
Thematic Apperception Test (TAT)	Patient creates stories about ambiguous pictures Appropriate for children, adolescents, and adults

TABLE 8-4 Frequently Used Tests of Intelligence, Achievement, and Aptitude

Test	Description
Intelligence	
Kaufman Adolescent and Adult Intelligence Test (KAIT)	Multiple subtest battery in which patient responds to questions and solves problems in a variety of visual and verbal formats Appropriate for ages 11–85 years
Kaufman Assessment Battery for Children (K-ABC)	Same as KAIT; appropriate for ages 2.5–12.5 years
Stanford-Binet Intelligence Scale, Fourth Edition	Multiple subtests yield norm-based scales that give information about intelligence and cognitive abilities Appropriate for ages 2 years through adulthood
Wechsler Adult Intelligence Scale, Third Edition (WAIS-III)	Multiple subtests in which patient responds to questions and solves problems in a variety of visual and verbal formats Appropriate for ages 16–89 years
Wechsler Intelligence Scale for Children, Third Edition (WISC-III)	Same as WAIS-III; appropriate for ages 6–16 years
Wechsler Preschool and Primary Scale of Intelligence, Third Edition (WPPSI-III)	Same as WAIS-III; appropriate for ages 2–7 years
Aptitude	
Detroit Tests of Learning Aptitude, Fourth Edition (DTLA-4)	Multiple subtest measure of general intelligence and discrete ability areas Appropriate for ages 6–17 years
Achievement	
Wide Range Achievement Test 3 (WRAT-3)	Assesses reading, spelling, and arithmetic skills Appropriate for ages 5–75 years

Mean IQ = 100

b. An individual's **intelligence quotient** (IQ) score generally is **stable throughout adulthood.**

c. **IQ score** is derived by the following formula:

$$IQ = \frac{\text{Mental age}}{\text{Chronological age}} \times 100$$

    (1) **Mental age:** performance on intelligence test items compared with the typical performance of individuals in the same age group (e.g., a 10-year-old child whose performance is found to be about the same as the typical performance of 7-year-old children has a mental age of 7)

    (2) **Chronological age:** the number of years that have elapsed since birth

d. **IQ ranges:** the mean score is 100.

    (1) ≥ 130: very superior

    (2) 120–129: superior

    (3) 110–119: bright normal

    (4) 90–109: normal

    (5) 80–89: dull normal

    (6) 70–79: borderline

    (7) ≤ 70: mental retardation (see Chapter 22)

3. **Aptitude tests** measure probable future performance fol-

TABLE 8-5   Commonly Used Neuropsychological Batteries and Tests

Battery	Description
Halstead-Reitan Neuropsychological Battery (HRNB)	Multitest assessment of selected perceptual and cognitive functions Appropriate for ages 16–79 years
Luria's Neuropsychological Investigation	Systematic assessment of neuropsychological signs and symptoms of brain injury Appropriate for adults

Test	Description
Attention	
Paced Auditory Serial Addition Test (PASAT)	Measures ability to divide attention between similar tasks Appropriate for adults
Memory	
California Verbal Learning Test, Second Edition (CVLT-II)	Assesses verbal learning and memory Appropriate for ages 16–89 years
Wechsler Memory Scale, Third Edition (WMS-III)	Assesses memory for both verbal and nonverbal material Appropriate for ages 16–89 years
Speech/Language	
Boston Diagnostic Aphasia Examination (BDAE), Third Edition	Assesses speech and language impairments Appropriate for adults
Visuospatial Abilities	
Rey Complex Figure Test and Recognition Trial (RCFT)	Measures visuospatial constructional ability and visuospatial memory Appropriate for ages 6–89 years
Executive Functions	
Wisconsin Card Sorting Test (WCST)	Measures ability to form abstract concepts from visual material and to shift concepts as appropriate Appropriate for adults

lowing additional training or maturation. They are often used interchangeably with tests of intelligence.

4. **Achievement tests** measure information attained through educational activities.
5. **Neuropsychological tests** measure the behavioral expression of neurologic impairment, assessing brain-behavioral relationships (Table 8-5).
   a. **Batteries** of neuropsychological tests usually include measures of attention, memory, speech/language, visuospatial abilities, and executive functions.
   b. These batteries often include **personality**, **intelligence**, **aptitude**, and **achievement** tests.

IV.   Treatment Planning
A.   **Assessment summary**
   • A summary of the patient's psychosocial strengths and weaknesses, compiled from the clinical interview, the mental status examination, and psychological testing, is combined with findings from the physical examination and laboratory and diagnostic studies to provide the **basis for treatment planning.**

Screening for psychiatric illness should always include a thorough physical evaluation to rule out organic etiologies of symptoms.

TABLE 8-6   DSM-IV-TR Multiaxial Classification

Axis	Axial Format	Examples*
I	Clinical disorders Other conditions that may be the focus of clinical attention	Major depressive disorder Bipolar disorder Schizophrenia Cocaine dependence
II	Personality disorders	Borderline personality disorder Narcissistic personality disorder
	Mental retardation	Mental retardation (mild, moderate or severe)
III	General medical conditions	Acute and chronic illnesses
IV	Psychosocial and environmental problems	Occupational problem (e.g., unemployment) Family problem (e.g., illness) Marital problem (e.g., separation) Financial problem (e.g., bankruptcy) Other social problem (e.g., arrest)
V	Global assessment of functioning (Usually given for current functioning and for level of functioning over the past year)	Numerical description of an individual's functioning on a scale from 0 to 100

*May list more than one diagnosis in order of importance.

B. Diagnosing psychiatric disorders

   1. The *Diagnostic and Statistical Manual of Mental Disorders,* 4th edition, text revision (DSM-IV-TR) uses a **multiaxial classification system** to classify psychiatric disorders, incorporating psychiatric diagnosis, medical conditions, and psychosocial factors (Table 8-6).

   2. The five axes from the DSM-IV-TR can be used to provide a full description of the **biopsychosocial components** of a patient's illness.

C. Treatment: incorporates various levels of care and may include the following components:

   1. Pharmacotherapy

   2. Psychotherapy

   3. Laboratory and diagnostic studies

   4. Inpatient treatment

   5. Support groups

D. Indications for mental health consultation or patient referral

   1. Psychiatric disorder with severe impairment

   2. Risk of suicide or homicide

   3. Treatment by primary care physician has been ineffective

   4. Need for specific treatment (e.g., psychotherapy)

Adequate patient follow-up and documentation of treatment outcomes are essential.

9

Biological Assessment

Target Topics

▶ Physical examination and neuroimaging in psychiatric evaluation
▶ Underlying diseases associated with psychiatric symptoms
▶ Laboratory screening tests and therapeutic drug monitoring

I. Physical Examination of Patients With Psychiatric Symptoms

A. A physical examination is an often overlooked but highly important part of the evaluation of individuals with psychiatric symptoms.

B. Patients with psychiatric illnesses often **lack access to appropriate health care;** therefore, every opportunity should be taken to intervene with a thorough physical examination.

C. A physical examination often **unmasks comorbid illnesses** and biological alterations that produce psychiatric symptoms (Table 9-1).

  1. **Underlying medical illnesses must be ruled out** when patients with psychiatric disorders report somatic complaints in the review of systems.

  2. In patients **older than 50 years of age** with onset of new psychiatric complaints, an **underlying medical etiology** is highly likely (see Table 9-1).

D. **Pharmacologic agents** used to treat psychiatric or medical disorders can cause **serious side effects** that require a thorough medical workup.

  • Any pharmacologic agent used to treat a variety of diseases may cause side effects, manifested as **mental status changes** or **psychiatric symptoms,** particularly in the elderly or in those taking multiple medications (Table 9-2).

Careful physical examination of patients with psychiatric symptoms may lead to diagnosis of underlying medical illnesses that produce behavioral symptoms.

Pharmacotherapy with multiple drugs may cause psychiatric symptoms in elderly patients.

TABLE 9-1 Diseases That Manifest With Psychiatric Symptoms

Disease	Anxiety	Depression	Mania or Excitement	Delirium or Confusion	Dementia	Psychosis	Personality Change
Acute intermittent porphyria		+					
Adrenocortical insufficiency		+	+			+	
AIDS		+	+		+	+	+
Brain tumors		+	+	+		+	+
Cerebrovascular disease		+		+	+		
Cushing's syndrome		+	+	+			
Encephalitis				+		+	
Epilepsy or seizures		+				+	+
Hepatic encephalopathy		+	+				
Huntington's disease		+			+	+	+
Hyperglycemia				+			
Hyperparathyroidism		+		+		+	
Hyperthyroidism	+	+	+			+	
Hypoglycemia	+			+			
Hyponatremia				+		+	
Hypoparathyroidism	+	+	+	+			
Hypothyroidism		+				+	
Hypoxia	+			+		+	
Multiple sclerosis	+	+	+				
Normal pressure hydrocephalus					+		
Pancreatic cancer		+					
Pheochromocytoma	+						
Systemic lupus erythematosus	+	+				+	
Tertiary syphilis					+	+	
Vitamin B$_{12}$ deficiency		+			+		+
Wilson's disease		+				+	+

TABLE 9-2   Some Psychiatric Symptoms Associated With Toxicity
or Reactions to Drugs

Drug	Psychiatric Symptoms
Amantadine	Delirium, hallucinations
Aminophylline	Delirium
Amphetamines	Paranoia, mania
Anticholinergics	Delirium, confusion
Antidepressants	Mania
Benzodiazepines	Drowsiness, disinhibition
Beta-blockers	Depression, hallucinations
Cimetidine	Delirium, confusion
Clonidine	Depression, drowsiness
Digitalis	Delirium, confusion
Glucocorticoids	Delirium, mania
Interferon	Depression
Isoniazid	Delirium, confusion
Levodopa	Delirium, psychosis, mania
Methyldopa	Delirium
Monoamine oxidase inhibitors	Mania, excitation, confusion
Opiates	Confusion, drowsiness, hallucinations
Phenothiazines	Delirium, drowsiness
Reserpine	Depression
Sedative hypnotics	Delirium, confusion
Steroids	Excitation, mania, insomnia, psychos s
Sympathomimetics	Insomnia, mania, excitation
Tricyclic antidepressants	Anticholinergic delirium, mania

II. **Laboratory Evaluation**
   A. **Screening tests used during the initial psychiatric
      evaluation**
      • The following **laboratory studies** provide basic screening
        for **metabolic** and **endocrine problems** that may cause psy-
        chiatric symptoms:
      1. **Complete blood count**
      2. **Blood chemistry panel**, including electrolytes, glucose,
         creatinine, liver enzymes, and calcium
      3. **Urinalysis**
      4. **Thyroid hormone levels:** thyroid-stimulating hormone
         (TSH) usually is used for screening.
   B. **Therapeutic drug monitoring**
      1. **Plasma drug levels** are routinely measured, if indicated,
         for each prescribed medication to determine patient
         adherence and **therapeutic dosage.**
      2. Plasma levels are checked in patients with an **exacerba-
         tion of psychiatric symptoms** or a **suspected overdose.**
   C. **Additional laboratory testing:** findings from the physical ex-
      amination or initial laboratory screening may indicate the
      need for further testing.
      Example: Physical examination of a depressed 35-year-old
      woman indicates a butterfly rash and joint pain. These find-
      ings prompt the physician to order the following labora-

Laboratory studies
help to rule out
underlying medical
etiologies of psychi-
atric complaints.

tory studies: erythrocyte sedimentation rate, antinuclear antibody and subtypes, complement levels, VDRL (for syphilis), prothrombin time, partial thromboplastin time, and anticardiolipin antibody. The results confirm the diagnosis of systemic lupus erythematosus.

D. Tests used for specific psychiatric disorders
   1. The following tests may help to clarify diagnosis, but they are rarely used in practice because of the reliability of diagnosis based on the clinical presentation.
      a. The **dexamethasone suppression test** (DST) demonstrates the failure to suppress secretion of cortisol after administration of dexamethasone in about 50% of patients with **major depression.** However, findings are not specific—they occur in the presence or absence of depression but are seen more often in symptomatic than in asymptomatic individuals.
      b. **Intravenous administration of sodium lactate** or **inhalation of carbon dioxide** can elicit a **panic attack** in patients with panic disorder, but these tests are not confirmatory.
   2. **Neurotransmitter levels** can be obtained from cerebrospinal fluid analysis and, experimentally, using functional imaging studies, but this information does not alter treatment and involves risks to the patient.

Neuroimaging studies should be performed in patients with mental status changes.

III. Neuroimaging Studies and the Electroencephalogram (EEG)
   • Neuroimaging studies are routinely performed when patients exhibit **onset of new psychiatric symptoms,** particularly **psychosis** and **confusion.**
   A. Magnetic resonance imaging (MRI) and **computed tomography** (CT) are the studies most often used to observe abnormalities of brain anatomy or activity in psychiatric patients (Table 9-3).
      1. MRI visualizes **anatomic brain lesions, soft tissue,** and **water.** Contrast agents can be used for vascular visualization and tumor enhancement.
         a. MRI is a **more definitive** study than CT.
         b. MRI is limited by the patient's tolerance for the enclosed area and **contraindicated in patients with metal implants,** such as pacemakers.
      2. CT visualizes **anatomic brain lesions, bone, air,** and **blood.** Contrast agents may be used to enhance visualization of vascular lesions.
   B. Single photon emission computed tomography (SPECT), **positron emission tomography** (PET), and **magnetic resonance spectroscopy** (MRS) reveal **abnormalities of brain function.**
      1. **SPECT** measures blood flow as well as receptor binding using neurotransmitter compounds or agonists.
      2. **PET** assesses dysfunction of various brain locations by measuring decreased or increased brain activity.

TABLE 9-3   Diagnostic Tests Used to Assess Brain Anatomy and Function in Patients With Psychiatric Symptoms

Test	Description	Examples of Pathologic Findings
Computed tomography (CT)	Uses a computer to process x-rays emitted and detected on a transaxial axis	Hemorrhage Abscess Tumors Ventricular changes Dementias
Electroencephalography (EEG)	Measures brain activity via differences in electrical potential between scalp electrodes	Seizure activity Localized areas of dysfunction Generalized dysrhythmia or slow pattern (delirium)
Evoked potentials	Measures standard stimuli, such as clicks or lights	Infantile hearing and vision loss Changes in response patterns (comatose patients)
Magnetic resonance imaging (MRI)	Measures radio waves emitted by magnetically aligned nuclei passing between excited and relaxed states	Dementias White plaques (multiple sclerosis) Arteriovenous vascular malformation Reduced or increased cortical volume Previous hemorrhage Posterior fossa and brainstem abnormalities Abnormal deposition of iron (hemochromatosis) and copper (Wilson's disease)
Functional MRI (fMRI)	Detects levels of oxygenated hemoglobin, which rise in the brain with brain activity	Localized areas of dysfunction Same pattern of brain activation for hallucinations and actual verbal stimuli (schizophrenia)
Magnetic resonance spectrography (MRS)	Produces an image of phosphorus-31– and hydrogen-1–containing compounds in cell nuclei	Lithium and paroxetine steady-state levels Tumor growth and remission Neural death and repair (stroke)
Positron emission tomography (PET)	Measures brain activity during a cognitive task, using a radionuclide-labeled, positron-emitting substance (e.g., glucose or a neurotransmitter)	Increased activity in frontal cortex and basal ganglia (obsessive-compulsive disorder) Diffuse reduced metabolism (Alzheimer's dementia) Deficits in radionuclide uptake (traumatic brain injuries) Reduced anterior-to-posterior ratios (schizophrenia)
Single photon emission computed tomography (SPECT)*	Uses single photon–emitting radionuclides as tracers to produce images of brain	Bilateral parietal lobe deficits (Alzheimer's type dementia) Frontal lobe deficits (Pick's disease)

*Normal findings are seen in patients with pseudodementia.

    3. **MRS** is used mainly in research settings to measure adenosine triphosphate (ATP), phosphocreatine, GABA, glutamate, and certain drug pharmacokinetics.

  C. **EEG** and **evoked potentials** measure **electrical activity** in the brain.

    1. EEG measures **disruption** in amplitude, frequency, and rhythm in α, β, δ, or θ **bands**.

    2. EEG should be performed if **seizure activity** or **delirium** is suspected.

10

Pharmacologic and Biological Therapies

Target Topics

▶ Psychotropic drugs: classes, mechanisms of action, and adverse effects
▶ Electroconvulsive therapy and phototherapy

I. Overview

A. Neurotransmitter dysfunction is often indicated by symptoms such as depression, anxiety, and psychosis that occur in patients with psychiatric disorders.

B. Psychotropic drugs act at the neuronal level of the central nervous system (CNS) to **restore homeostatic function** to neurotransmitters.

C. Classes of drugs used to treat psychiatric symptoms
1. Antipsychotics
2. Antidepressants
3. Mood stabilizers
4. Antianxiety agents
5. Stimulants

D. Before initiating pharmacologic therapy, any general medical conditions, use of other medications, and potential for pregnancy must be considered.

E. Other treatments for psychiatric disorders include **electroconvulsive therapy** (ECT) and **phototherapy.**

II. Antipsychotics

A. General considerations
1. Antipsychotic drugs (formerly referred to as neuroleptics) are classified as **typical** or **atypical** (Table 10-1).
2. Use
   a. Schizophrenia

> Psychotropic drugs may cause significant adverse effects and drug interactions.

TABLE 10-1   Some Atypical and Typical Antipsychotic Drugs

Classification	Drug
Atypical antipsychotics	Aripiprazole
	Clozapine
	Olanzapine
	Quetiapine
	Risperidone
	Ziprasidone
Typical antipsychotics	
Low potency	Chlorpromazine
	Thioridazine
High potency	Fluphenazine
	Haloperidol
	Loxapine
	Molindone
	Pimozide
	Thiothixene
	Trifluoperazine

   b. **Manic phase of bipolar disorder**
   c. Other psychotic disorders (e.g., schizoaffective disor-
       der, delusional disorder, brief psychotic disorder)
   d. **Psychotic symptoms** resulting from substances (e.g.,
       cocaine-induced psychotic disorder) and general
       medical conditions (e.g., delirium resulting from
       hypoxia)
 3. Metabolism
   a. Antipsychotic drugs are metabolized by multiple
       routes.
   b. Although drug interactions via cytochrome P450
       isoenzymes *do not* have a significant impact on the
       metabolism of these drugs, the clinical significance of
       potential interactions should be assessed in each
       patient and dosages adjusted, if necessary.
 B. **Typical (conventional) antipsychotics**
   • Are highly effective in treating psychosis but have **poten-
     tially serious adverse effects**
 1. **Mechanism of action**
   a. **Block dopamine (D$_2$) receptors** in the mesolimbic
       and mesocortical pathways of the brain, thereby
       reducing the occurrence of psychotic symptoms
   b. **Affect other dopamine pathways and neurotrans-
       mitters,** increasing the potential for adverse effects
 2. Adverse effects of typical antipsychotics (Table 10-2)
   a. **Low-potency** drugs are more likely to **cause hypo-
       tension** and **cardiac effects.**
   b. **High-potency** drugs cause more extrapyramidal side
       effects but tend to be **less sedating** and have **fewer
       anticholinergic effects.**

Thioridazine: *do not* use in combination with other drugs (e.g., cimetidine) that prolong the QT interval.

Antipsychotic drugs act by blocking dopamine receptors.

TABLE 10-2   Adverse Effects of Antipsychotic Drugs

Adverse Effects	Treatment
Associated With Dopamine Blockade	
Extrapyramidal Effects	
Dystonia (severe muscle spasm), parkinsonian symptoms, akathisia (internal restlessness)	Use an anticholinergic, such as benztropine or diphenhydramine
Tardive Dyskinesia	
Choreoathetotic, irregular movements of face, tongue, and body that occur after 3 or more months of treatment; symptoms may be permanent	Gradually reduce and eliminate drug or switch to an atypical antipsychotic
More frequent in women and in individuals with mood disorders	
Incidence increases with each year of use	
Prolactin Elevation	
Galactorrhea, amenorrhea	Switch to an atypical antipsychotic
Neuroleptic Malignant Syndrome	
Hyperthermia, muscle rigidity, delirium, autonomic dysfunction, elevated creatine phosphokinase	Withdraw antipsychotics
	Treat with bromocriptine and supportive therapy
Associated With Other Neurotransmitters	
Anticholinergic Effects	
Blurred vision, constipation, urinary retention, confusion	Switch to another antipsychotic drug with a different side-effect profile
Antihistaminic Effects	
Weight gain, dry mouth, sedation	Switch to another antipsychotic with a different side-effect profile
α_1 **Blockade**	
Hypotension	Switch to another antipsychotic with a different side-effect profile
Cardiac Effects	
Prolonged QT interval, seen particularly with thioridazine	Switch to another antipsychotic with a different side-effect profile
Sexual Dysfunction	
Erectile and orgasmic dysfunctions, loss of libido	Switch to another antipsychotic with a different side-effect profile or add a medication such as sildenafil
Lipid and Liver Changes	
Elevated liver function tests, drug-induced hepatitis, hypercholesterolemia	Withdraw drug until liver function returns and restart with a different medication
Ophthalmologic Changes	
Cornea and lens changes	Switch to another antipsychotic
Most serious is retinal pigmentation seen with thioridazine at doses > 800 mg	
Agranulocytosis	High risk with clozapine; check complete blood count weekly
Seizures	
Decreased seizure threshold	Use a higher potency antipsychotic with less potential for seizure
Skin Changes	
Photosensitivity and rash	Switch to another antipsychotic

        c. **Neuroleptic malignant syndrome** (NMS) is a potentially lethal adverse effect associated with typical antipsychotics.

    3. Clinical considerations

        a. **Haloperidol** and **fluphenazine:** available in **long-acting depot injections,** which may be beneficial in cases of patient nonadherence

        b. **Haloperidol** and **pimozide:** other uses include treatment of **Tourette's disorder.**

C. Atypical antipsychotics

    • Are the **first line of treatment** because they have **fewer adverse effects** than typical antipsychotics

    1. **Mechanism of action:** act on **serotonergic neurons,** and D_4 and D_2 receptors

    2. Adverse effects of atypical antipsychotics (see Table 10-2)

        a. **Fewer extrapyramidal side effects** occur than with typical antipsychotics.

        b. Risk of **NMS** or **tardive dyskinesia** is **minimal.**

    3. Clinical considerations

        a. **Newer atypical drugs** (e.g., olanzapine) have **mood-stabilizing qualities** in addition to antipsychotic effects.

        b. Atypical drugs improve both negative and positive symptoms of **schizophrenia** (see Table 12-1).

        c. **Clozapine** is **not prescribed** unless treatment with other drugs has been unsuccessful, because it can **cause agranulocytosis** and other adverse effects, such as drowsiness, weight gain, and seizures. Its use has proven effective in many otherwise refractory patients.

III. **Antidepressants**

    • This drug class includes **selective serotonin reuptake inhibitors** (SSRIs), **tricyclic antidepressants** (TCAs), and **monoamine oxidase inhibitors** (MAOIs).

A. Use

    1. Most commonly used in the treatment of **depressive disorders, depressed phases of bipolar disorder,** and specific **anxiety disorders** (Box 10-1)

    2. Indications for use, other than for depression, are listed in Table 10-3.

    3. The newer classes of antidepressants, such as **SSRIs,** have become the **initial treatment of choice** because of the increased incidence and seriousness of adverse effects associated with MAOIs and TCAs. **MAOIs** and **TCAs** are used **after** an **unsuccessful course of treatment** with the newer drugs.

B. Mechanism of action

    1. Antidepressant response depends on returning neurotransmitter levels to normal at the synaptic cleft (Figure 10-1).

Typical antipsychotics are associated with extrapyramidal side effects, tardive dyskinesia, and NMS.

Clozapine: effective in otherwise refractory patients.

Newer classes of antidepressants (e.g., SSRIs) are the initial treatment of choice for depression and anxiety disorders.

All antidepressants (except MAOIs) block neurotransmitter reuptake into the presynaptic neuron.

BOX 10-1	Treatment of the Patient With Depression

A 48-year-old woman sees her physician because she is always tired, frequently cries, and believes that her life will not improve. She has lost 15 pounds (7 kg) in the past 2 months and has stayed in bed for several days this week. Her job performance is suffering because she is unable to focus on work. The physician diagnoses major depression, prescribes a selective serotonin reuptake inhibitor (SSRI), and refers the patient to a psychologist for therapy. The patient returns 3 weeks later and says her mood, energy, and ability to function at work have improved. The physician then recommends continuing the SSRI regimen for 1 year.

TABLE 10-3   Other Uses of Antidepressant Drugs in Addition to Depression

Drug	Use
Selective serotonin reuptake inhibitors (SSRIs)	Obsessive-compulsive disorder Bulimia nervosa Panic disorder Social anxiety disorder Generalized anxiety disorder
Tricyclic and tetracyclic antidepressants (TCAs)	Chronic pain Obsessive-compulsive disorder (clomipramine only) Panic disorder
Monoamine oxidase inhibitors	Bulimia nervosa Panic disorder

Other antidepressants
  Bupropion
  Nefazodone, venlafaxine
  Trazodone
	
	Smoking cessation
	Generalized anxiety disorder
	Sleep induction

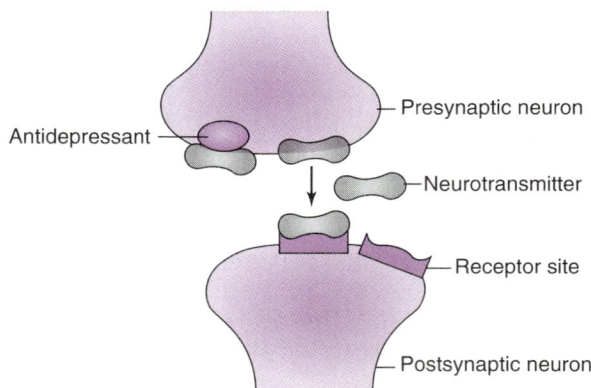

Figure 10-1 Antidepressants block reuptake of neurotransmitter into presynaptic neurons, thereby increasing the amount of neurotransmitter available to react with postsynaptic receptor sites.

   a. **Upregulation** is an increase in the number and sensitivity of postsynaptic receptor sites and is caused by a decrease in neurotransmitter at the synapse, which occurs in **depression.**

   b. **Downregulation** is a decrease in the number of receptor sites and occurs after treatment with antidepressant drugs or ECT and correlates with **improvement in mood.**

   2. **Onset** of the antidepressant effect usually occurs **after 2–4 weeks of therapy,** a delay that represents the time required for intracellular, genetic, and protein synthesis changes to occur.

C. **Adverse effects** (Table 10-4)

   1. Antidepressants may trigger a switch to **mania** in susceptible individuals with bipolar disorder.

   2. **Abrupt discontinuance** of antidepressants can lead to **withdrawal symptoms,** particularly for newer drugs with shorter half-lives.

   3. **Nefazodone, mirtazapine,** and **bupropion** are recommended for patients who experience sexual dysfunction with use of other antidepressants.

   4. **Bupropion** *should not* be used in patients with a history of seizures or bulimia nervosa.

D. **Clinical considerations**

   1. **MAOIs** have potentially **serious interactions when taken with other drugs** (e.g., levodopa, sympathomimetics, other antidepressants) and with **foods high in tyramine** (e.g., cheeses, wines, preserved meats).

   2. **Serotonin syndrome** (tremor, myoclonus, hyperthermia, delirium, and possibly death) may occur when **SSRIs** are **combined with MAOIs.**

   3. **Blood plasma levels of TCAs** (e.g., amitriptyline, nortriptyline, desipramine) should be monitored to ensure safe, therapeutic levels.

   4. Elevated levels of TCAs may occur when these drugs are used in combination with SSRIs.

IV. **Mood Stabilizers** (Table 10-5)

A. **General considerations**

   1. **Mood-stabilizing drugs** (e.g., lithium, valproic acid, carbamazepine) are used in the treatment of:

   a. **Mania:** acute and long-term treatment

   b. **Bipolar disorder:** to prevent mood cycling (switching between depressive and hypomanic or manic phases)

   2. **Antidepressants** and **antipsychotics** also are used for mood stabilization.

B. **Lithium**

   1. Used in the treatment of **manic** and **depressive phases** of **bipolar disorder**

   2. **Reduces suicidal ideation** in patients with **bipolar disorder**

Whenever possible, antidepressants should be withdrawn by tapering dosage.

Foods high in tyramine may induce hypertensive crisis in patients taking MAOIs.

Mood-stabilizing drugs are the primary treatment for bipolar disorder.

TABLE 10-4   Adverse Effects of Antidepressant Drugs

Drug	Adverse Effects
Dopamine Reuptake Inhibitor	
Bupropion	Agitation, seizures, nausea, insomnia
Monoamine Oxidase Inhibitors (MAOIs)	
Phenelzine	Hypotension, neurologic symptoms, weight gain, sexual
Tranylcypromine	dysfunction, seizures, myoclonic jerking, hypertensive crisis
Nonselective Serotonin Reuptake Inhibitor	
Trazodone	Priapism (sustained erection), syncope, drowsiness
Noradrenergic and Specific Serotonergic Inhibitor*	
Mirtazapine	Agranulocytosis, somnolence, dry mouth, weight gain, constipation, dizziness, flu symptoms, urinary frequency
Norepinephrine and Serotonin Reuptake Inhibitors	
Nefazodone	Headache, nausea, somnolence, weight loss, constipation,
Venlafaxine	dizziness, insomnia, sweating, orthostatic hypotension (nefazodone only)
Selective Serotonin Reuptake Inhibitors (SSRIs)	
Citalopram	Gastrointestinal distress, jitteriness, headache, insomnia,
Fluoxetine	sexual dysfunction, akathisia, agitation, sweating,
Fluvoxamine	somnolence, tremor, fatigue
Paroxetine	
Sertraline	
Tricyclic and Tetracyclic Antidepressants (TCAs)†	
Amitriptyline	Dry mouth, blurred vision, constipation, urinary retention,
Amoxapine	orthostatic hypotension, reflex tachycardia, dizziness,
Clomipramine	weight gain, drowsiness, heart block, seizures, sexual
Desipramine	dysfunction
Doxepin	Neuroleptic malignant syndrome and tardive dyskinesia
Imipramine	(amoxapine only)
Maprotiline	
Nortriptyline	

*Blocks α_2, 5-HT$_2$, and 5-HT$_3$ receptors, stimulates 5-HT$_{1A}$ receptors, and promotes norepinephrine release.
†Nonselective norepinephrine and serotonin reuptake inhibitors.

3. May be used to **augment the action of antidepressants** in patients with symptoms of depression that are resistant to other treatment
4. **Therapeutic level:** 0.5–1.3 mEq/L
   a. Usually not achieved until **6–10 days after treatment is initiated**
   b. **Higher levels** produce symptoms of **toxicity** (slurred speech, ataxia, altered consciousness, arrhythmias)
   c. After initiating or changing dosage, serum levels should be obtained every 3–4 days until a therapeutic level is sustained.
C. **Anticonvulsants**
   • Most commonly used are valproic acid and carbamazepine

TABLE 10-5   Adverse Effects of Mood-Stabilizing Drugs

Drug	Adverse Effects	Comments
Carbamazepine	Aplastic anemia, agranulocytosis, thrombocytopenia, rash, hyponatremia, liver dysfunction, drowsiness, dizziness Associated with **neural tube defects** and other malformations	Potential for overdose Monitor serum levels, complete blood count (CBC), liver function tests, and blood chemistries
Lithium	**Renal dysfunction,** hypothyroidism, tremor, acne, gastrointestinal distress, cognitive abnormalities, increased appetite First-trimester **teratogenic cardiovascular effects (Ebstein's anomaly)**	Potentially lethal in overdose Treat toxicity with discontinuance, hydration, and possibly dialysis (> 1.8 mEq/L) Monitor serum levels, thyroid-stimulating hormone, CBC, and blood chemistries Screen for ECG abnormalities in older patients or those with a history of cardiac disease
Olanzapine	Hyperglycemia, somnolence, weight gain, hypotension, gait abnormalities Potential for extrapyramidal side effects and tardive dyskinesia is less than with typical antipsychotics	Class C drug (**safer for pregnant patients** than lithium and valproic acid, which are category D)
Valproic acid	Gastrointestinal complaints, increased appetite, **liver dysfunction,** bone marrow suppression, thrombocytopenia, dizziness Teratogenic **neural tube defects**	Potentially lethal in overdose Monitor serum levels, CBC, liver function tests, and blood chemistries

1. Valproic acid
   a. Highly efficacious, particularly for **rapid cycling and mixed episodes** in patients with **bipolar disorder**
   b. Also indicated in **migraine prophylaxis**
   c. Therapeutic level: 50–100 μg/mL
2. Carbamazepine
   a. Used in patients with **bipolar disorder**
   b. Also used in the treatment of **trigeminal neuralgia, chronic pain,** and **neuropathy**
   c. Therapeutic level: 6–12 mg/mL
3. **Newer anticonvulsants** (e.g., gabapentin, lamotrigine, oxycarbazepine, topiramate) are used as monotherapy for mood stabilization or as adjunctive therapy to augment the action of the more commonly used mood stabilizers.
D. Antipsychotics
   1. Indicated in the treatment of **mania when psychosis and agitation are present**
   2. Newer, atypical antipsychotic drugs are being studied for their mood-stabilizing qualities in patients with bipolar disorder. **Olanzapine** has been approved for the treatment of **all phases of bipolar disorder.**

TABLE 10-6   Adverse Effects of Antianxiety Drugs

Drug	Duration of Action	Adverse Effects
Benzodiazepine Anxiolytics		
Alprazolam	Short	Sedation, dizziness, nausea,
Chlorazepate	Long	hypotension, weakness,
Chlordiazepoxide	Long	ataxia, decreased motor
Clonazepam	Long	performance, anterograde
Diazepam	Long	amnesia, syncope, dry
Lorazepam	Short	mouth, and blurred vision
Benzodiazepine Hypnotics		
Temazepam	Short	Same as for benzodiazepine anxiolytics
Nonbenzodiazepine Anxiolytics		
Beta-blockers (e.g., propran-olol, timolol)	Variable	Bradycardia, broncho-spasm, and congestive heart failure
Buspirone	Short half-life, but long-term neurotransmitter changes	Headache, nausea, dizzi-ness, dysphoria, fatigue, and dry mouth
Nonbenzodiazepine Hypnotics		
Zaleplon	Short	Lethargy, dry mouth, phar-yngitis, depression, head-ache, and myalgias
Zolpidem	Short	Drowsiness, headache, nausea, and visual changes

V.   **Antianxiety Agents** (Table 10-6)
  A.   **Benzodiazepines**
    1.   **Use**
      a.   Provide effective **initial treatment** of **moderate to severe anxiety**
      b.   **Vary** in **half-life** and **potency**, which determines their usefulness in the treatment of specific anxiety symptoms and insomnia
      c.   Have **anticonvulsant** and **muscle relaxant** effects and can be used to **decrease agitation** and symp-toms of **substance withdrawal**
    2.   **Mechanism of action**
      a.   **Bind to the GABA receptor site** and increase the af-finity of the receptor for GABA, the inhibitory neurotransmitter
      b.   GABAergic action reduces neurotransmission by **opening chloride channels** and causing **hyperpo-larization** (Figure 10-2).
      c.   Have a **rapid onset**
    3.   **Clinical considerations**
      a.   Are **safer than barbiturates** and usually are not

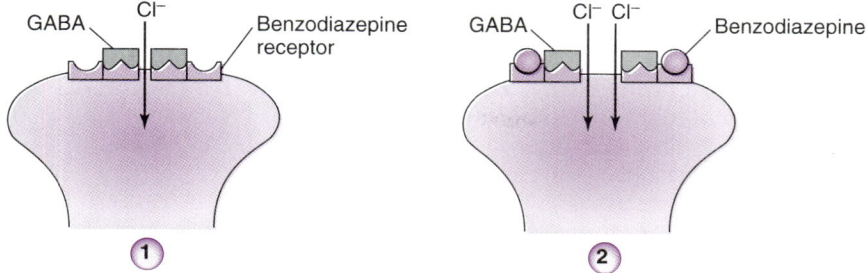

Figure 10-2   Benzodiazepine receptors are bound to the GABA receptor site **(1)**. Benzodiaz-epines enhance GABAergic action to open chloride channels and hyperpolarize the neuron **(2)**.

lethal except when taken in combination with other CNS-depressant drugs or alcohol

b.   Short-term use at the lowest effective dose is pre-ferred because of the **potential for tolerance, abuse, and withdrawal symptoms** (see Chapter 16).

c.   **Elderly patients** are more likely to have more **severe adverse effects** such as confusion, unsteadiness, and sedation.

d.   To prevent oversedation or other adverse effects, **longer-acting drugs** must be **used with caution** in the **elderly** and in patients with **impaired liver function.**

B.   **Nonbenzodiazepine antianxiety drugs**

1.   **Zolpidem** and **zaleplon** act on the **GABA receptor** and are used in the **short-term treatment of insomnia.**

2.   **Buspirone,** a **nonaddictive** drug, is used in long-term treatment of **generalized anxiety disorder.**

a.   The mechanism of action may involve stimulation of 5-HT_{1A} **receptors** in the raphe nucleus.

b.   **Onset** of action is **2–3 weeks** (compared with the im-mediate onset of benzodiazepines and sedative-hypnotic drugs).

VI.   **Stimulants**

A.   **Psychostimulants,** such as methylphenidate and dextroam-phetamine, are indicated in the treatment of **attention-deficit/hyperactivity disorder** and **narcolepsy.**

• **Modafinil,** which is *not* an amphetamine, increases alert-ness and is used in the treatment of **narcolepsy.**

B.   These drugs also are used to **augment the action of antide-pressants** in patients with depression.

VII.   **Electroconvulsive Therapy**

A.   **Use**

1.   Somatic treatment for **mood disorders** in which an **anes-thetized patient** undergoes brief pulse electrical stimu-lation that induces a generalized seizure lasting 20–60 seconds

Adverse effects of benzodiazepines are more severe in elderly patients.

ECT is highly effective in patients with life-threatening mood disorders or those unresponsive to other therapies.

2. **Highly effective** (80–90%) in **patients** who are **refractory to other treatments,** do not tolerate drugs, are actively **suicidal,** or are at medical risk of **deterioration.**
3. **Acute treatment** usually consists of three treatments per week, for a total of 6–12 treatments. Treatment may also follow a maintenance schedule, usually 1–2 times a month.

B. Complications
1. May include **short-term amnesia**, headache, myalgia, serious cardiovascular complications, and (rarely) death
2. In **severely depressed patients**, the benefits of treatment often outweigh the risk of complications.

VIII. Phototherapy
    A. Involves use of light of over 2500 lux
    B. Effective for patients whose **depression** has a **seasonal pattern**

11

Psychological Therapies

Target Topics

▷ Psychoanalytic therapies and techniques
▷ Cognitive and behavioral therapies and techniques
▷ Other therapies used in the treatment of emotional and behavioral problems

I. Overview

- Specific psychological therapies and techniques are effective in the treatment of **patients with mental disorders** and **nonpsychiatric patients** with emotional or behavioral problems.

II. Psychoanalytic Therapies

A. Psychoanalysis

1. **Sigmund Freud** developed the theory and practice of psychoanalysis.
2. The goal of this therapy is to **bring into awareness previously unconscious feelings** and **beliefs** from early developmental experiences that affect current psychological functioning. With insight into the influence of these previously unconscious forces, the patient is less likely to repeat maladaptive patterns of behavior.
3. Appropriate **candidates for psychoanalysis** include those with the following characteristics:
   a. Stable life circumstances
   b. History of positive relationships
   c. Average or above-average intelligence
   d. Motivation for self-understanding rather than for symptom relief
4. Psychoanalysis may be used in the treatment of patients with personality, anxiety, and dysthymic disorders.

Psychoanalysis seeks to bring into awareness unconscious feelings and beliefs.

Free association and dream interpretation are used to reveal patients' unconscious mental processes.

5. **Therapeutic techniques**
   a. **Free association:** the patient says everything that comes to mind. This enables the analyst to develop an understanding of the patient's unconscious thought processes.
   b. **Dream interpretation:** a method of learning more about the patient's unconscious wishes.
   c. **Interpretation of transference:** helping the patient understand his or her reactions to the analyst, as influenced by experiences with people who were important in the patient's early development. This process leads to insight regarding relationship patterns with others (see Chapter 1, III A 1).
   d. **Analysis of defense mechanisms:** commenting on mental processes used by the patient to keep anxiety-provoking feelings out of awareness (see Chapter 5, IV C).
6. **Structure of treatment**
   a. To facilitate free association, the patient **lies on a couch** and the analyst sits outside the patient's view.
   b. Treatment sessions are held **4–5 times a week** for **3–6 years.**
7. **Efficacy** of psychoanalytic therapy is **based mainly on clinical observation.**

B. **Other psychoanalytic therapies**
   1. Psychoanalytic, psychodynamic, and brief dynamic psychotherapies are based on theories derived from Freud and involve **modifications of classical psychoanalysis.**
   2. In these therapies, the **duration of treatment is shorter,** the therapist and patient sit facing each other, and the **therapist takes a more active role** in directly addressing the patient's problems.
   3. In general, these therapies are used in the treatment of a broader range of patients than is classical psychotherapy.
      a. Patients include those with severe disorders, such as **major depression** and **borderline personality disorder.**
      b. Brief dynamic psychotherapy typically *excludes* patients with severe chronic problems such as drug or alcohol dependence.

A basic tenet of behavior therapy is that adaptive behavior can be learned.

In vivo exposure and systematic desensitization are effective behavioral techniques for treating anxiety disorders.

III. **Cognitive and Behavioral Therapies**
   A. **Behavior therapy**
      1. A type of psychotherapy derived from principles of **learning theory** (see Chapter 5)
      2. Encompasses a **wide range of techniques** used in the treatment of patients with various psychiatric problems (Table 11-1).
      3. **Two of the most commonly used approaches** are:
         a. **In vivo ("real-life") exposure,** based on the concept

TABLE 11-1   Behavioral Techniques Used in the Treatment of Patients With Psychiatric Disorders

Technique	Therapeutic Process	Clinical Application	Example
Aversive conditioning	Repeated pairing of an aversive stimulus with an undesired behavior, resulting in its reduction	Sexual deviations Alcohol abuse	An alcoholic patient is given disulfiram, which makes him ill if he ingests alcohol.
In vivo exposure	Gradual real-life exposure to feared situations, using a behavioral hierarchy in which items are ranked in order of least anxiety-provoking to most anxiety-provoking	Specific and social phobias Agoraphobia Obsessive-compulsive disorder	An agoraphobic woman who is afraid to drive out of her neighborhood drives on a local highway and gets off at the first exit. Once she can drive this route with minimal anxiety, she drives to the next exit, progressively increasing her distance from home.
Flooding	A form of in vivo exposure in which exposure to the most feared situation occurs at the start of treatment, with the patient remaining in the situation until anxiety dissipates	Phobias	A man who is afraid of heights begins treatment by going to the top of a 100-story building and standing on the observation deck, until his anxiety subsides.
Implosion	Exposure to the most feared situation occurs, in imagination, at the start of treatment	Phobias	A woman who is afraid of heights starts treatment by imagining being in her most feared situation (e.g., standing on the edge of a cliff at the Grand Canyon).
Systematic desensitization	Gradual, imaginal exposure to feared situations, while pairing such exposure with relaxation	Specific and social phobias	A man who is afraid of flying learns a relaxation procedure. He relaxes and then imagines that he is driving to the airport. Once this image produces anxiety, he relaxes again. The process is repeated until he can keep the feared image in mind and remain relaxed. The procedure is repeated for each situation on the anxiety hierarchy.
Token economy	A reward system in which a token is given for displaying a desired behavior (or taken away for an undesired behavior). Tokens can later be "cashed" in for another reinforcer.	Mental retardation Psychiatric inpatients	A schizophrenic patient receives tokens for socializing with other patients. The tokens can later be exchanged for privileges on the unit.

that anxiety to a feared stimulus will eventually habituate (diminish) with repeated exposure.

    b. **Systematic desensitization**, based on the concept that by repeatedly pairing a feared stimulus with relaxation, a person learns a new response to the previously anxiety-provoking stimulus.

  4. **Behavioral techniques** are used in the treatment of patients with **nonpsychiatric conditions** (e.g., head-

TABLE 11-2   Behavioral Techniques Used in the Treatment of Patients With Psychiatric and Nonpsychiatric Problems

Technique	Therapeutic Process	Example
Goal-setting	Creating goals that are specific and realistic	A man who wishes to stop smoking agrees to reduce his cigarette consumption by 5 cigarettes in the next week.
Modeling (observational learning)	Observing others engaging in a desired behavior	A woman with a family history of breast cancer watches a videotape that shows a woman doing breast self-examination.
Positive reinforcement	Strengthening desired behaviors by providing positive consequences	An obese woman who has lost 20 pounds is genuinely praised by her physician for attaining her weight-loss goal. The patient says that she feels better since losing weight.
Self-monitoring	Recording occurrences of a targeted behavior to increase awareness and identify its antecedents	A woman with sleep difficulties is instructed to keep a record of when she falls asleep and to record how much sleep she gets each evening.
Shaping	Rewarding smaller approximations of a desired behavior	A man is encouraged to begin walking 10 minutes a day, 3 days a week. Upon reaching this initial goal, his physician praises him and recommends that he increase his walking time to 30 minutes, 5 days a week.
Relapse prevention	Identifying high-risk situations in which an undesired behavior might occur and developing plans for coping with such situations	A recovering alcoholic who recently lost his job is concerned that the stress may jeopardize his sobriety. He decides to increase his attendance at Alcoholics Anonymous meetings and to call a trusted friend when he feels tempted to drink.

aches) and in the **modification of health-risk behaviors** (Table 11-2).

B.   **Cognitive therapy**
   1.   Examines the **influences of thoughts, beliefs, and perceptions on emotions** and **behavior**
   2.   Seeks to **identify maladaptive thoughts** associated with emotional distress
       • Cognitive distortions are common in patients with **depression** (e.g., "I can't do anything right"; "Nothing will ever change") and those with **anxiety disorders** (e.g., "I'll never be able to handle these panic attacks").
   3.   **Attempts to correct maladaptive thoughts** by:
       a.   **Increasing** the patient's **awareness of the thoughts** (e.g., "Here I go again, jumping to conclusions.")
       b.   **Challenging distorted beliefs** (e.g., "What is the evidence for what I am thinking?")

Cognitive therapy aims to modify maladaptive thoughts that lead to emotional distress.

| BOX 11-1 | **The Patient Attending a Breast Cancer Support Group** |

A 56-year-old married woman who recently began treatment for breast cancer is encouraged by her physician to attend a local support group. He tells her that many women find the group to be a good source of both emotional support and medical information. He mentions that family members are welcome to attend some sessions, giving them an opportunity to learn more about the disease and share their own experiences. When the patient returns 1 month later, she reports that she attended the group and found it very comforting to talk with other women who "understand what she is going through."

       c. **Generating alternative thoughts** (e.g., "What are other explanations for this event?")

  C. **Cognitive-behavioral therapy (CBT)**
    1. Widely used psychotherapeutic approach in contemporary mental health treatment
    2. Involves the **integration of behavior and cognitive therapies** into a comprehensive treatment approach
    3. Effective treatment for **anxiety disorders** (e.g., panic disorder, phobias, obsessive-compulsive disorder), **major depression**, and **bulimia**

IV. Other Therapies
  A. **Group therapy** is a type of psychotherapy in which individuals (e.g., 8–10 people) meet under the supervision of a mental health professional to address **emotional problems** in a supportive environment.
  B. **Couples therapy** addresses problems within a partnered relationship and usually involves the therapist meeting jointly with the couple for treatment.
  C. **Family therapy**
    1. This therapy is derived from **family systems theory** (see Chapter 5).
    2. Family therapists view psychological symptoms in the **identified patient as representative of dysfunction in the family system.**
  D. **Interpersonal psychotherapy**
    1. Focuses on **current relationships** in the patient's life and addresses problems in interpersonal **interactions** as a means of alleviating psychological distress
    2. Effective in the treatment of **depression**
  E. **Supportive psychotherapy** provides emotional support and guidance to individuals who need assistance coping with **recent life crises** (e.g., bereavement) or ongoing assistance related to a **chronic illness** (e.g., schizophrenia, AIDS).
  F. **Support groups and self-help groups**
    1. **Support groups** provide **emotional support** and **information** in a **group format** (Box 11-1). These groups are *not* designed to offer psychotherapy.

Interpersonal psychotherapy is used in the treatment of depression.

    2. **Self-help groups** (e.g., 12-step programs such as Alcoholics Anonymous), although *not* professionally led, bring together individuals who share a common problem and provide a mechanism for support for **coping with life problems** or **maladaptive behaviors.**

  G. **Biofeedback**

    1. Biofeedback is a treatment modality that provides feedback about usually **involuntary physiologic processes,** with the goal of enabling a person to become more aware of and ultimately influence these processes.

    2. It is used in the treatment of a variety of conditions, including **Raynaud's syndrome, hypertension,** and **tension** or **migraine headache.**

    3. Biofeedback works through **operant conditioning** (see Chapter 5).

      a. Feedback about the physiologic state (e.g., muscle tension) serves as a **reinforcer,** signaling to the person whether the function is being influenced as desired.

      b. Feedback is usually given in the form of an **auditory tone** or **visual signal.**

    4. **Relaxation techniques,** such as progressive **muscle relaxation** and **relaxed breathing,** are often employed in biofeedback training.

Psychopathology and Other Clinical Conditions

12

Schizophrenia and Other Psychotic Disorders

Target Topics

▶ Epidemiology and neurobiology of schizophrenia
▶ Positive and negative symptoms of psychosis
▶ Features of other psychotic disorders
▶ Management of schizophrenia and other psychotic disorders

I. Schizophrenia
A. Overview
1. Is a **chronic, debilitating** mental disorder that results in impaired function
2. Involves **abnormal** or **bizarre behavior, thought,** and **speech** in the presence of intact memory and orientation
3. These abnormalities of thought and behavior are also present in other psychiatric disorders.
4. The *Diagnostic and Statistical Manual of Mental Disorders,* 4th edition, text revision (DSM-IV-TR), classification of psychotic disorders is listed in Box 12-1.

B. Epidemiology
1. Found in **1% of the population** regardless of socioeconomic class and sex

---

BOX 12-1 | **DSM-IV-TR Classification of Psychotic Disorders**

Schizophrenia
Schizophreniform disorder
Schizoaffective disorder
Brief psychotic disorder
Shared psychotic disorder
Delusional disorder
Psychotic disorder due to a general medical condition
Substance-induced psychotic disorder
Psychotic disorder not otherwise specified

Schizophrenia may affect as many as 50% of homeless individuals.

Schizophrenia is associated with an increased risk of suicide.

2. **Onset: earlier in males** (15–25 years of age) than in females (25–35 years of age)
3. Estimated to **affect 33–50% of homeless individuals**
   a. Individuals with schizophrenia tend to have residual symptoms and do not return to their original level of function after the onset of psychosis.
   b. The so-called "**downward drift**" in socioeconomic status is often experienced as a result of severely impaired function.
4. Compared with the general population, individuals with schizophrenia have higher mortality rates from accidents, natural causes, and suicide.
5. Dual diagnosis with **substance abuse** occurs in an estimated **50% of cases.**

C. **Etiology**
   • Schizophrenia has an **organic** basis, with a high degree of **heritability.**
   1. **Neurobiologic factors**
      a. Computed tomography (CT) and magnetic resonance imaging (MRI) show **enlarged ventricles** and **sulci** as well as **atrophy** in the **limbic** and **thalamic regions.** These anatomic changes are **more prevalent in males.**
      b. During cognitive testing, functional radiologic studies show decreased blood flow and decreased glucose consumption in the prefrontal cortex and reduced left and increased right temporal cortical response to speech perception.
      c. **Neurotransmitter dysfunction**
         (1) Increased dopaminergic activity may be a source of pathology.
            (a) **Dopaminergic agents** (e.g., cocaine) cause psychotic symptoms; **dopamine-blocking agents** have antipsychotic action.
            (b) **Homovanillic acid** (HVA), a metabolite of dopamine found in cerebrospinal fluid, is **increased.** After treatment with anti-

psychotic medication, HVA levels are reduced.

(2) An accelerated **loss of GABA neurons** occurs in the cingulate gyrus, with a subsequent increase in dopaminergic activity that GABA would have inhibited.

(3) **Serotonergic activity** (particularly 5-HT_2) is associated with **hallucinations** and **mood-related symptoms.**

2. **Genetic factors**

   a. Prevalence: approximately **50% in monozygotic twins**

   b. Restriction fragment length polymorphisms segregate to long arms of chromosomes 5, 11, and 18 and the short arm of chromosomes 19 and X, indicating a **heterogeneous inheritance.**

3. **Environmental factors**

   a. **Stress** may cause **earlier onset.**

   b. Incidence of schizophrenia is higher in individuals born in the winter or early spring, possibly because of a higher prevalence of viral illness in utero.

D. **Clinical presentation** (Table 12-1)

   1. **Positive symptoms:** active-phase symptoms that occur in addition to behavior or thought, such as hallucinations or delusions

   2. **Negative symptoms:** deficits of behavior and thought, such as social withdrawal or poverty of thought and speech

   3. Subtypes of schizophrenia are based on the nature of the predominant symptoms (Table 12-2).

   4. **Course**

      a. A **prodromal period** of bizarre or withdrawn behavior often precedes the initial psychotic episode.

      b. **Multiple exacerbations** and **remissions of psychosis** generally occur.

      c. **Behavioral** and **cognitive deterioration** and **residual negative symptoms** are common.

E. **Key features**

   1. **Symptoms that last for at least 6 months** and may include:

      a. Prodromal period

      b. Period of actual psychotic symptoms

      c. Residual period, in which odd behavior or thought does not completely resolve

   2. **Psychotic symptoms:** hallucinations, delusions, disorganization of speech or behavior, or negative symptoms (Box 12-2)

Bleuler's "4 As":
Ambivalence (indecisive)

Autism (self-preoccupied)

Affect (blunted)

Associations (disorganization)

TABLE 12-1 Manifestations of Schizophrenia

Manifestation	Type of Symptom	Description
Positive		
Hallucinations or illusions	Perceptual	Hallucinations: false perceptions that may be auditory (most common), somatic, visceral, olfactory, or visual; voices may comment or command Illusions: fleeting images seen out of the corner of the eye
Delusions	Thought content	Falsely held beliefs maintained despite obvious proof to the contrary; often persecutory, but jealous, religious, and grandiose delusions are also common
Ideas of reference	Thought content	Delusions that the individual is the center of widespread media or community concern and comment
Thought broadcasting, withdrawal, or insertion	Thought content	Belief that one's thoughts are evident to all or that thoughts may be inserted or withdrawn from one's mind
Bizarre behavior	Behavioral	Agitated, aggressive, or repetitive behavior; odd-appearing clothing, appearance, and social interactions; inappropriate affect or incongruent with mood
Catatonia	Behavioral	Mutism, peculiar body posturing, waxy flexibility, and rigidity
Tangentiality	Form of thought	Straying from topic so point or conclusion is not reached
Circumstantiality	Form of thought	Speech rambles around general topic in expanded way but may eventually address the issue at hand
Word salad	Form of thought	Incoherent, disjointed speech
Loose associations	Form of thought	Topics of speech shift and are not necessarily connected
Perseveration	Form of thought	Repeating a phrase again and again
Echolalia	Form of thought	Mimicking words of another
Neologisms	Form of thought	Effortlessly creating new words
Negative		
Thought blocking	Thought process	Interrupted or halting thought due to hallucinations
Impaired abstraction	Thought process	Difficulty determining meaning beyond concrete or superficial ideas
Poverty of speech or content of speech	Thought content	Use of few words or words with little meaning that relay little information
Avolition	Behavioral	Reduced physical activity, grooming, and hygiene
Affective flattening	Behavioral	Unchanging facial expression, decreased spontaneity, lack of vocal inflection, and eye contact
Anhedonia	Behavioral	Reduced activities, social interactions, and intimacy

TABLE 12-2 DSM-IV-TR Subtypes of Schizophrenia

Subtype	Description	Example
Paranoid	Persecutory delusions More organized behavior and thought than other subtypes	A man believes that his neighbors are plotting against him
Disorganized	Early onset with deterioration of organization, appearance, and bizarre behavior	Despite 90-degree heat, a woman is dressed in a winter coat and is incoherently mumbling to herself
Undifferentiated	Symptoms of more than one subtype	A man refers to himself as God in a rambling discourse
Catatonic	Muteness and posturing May alternate between stupor and lability	A woman with no language deficits stops talking and assumes unusual postures (e.g., standing like the Statue of Liberty) for lengthy periods of time
Residual	Residual symptoms of schizophrenia (usually negative or odd) No active psychosis	Despite treatment for schizophrenia, a young man is socially withdrawn and shows little emotional expression

BOX 12-2	**The Patient With Schizophrenia of the Paranoid Type**

A 19-year-old college student is brought to the physician's office by his parents, who have noticed that he has been avoiding friends and family members for the past 6 months. His grades have been falling, and he has stopped attending classes. He says that his classrooms are bugged and that the faculty and dean are part of a government conspiracy to control his mind. A psychiatrist rules out physical causes for the patient's psychotic behavior. He is started on olanzapine and shows a gradual resumption of reality-based thought, although his symptoms of social withdrawal do not resolve completely. The patient is referred for supportive counseling.

- F. Management
  - 1. At the initial onset of symptoms, a medical workup is necessary to rule out other medical etiologies for psychotic symptoms. This includes a **physical examination** and the **following studies:**
    - a. Complete blood count and blood chemistries (glucose, creatinine, electrolytes, liver function)
    - b. Thyroid-stimulating hormone level
    - c. Urine drug profile
    - d. CT or MRI of head
  - 2. **Pharmacologic treatment:** antipsychotic drugs, which block dopamine (D_2) receptors (see Chapter 10)
    - a. **Atypical antipsychotics** (e.g., olanzapine, quetiapine, risperidone)
      - (1) Act on the serotonergic system and block dopamine receptors, resulting in improvement in mood and negative symptoms
      - (2) Have fewer extrapyramidal effects and negative symptoms than typical antipsychotics
    - b. **Long-acting depot injectable drugs** may be used when medication adherence is a concern.
  - 3. **Psychological intervention:** case management, individual and group supportive therapy, and family involvement
  - 4. **Prognosis:** improved in association with the following factors:
    - a. Later disease onset
    - b. Female
    - c. More positive symptoms
    - d. Mood-related symptoms
    - e. History of supportive relationships

- II. **Other Psychotic Disorders** (see Box 12-1)
  - A. Overview
    - 1. Other psychotic disorders differ from schizophrenia in severity, character, and duration of symptoms.
    - 2. **Treatment** of psychotic symptoms requires **antipsychotics**, perhaps for a shorter period than in schizophrenia.

TABLE 12-3   Types of Delusions That Occur in Delusional Disorder

Type of Delusion	Example of Patient Statement
Erotomanic	"The DJ on the radio is sending me romantic messages"
Grandiose	"I am more gifted than other workers, and I will be selected for special treatment"
Jealous	"Those telemarketing calls are really messages from my husband's lover"
Persecutory	"My fellow workers are sabotaging my work production"
Somatic	"The fungus on my foot has invaded my entire body, causing a strange odor"

Schizophreniform disorder may precede schizophrenia.

B. Schizophreniform disorder
1. Has the same **symptoms and diagnostic criteria as schizophrenia** with the following **exceptions:**
   a. **Duration** is **less than 6 months**
   b. More often associated with a specific stressor
   c. Has a **more favorable outcome** than schizophrenia
2. **May be the precursor of schizophrenia:** diagnosis is considered provisional until 6 months of treatment have elapsed
C. Schizoaffective disorder
1. Satisfies the criteria for both **schizophrenia** and **mood disorder.** At times, psychotic features occur in the absence of mood symptoms.
2. Depending on the presenting mood symptoms, schizoaffective disorder is classified as either **bipolar** or **depressive.**
D. Brief psychotic disorder
1. Characterized by **psychotic** and **residual symptoms** that last **1 month or less**
2. Generally, an environmental trigger or stress (e.g., divorce, death, or job stress) causes the condition.
3. Functioning before and after the episode is good.
E. Shared psychotic disorder (also known as folie à deux)
1. Involves the development of a delusion **shared between two close, interdependent individuals**
2. After separation of the individuals, the psychosis resolves in the more dependent of the two but persists in the inducer of the delusion.
F. Delusional disorder
1. Characterized by **nonbizarre, fixed delusions**
2. Delusions may be erotomanic, grandiose, jealous, persecutory, or somatic (Table 12-3).

Mood Disorders and Suicide

Target Topics

▸ Epidemiology and etiology of mood disorders
▸ Symptoms and differential diagnosis of mood disorders
▸ Management of mood disorders
▸ Assessment and management of patients at risk for suicide

I. Overview

A. General characteristics of mood disorders

 1. Mood disorders are characterized by **elevated, expansive, irritable,** or **depressed** moods.

 a. **Depressive disorders** (unipolar disorders) involve depressed mood only, frequently with loss of interest.

 b. **Manic-depressive disorders** (bipolar disorders) involve elevated, expansive, or irritable moods, usually in combination with depressed mood.

 2. Symptoms of mood disorders cause **emotional distress** and/or **impairment in daily activities.**

B. The *Diagnostic and Statistical Manual of Mental Disorders,* 4th edition, text revision (DSM-IV-TR), classification of mood disorders is listed in Box 13-1.

C. Mood and affect

 1. Mood

 a. **Pervasive, sustained emotion** that influences an individual's perceptions and outlook

 b. Subjective emotional experience

 c. Information obtainable from patient reports

 2. Affect

 a. More **transient pattern** of emotional expression

> Unipolar disorders: depressed mood.

> Bipolar disorders: elevated expansive or irritable mood, typically in combination with depressed mood.

b. Objective, behavioral expression of emotion
c. Information obtainable from observing patient actions

II. Epidemiology and Etiology of Mood Disorders
A. Epidemiology
1. **Lifetime prevalence rates:** highest for major depressive disorder (10–25% for females, 5–12% for males), followed by dysthymic disorder (6%), bipolar I (1%), bipolar II (1%), cyclothymic disorder (1%)
2. **Risk factors**
   a. **Female** and **adolescent** or **young adult** (Table 13-1)
   b. Previous or concurrent psychiatric illness (e.g., schizophrenia, posttraumatic stress disorder)
   c. Chronic or severe medical illness (e.g., stroke that causes disability, life-threatening cancer)
   d. Adverse life events (e.g., loss of job, victim of crime)
   e. Divorced, separated, or widowed
   f. Substance abuse; history of smoking
   g. Low socioeconomic status
3. **Morbidity and mortality**
   a. **Disabilities associated with chronic mood disor-**

Major depressive disorder is more common in females.

Up to 15% of individuals with untreated depression commit suicide.

BOX 13-1 DSM-IV-TR Classification of Mood Disorders

Depressive Disorders
  Major depressive disorder
  Dysthymic disorder
  Depressive disorder not otherwise specified
Bipolar Disorders
  Bipolar I disorder
  Bipolar II disorder
  Cyclothymic disorder
  Bipolar disorder not otherwise specified
Other Mood Disorders
  Mood disorder due to a general medical condition
  Substance-induced mood disorder
  Mood disorder not otherwise specified

TABLE 13-1 Risk Factors of Gender and Age for Selected Mood Disorders

Mood Disorder	Gender	Typical Age of Onset
Major depressive disorder	Two times as likely in females	Mid 20s
Dysthymic disorder	Two to three times as likely in females	Childhood, adolescence, early adulthood
Bipolar I	Equally common in males and females	Early 20s
Bipolar II	More common in females	Early 20s
Cyclothymic disorder	Equally common in males and females	Adolescence and early adulthood

ders may be as great or greater than problems associated with major diseases (e.g., diabetes mellitus,
hypertension, and arthritis).
   b. Most individuals who attempt suicide are suffering
      from a **mood disorder.**
   B. Etiology
      1. Neurobiologic factors
         a. **Dysfunction** of **norepinephrine, serotonin,** and **do-
            pamine** is implicated in the pathology of mood
            disorders.
         b. **Neuroendocrine dysfunction,** especially involving
            cortisol and thyroid hormones, is linked to mood
            abnormalities.
      2. **Genetic factors:** as shown by family, adoption, and twin
         studies
      3. **Environmental factors:** stress may precipitate mood
         episodes.
      4. **Cognitive factors**
         a. **Learned helplessness** is a habitual passive response
            to conflicts that may place individuals at risk for
            depression.
         b. Certain **cognitive patterns** (e.g., viewing events
            and oneself in a negative light, having a negative
            outlook of the future) are associated with depression.

Depression is asso-
ciated with de-
creased levels of
norepinephrine,
serotonin, and
dopamine.

III. **Mood Episodes**
   A. Overview
      1. Mood episodes are **distinct periods** during which a **char-
         acteristic mood** and **specific symptoms** are **identified**
         by the patient or readily inferred by family or friends.
      2. Mood episodes are **prerequisites** ("building blocks") **for
         several diagnoses.** Thus, recognition of mood episodes is
         fundamental to making an accurate diagnosis.
   B. **Type of episodes:** major depressive, manic, hypomanic, and
      mixed (Table 13-2)
   C. **Key features of major depressive episodes** (Box 13-2)
      1. Depressed mood
      2. Loss of interest in normal activities
      3. Sleep disturbance (e.g., early morning wakening)
      4. Excessive guilt about past mistakes; feelings of
         worthlessness
      5. Decreased energy; fatigue
      6. Difficulty concentrating; poor memory
      7. Appetite change or weight loss or gain
      8. Psychomotor agitation or retardation
      9. Suicidal thoughts
   D. **Key features of manic/hypomanic episodes** (see Box 13-2)
      1. **Elevated, expansive, or irritable mood**
      2. Flight of ideas
      3. Increase in goal-directed activity
      4. Sleep (decreased need)
      5. Talkative (more than usual)

TABLE 13-2   Types of Mood Episodes

Type of Episode	Minimal Duration	Key Features
Major depressive	2 weeks	Depressed mood (dysphoria) or lack of interest in formerly enjoyable activities (anhedonia)
Manic	1 week (less if hospitalization is necessary)	Elevated, expansive, or irritable mood
		Markedly impaired social or occupational functioning, psychotic features, or need for hospitalization to protect from harm
Hypomanic	4 days	Elevated, expansive, or irritable mood
		May have some impaired functioning but not marked amount
		No psychotic features and no need for hospitalization to protect from harm
Mixed	Both major depressive and manic episodes almost every day for at least 1 week	Features of both depression and mania
		Markedly impaired social or occupational functioning, psychotic features, or need for hospitalization to protect from harm

---

BOX 13-2   **Mnemonics: Symptoms of Major Depressive and Manic Episodes**

Major Depressive Episode:
"SIG E CAPS"
Sleep disturbance
Interest (loss of)
Guilt
Energy (loss of)
Concentration difficulties
Appetite change
Psychomotor agitation or
   retardation
Suicidal thoughts

Manic Episode:
"FAST PED"
Flight of ideas
Activity (increased, goal-directed)
Sleep (decreased need)
Talkative (more than usual)
Pleasure (seeks gratification without
   regard for harmful consequences)
Self-Esteem (increased)

Distractibility

---

   6. Pleasure (seeks gratification without regard for harmful consequences)
   7. Inflated self-esteem
   8. Distractible

IV.   Clinical Presentation of Mood Disorders
   A.   Classification, based on key features and course (Table 13-3):
      1. Depressive disorders
      2. Bipolar disorders
      3. Disorders due to physiologic agents

TABLE 13-3   Features of Mood Disorders

Diagnosis	Key Features	Typical Course
Depressive Disorders		
Major depressive disorder	Occurrence of major depressive episode(s) No evidence of manic, hypomanic, or mixed episode	Recurrence in 60% of patients who have one episode Recurrence in 70% of patients who have two episodes
Dysthymic disorder	Depressed mood occurs for most of day, for more days than not, for ≥ 2 years Accompanied by at least two of the following factors: hopelessness, low self-esteem, sleep disruption (insomnia), poor appetite or overeating, decision-making difficulty, low energy	Chronic course
Bipolar Disorders		
Bipolar I	History of manic or mixed episodes alternating with depressive episodes (usually major depression)	Recurrence in 90% of patients who have one episode Interval between episodes tends to decrease with advancing age
Bipolar II	History of hypomanic episode(s) alternating with major depressive episode(s)	Most patients return to fully functional level between episodes Interval between episodes tends to decrease with advancing age
Cyclothymic disorder	Hypomanic symptoms/episode alternating with depressive symptoms (no episode) for ≥ 2 years	Insidious onset Chronic course
Disorders Due to Physiologic Agents		
Substance-induced mood disorder	Direct physiologic consequence of exposure to drug of abuse, medication, or toxic substance	Mood symptoms subside as substance levels return to normal
Mood disorder due to general medical condition	Direct physiologic consequence of illness	Mood symptoms subside as medical condition improves

    B.   Presenting symptoms (Box 13-3)
       1.   Emotional distress (e.g., dysphoria, anhedonia)
       2.   Physical symptoms (e.g., decreased libido, pain, fatigue)
         • **"Masked depression"** describes a presentation of physical symptoms while being unaware of emotional distress.
       3.   Cognitive changes (e.g., trouble concentrating, hopelessness)
         • **Pseudodementia** refers to memory loss or confusion that resolves with improvement in symptoms of depression (see Chapter 20).
       4.   Behavioral changes (e.g., social withdrawal)
    C.   Specifiers used in the DSM-IV-TR to describe the most recent mood episode or the course of certain mood disorders:
       1.   "With melancholic features": severe depressive episode; characterized by the loss of pleasure in almost all activities or by loss of reactivity (e.g., mood does not brighten in response to positive events)

BOX 13-3	The Patient With Bipolar II Disorder

A 22-year-old woman sees her physician because of chronic nausea and lower abdominal bloating. She displays a flat affect and psychomotor slowing, prompting the physician to ask her about her mood. She admits to feeling depressed and fatigued, experiencing hypersomnia and anhedonia, and having difficulty concentrating over the past few months. She denies suicidal thoughts or use of alcohol or drugs during this time. Suspecting a mood disorder, the physician asks if she has had times when her mood is especially good. She reports a 2-week period during the past year when she felt great and had lots of energy. She acknowledges that racing thoughts, pressured speech, distractibility, and a decreased need for sleep were also present, but she denies any disruption in her job or relationships at the time. Based on this history of a hypomanic episode and current depressive episode, the physician diagnoses bipolar II disorder. He discusses a plan for treating her gastrointestinal complaints and expresses concern about her mood symptoms. She agrees to see a psychiatrist and to return for follow-up for her gastrointestinal complaints.

2. **"With postpartum onset"**: episode that occurs within 4 weeks of giving birth; occurs in **5–10%** of postpartum women. In contrast, **"baby blues"** is a mild transient mood change that resolves within about 10 days of delivery. It is seen in up to **70% of mothers**, but it is not a mood episode.

3. **"With seasonal pattern"**: major depressive episodes involving a temporal relationship between the onset and remission of the episodes and a particular time of year (e.g., seasonal affective disorder)

4. **"Severe with psychotic features"**: hallucinations or delusions that accompany a depressive episode

5. Other specifiers refer to **catatonic, atypical,** and **rapid cycling** conditions.

V. **Differential Diagnosis of Mood Disorders**

A. **Conditions that cause mood symptoms** and that must be differentiated from primary mood disorders include:

1. **Medical conditions** (e.g., hypothyroidism)

2. **Substance use** (e.g., alcohol dependence): mood disturbances that persist after detoxification has occurred may result in diagnosis of a primary mood disorder.

3. Other **psychiatric conditions** (e.g., schizoaffective disorder, adjustment disorders)

4. **Bereavement**

B. **Depression and anxiety** (Table 13-4)

1. Depressive and anxiety disorders **share** some **common features**, but certain characteristics are clinically useful in differentiating between these types of disorders.

2. **Depression** is commonly **comorbid with anxiety disorders.**

TABLE 13-4   Distinguishing Features of Depression and Anxiety

Feature	Depression	Anxiety
Motivation or "drive"	Helplessness and hopelessness	Driven to anticipate and prepare for next event
Insomnia	Initial, middle, and terminal insomnia	More likely to have difficulty falling asleep
Pleasure	Little or none	More often
Thought content	Suicidal or depression-generating	Involving questioning and worry
Emotion	Sad	Anxious or worried
Behavior	Flat affect Psychomotor retardation	Agitation

C.   Depression and medical illness
1.   Depression in medically ill patients is often difficult to detect because patients' **psychological** and **medical symptoms** often **overlap** (e.g., poor appetite may be a symptom of either depression or pneumonia).
2.   **Cognitive symptoms** (e.g., thoughts of hopelessness, worthlessness) and **suicidal thoughts** may indicate a clinically significant depression in patients with medical illness.
3.   **Higher rates of depression** are observed among individuals who **suffer from a variety of physical disorders** (e.g., at least 40% of patients with acute stroke have diagnosable depression).

D.   Depression and bereavement
1.   Many **symptoms** of **depression** and **bereavement are similar** (e.g., insomnia, sadness), but if symptoms of a major depressive disorder **persist 2 months after** the **loss of a loved one**, the presence of this disorder, rather than bereavement, should be considered.
2.   The occurrence of certain symptoms at any time following the loss of a loved one signals a **diagnosis of depression.** Symptoms include:
    a.   Persistent and markedly **impaired functioning**
    b.   Significant **psychomotor retardation**
    c.   Excessive preoccupation with **feelings of worthlessness**
    d.   **Feelings of guilt** (other than guilt about events related to the death of a loved one)
    e.   **Hallucinations** (other than thinking that one has briefly seen or heard the deceased)
    f.   **Suicidal thoughts** (except those related to the belief that a survivor should have died with the deceased or would be better off deceased themselves)

VI.   Management of Mood Disorders
   • Treatment of mood disorders may involve pharmacotherapy and/or psychotherapy.
   • Drugs are the treatment of choice for bipolar disorders.

Depressive and anxiety disorders often occur at the same time.

Indicators of depression in bereavement: "DIP HUG"

Death (thoughts of)
Impairment
Psychomotor retardation

Hallucinations
Unworthiness
Guilt

A. **Pharmacologic therapy and other medical therapies** (see Chapter 10)
  1. **Antidepressant drugs**
     a. Primary pharmacologic treatment for **depressive (unipolar) disorders**
     b. Used in the treatment of the depressive phases of manic-depressive (bipolar) disorder after the initiation of mood-stabilizing drugs.
  2. **Antipsychotic drugs:** used to treat mood disorders accompanied by **psychotic symptoms**
  3. **Antianxiety drugs:** often indicated in combination with antidepressants, because of the **high comorbidity of depression and anxiety disorders**
  4. **Electroconvulsive therapy (ECT):** indicated in the treatment of mood disorders in cases of severe life-threatening symptoms or lack of response to drugs

B. **Psychotherapy**
  1. Behavior, cognitive-behavioral, interpersonal, and family therapies are **effective treatments for major depressive disorder** (see Chapter 11).
  2. A combination of **psychotherapy and antidepressant medication** is more effective in treating major depressive disorder than using either form of treatment alone.
  3. An important aspect of psychotherapy for **bipolar disorder** is its focus on **adherence to medication** schedules.

C. **Patient education** is a high-yield **intervention strategy.**
  1. Education fosters a **collaborative relationship** that encourages the patient to become an active participant rather than a passive recipient in his or her care.
  2. Learning about the **flawed thinking patterns** that are associated with mood disorders often helps the patient **avoid making poor decisions** during a mood episode.
  3. Education about symptom detection, intervention options, and anticipated treatment outcomes usually produces an **improved sense of personal control.**

VII. **Suicide**

A. **Epidemiology and etiology**
  1. Suicide is the eleventh leading cause of death in the United States.
  2. Suicide rates are highest in the **elderly.**
  3. Females are more likely to attempt suicide, but male suicide attempts more often result in death because males tend to use more lethal methods. **White males** account for **70%** of all suicides.

B. **Suicide risk** is associated with several demographic, genetic, psychiatric, physical, and psychosocial factors (Table 13-5; Box 13-4).
  1. **Most individuals** who **commit suicide** have a **diagnosable psychiatric disorder.**
  2. Many individuals who commit suicide have visited a physician in the month preceding the event.

Indicators of suicide risk: "SAD PERSONS"

Sex
Age
Depression
Previous attempts
Ethanol abuse
Rational thinking (loss of)
Social support (lacking)
Organized plan
No spouse
Sickness

TABLE 13-5   Risk Factors for Suicide

Category	Risk Factor
Demographic	Sex: male Age: 15–24 years, > 65 years Marital status: widowed or divorced Race: white, Native American Religion: Protestant, Jewish Occupation: physician, dentist, police officer, attorney, musician, writer Unemployed
Genetic	Family history of suicide
Psychiatric	Major depression, bipolar disorder Schizophrenia Substance abuse and dependence Borderline and antisocial personality disorders, panic disorder, anorexia nervosa
Physical	Chronic or terminal illness (e.g., AIDS, cancer, chronic renal failure) Prolonged pain, loss of function, disfigurement
Psychosocial Current	Hopelessness Suicidal ideation, plan for suicide Access to firearms High levels of stress, recent loss Lack of social support, lives alone Impulsiveness
Past	Previous suicide attempts Personal knowledge of suicide victim

BOX 13-4   The Patient at High Risk for Suicide

A 68-year-old recently widowed white man seeks help for chronic pain related to an automobile accident. He reports that the pain has been worse than usual and that he has been drinking more alcohol to help him sleep. When the physician suggests placing him on a different pain medication, the patient replies, "What's the use? It doesn't matter." The physician asks if he has ever considered suicide, and the patient admits that he has been thinking about suicide frequently. The previous evening, he loaded a gun but put it away after thinking about the effect that his death would have on his children. The physician expresses great concern for the patient's safety and recommends admission to a hospital. The patient admits that he needs help and agrees to be hospitalized.

    3. **Decreased cerebrospinal fluid levels of 5-hydroxyindoleacetic acid,** a metabolite of serotonin, have been observed in individuals who have committed or attempted suicide.

  C. **Management of patients at risk for suicide** depends on knowledge of general suicide risk factors and a thorough assessment of the degree of risk (see Table 13-5).

14

Anxiety Disorders

▶ Biological and psychological aspects of anxiety disorders
▶ Symptoms and differential diagnosis of anxiety disorders
▶ Management of anxiety disorders

I. **Overview**
   A. **Anxiety** is a **normal** and **adaptive emotion** that helps individuals meet the challenges of daily life. Moderate levels of anxiety enhance performance, whereas too little or too much anxiety may impair performance.
   B. **Anxiety** becomes **problematic** when **symptoms are excessive**, negatively **affect functioning**, or cause **marked distress.**
      1. **Anxiety disorders** are generally **chronic** and **recurrent.** They are among the **most common mental health problems** and are **usually treatable.**
      2. For some conditions, such as posttraumatic stress disorder (PTSD), generalized anxiety disorder, and obsessive-compulsive disorder (OCD), treatment usually results in improvement but does not eliminate symptoms.
      3. **Manifestations of anxiety** (Table 14-1)
   C. The *Diagnostic and Statistical Manual of Mental Disorders,* 4th edition, text revision (DSM-IV-TR), classification of anxiety disorders is listed in Box 14-1.
   D. **Etiology**
      1. **Neurobiologic factors**
         a. **Structures of the brain associated with anxiety disorders** include the locus ceruleus, raphe nucleus, limbic system, frontal cortex, and caudate nucleus.
         b. **Neurotransmitters** implicated in the neurobiology

TABLE 14-1 Manifestations of Anxiety

Physical Symptoms	Psychological Symptoms
Palpitations	Worry
Increased heart rate	Apprehension, feeling of unease
Chest pain or discomfort	Irritability
Abdominal distress	Difficulty relaxing
Nausea	Vigilance
Shortness of breath	Exaggerated startle response
Dizziness	Feelings of unreality (derealization)
Hot flashes or chills	Feeling detached from oneself (depersonalization)
Trembling or shaking	
Fatigue	
Paresthesias	
Muscle tension	
Sleep disturbance	

BOX 14-1   DSM-IV-TR Classification of Anxiety Disorders

Generalized anxiety disorder
Panic disorder with agoraphobia
Panic disorder without agoraphobia
Agoraphobia without a history of panic disorder
Social phobia
Specific phobia
Obsessive-compulsive disorder
Posttraumatic stress disorder
Acute stress disorder
Anxiety disorder due to a general medical condition
Substance-induced anxiety disorder
Anxiety disorder not otherwise specified

---

of anxiety disorders include norepinephrine, serotonin, and GABA.

2. **Genetic factors:** increased rates of anxiety disorders occur in family members of individuals with such disorders.

3. Anxiety disorders develop when **environmental factors** act on **biologically vulnerable** individuals.

E. Differential diagnosis

1. **Conditions that may produce** anxiety symptoms **or mimic** anxiety disorders include:

a. **Medical disorders** (e.g., hyperthyroidism, hypoglycemia, pheochromocytoma, cardiac arrhythmias)

b. **Substance use** (e.g., amphetamines, caffeine, medications, toxins)

c. **Other psychiatric conditions** (e.g., depression, psychosis, adjustment disorder, drug and alcohol withdrawal, drug intoxication)

2. Table 14-2 lists key features used to differentiate anxiety disorders.

TABLE 14-2   Key Features of Anxiety Disorders

Disorder	Key Feature	Example
Generalized anxiety disorder	Chronic uncontrollable worry about everyday life	Constant worrying about health, finances, and job, although concerns are unwarranted
Panic disorder (with or without agoraphobia)	Episodic attacks associated with fear and physical symptoms, with or without agoraphobia	Fear of having a panic attack
Social phobia	Distress about possible scrutiny by others and possible embarrassment or humiliation	Fear of public speaking
Specific phobia	Fear of a specific object or situation, with anxiety diminishing once exposure or anticipated exposure has passed	Fear of heights (acrophobia) Fear of enclosed spaces (claustrophobia)
Obsessive-compulsive disorder	Distress related to specific themes, which is temporarily relieved by engaging in certain repeated activities	Obsession: fear of contamination Compulsion: excessive handwashing
Posttraumatic stress disorder	Distress after exposure to a traumatic event involving actual or threatened death or serious injury	Reexperiencing trauma in nightmares

    F.   Comorbidity: comorbid conditions include depression, substance abuse, and anxiety disorders other than the one diagnosed.

II.   Generalized Anxiety Disorder
  A.   Epidemiology
    1.   Onset: usually in **early adulthood** (can occur in childhood)
    2.   More common in **females**
    3.   Course: chronic, fluctuating, exacerbated by stress
  B.   Clinical presentation
    1.   Patients with generalized anxiety disorder may not spontaneously report their worries to a physician and may instead focus on physical complaints when seeking medical care.
    2.   Excessive anxiety and worry occurs for at least 6 months, more days than not.
      a.   Worries are about numerous events and focus on everyday life circumstances (e.g., health, finances).
      b.   Worries are **out of proportion to the situation** and are **difficult to control.**
    3.   Diagnosis: At least **three** of the following **additional symptoms** must also be present for the diagnosis of generalized anxiety disorder:
      a.   Restlessness, feeling on edge or "keyed up"

Generalized anxiety disorder: excessive worry that is difficult to control and lasts for at least 6 months.

TABLE 14-3   Drugs Used To Treat Anxiety Disorders

Anxiety Disorder	Drug	Use
Generalized anxiety disorder	Buspirone Benzodiazepines Antidepressants: SSRIs,* venlafaxine	Short-term
Panic disorder (with or without agoraphobia)	Antidepressants: SSRIs	TCAs and MAOIs in resistant cases
	Benzodiazepines	Short-term
Social phobia	Antidepressants: SSRIs	TCAs and MAOIs in resistant cases
	Benzodiazepines and beta blockers	Prior to exposure
Specific phobia	Benzodiazepines	Prior to exposure
Obsessive-compulsive disorder	Antidepressants: SSRIs, clomipramine	Usually require higher doses and up to 12-week trials
	Benzodiazepines	During initial treatment
	Antipsychotics	If obsessions reach delusional level
Posttraumatic stress disorder	Antidepressants: SSRIs and other newer antidepressants	TCAs and MAOIs in resistant cases
	Mood stabilizers: lithium, valproate, and carbamazepine	For explosive symptoms and mood instability
	Clonidine or beta blockers	For increased startle reflex
	Antipsychotics	For severe flashbacks or psychotic symptoms
Acute stress disorder	Benzodiazepines	Short-term use for anxiety and insomnia
Anxiety disorder due to a general medical condition	—	Use drugs as indicated to treat anxiety symptoms, but find and treat underlying medical etiology

MAOI, monoamine oxidase inhibitor; *SSRI,* serotonin specific reuptake inhibitor; *TCA,* tricyclic antidepressant.
*Although not every SSRI has a US FDA indication for every disorder mentioned in the table, in practice, all SSRIs are used for all disorders.

    b. Fatigue
    c. Difficulty concentrating
    d. Irritability
    e. Difficulty sleeping
    f. Muscle tension
  4. **Associated physical complaints** include:
    a. Dry mouth
    b. Headache
    c. Sweating
    d. Trembling
    e. Gastrointestinal symptoms (difficulty swallowing, nausea, diarrhea, and irritable bowel syndrome)
C. **Management**
  1. **Pharmacologic agents** (Table 14-3)
    a. Anxiety and depression result from **disruption of** the

same **neurotransmitter systems.** Many of the same drugs are used to treat both disorders in an attempt to restore **homeostasis.**

  b. **Tricyclic antidepressants** (TCAs) and **monoamine oxidase inhibitors** (MAOIs) are second- and third-line choices because of the potential for **adverse effects.**

 2. **Cognitive-behavioral therapy,** which focuses on:
  a. Helping patients learn to **reduce physiologic arousal** (e.g., relaxation skills)
  b. **Modifying maladaptive thinking patterns** that contribute to excessive anxiety (see Chapter 11)

 3. **Lifestyle modification** (e.g., reducing or eliminating caffeine intake)

III. **Panic Disorder (With or Without Agoraphobia)**
  A. **Epidemiology**
   1. **Onset:** typically in **late adolescence** and **early adulthood**
   2. More common in **females**
   3. **Course: chronic** and **fluctuating**
   4. **Stressful events** are associated with the onset and exacerbation of symptoms.
  B. **Panic attacks**
   1. **Distinct periods of intense fear or discomfort** that are often accompanied by:
    a. Feelings of **terror** or **impending doom**
    b. **Desire to escape** the situation in which the attack is occurring
   2. **Attacks occur spontaneously** ("out of the blue"), in expected situations (cued), or during sleep (nocturnally) and are accompanied by **strong physical sensations** and **distress.**
   3. **Symptoms**
    a. May include **shortness of breath, chest pain** or discomfort, **palpitations, sweating, lightheadedness,** and fear of losing control
    b. **Develop suddenly** and reach their peak intensity within 10 minutes
   4. Panic attacks may occur **in other anxiety disorders** (e.g., generalized anxiety disorder, PTSD, phobias) and **other psychiatric conditions** (e.g., depression).
  C. **Clinical presentation** (Box 14-2)
   1. **Recurrent, unexpected** panic attacks
   2. In addition, **at least one of the following conditions must be present for at least 1 month:**
    a. **Anticipatory anxiety:** concern about having additional attacks
    b. **Change in behavior** associated with the attacks
    c. **Worry about the implications or consequences** of the attacks (e.g., fear of illness)

Panic disorder: typically develops in late adolescence and early adulthood; more common in females.

Panic disorder: recurrent, spontaneous panic attacks.

BOX 14-2	The Patient With Panic Disorder

A 24-year-old woman experiences the sudden onset of shortness of breath, palpitations, chest pain, sweating, and dizziness when she is at a shopping mall. Terrified that she is having a heart attack, she seeks help at a nearby emergency facility. She reports having five similar episodes in the past month and fears repeated episodes. She has no known cardiac risk factors. Her family history is remarkable for a mother who has "nerve" problems and refuses to travel. After ruling out an underlying medical condition, the emergency department physician diagnoses panic disorder. The patient is briefly educated about panic attacks (i.e., panic attacks are frightening but will pass) and is advised to continue to frequent places where the attacks occurred. The patient receives a prescription for paroxetine (an SSRI), a referral for cognitive-behavioral therapy; and instructions to follow up with her primary care physician. Six months later, the patient is symptom-free and confident about managing future symptoms.

3. **Fear of dying** or of having a heart attack may prompt patients to seek emergency medical care.
4. Panic attacks are *not* the result of a medical condition or substance use.

D. Agoraphobia
   1. Characterized by fear of situations in which **escape may be difficult** or **help is unavailable** if panic symptoms develop
   2. Develops in many patients **with panic disorder**
   3. **Common agoraphobic fears**
      a. **Traveling** away from home
      b. Being in **crowds**
      c. **Standing in line**
      d. **Crossing bridges**
      e. Using **public transportation**

E. Management
   1. **Pharmacologic therapy** (see Table 14-3)
   2. **Cognitive-behavioral therapy**
      a. **Patient education**
      b. Development of **skills for managing anxiety** (e.g., relaxation skills, diaphragmatic breathing, cognitive self-talk)
      c. **In vivo exposure** (desensitization) **to feared situations** when agoraphobia is present (see Chapter 11)

IV. **Phobias**
   A. **Clinical presentation**
      1. Phobic individuals typically **avoid exposure** to feared objects or situations, if possible, or **endure exposure with distress.**
      2. Distress increases when the patient is **exposed to the feared object** or in **anticipation of such exposure.**

Phobias: most frequently occurring anxiety disorders.

| BOX 14-3 | The Patient With Specific Phobia |

A 29-year-old pregnant woman is brought to the clinic by her husband for a prenatal visit after she has canceled several previous appointments. The woman appears very anxious and concerned about the type of evaluation that she will undergo. She learns that she needs to be screened for gestational diabetes mellitus, which involves having her finger pricked to obtain a blood sample. She becomes distressed and pleads to have the test postponed, saying that she "just can't manage it." The physician calmly asks the patient whether the sight of blood or the idea of receiving injections distresses her. The patient, who seems relieved that someone understands, responds "How did you know?" The physician refers the patient to a psychologist for behavioral treatment of her phobia, and after four visits, she is able to undergo the screening procedure.

B. Social phobia

Social phobia: fear of exposure to possible scrutiny.

1. Fear of **social or performance situations** that involve exposure to **unfamiliar persons** and **possible scrutiny**
2. Distress about **being embarrassed or humiliated**
3. May be either **specific** to a situation (e.g., public speaking) or **generalized** across many social situations
4. **Blushing** and other symptoms of anxiety may occur with exposure to the feared situation.
5. **Commonly feared situations** include:
   a. Eating or drinking in public
   b. Public speaking, writing in public
   c. Using public restrooms
   d. Talking with authority figures
   e. Dating

C. Specific phobia
1. **Intense and persistent fear of specific objects or situations** (Box 14-3; see Table 14-2)
2. In medical settings, **uncooperative patient behavior** may be a sign of an **undisclosed phobia** (e.g., a patient with claustrophobia who refuses to have a magnetic resonance imaging scan).

D. Management
1. **Pharmacologic therapy** may be prescribed when patients anticipate exposure to feared situations (see Table 14-3).
2. **Cognitive-behavioral therapy** involves gradually exposing patients to feared situations (e.g., fear of flying). If "real life" exposure is not practical, **systematic desensitization** is used (see Chapter 11).
3. **Social skills training** may be used as an adjunct treatment for patients with **social phobia** who have social skills deficits.

V. **Obsessive-Compulsive Disorder (OCD)**
A. **Epidemiology**
1. Estimated lifetime **prevalence** in the United States: **2–3%**

| BOX 14-4 | The Patient With Obsessive-Compulsive Disorder |

A 14-year-old boy with red, severely chapped hands is diagnosed with contact dermatitis. When the physician asks him about his use of soaps and other possible skin irritants, the boy says that he uses alcohol wipes and household cleansers on his hands several times daily to keep them clean. He admits to worrying a great deal about whether his hands are contaminated with "germs." In addition, he says that using cleansers eliminates his need for frequent handwashing. The patient's mother, who knows that her son likes to take lengthy showers, is unaware that he has been engaging in these behaviors. The physician diagnoses OCD and starts the patient on sertraline (an SSRI) and refers him for cognitive-behavioral treatment.

    2. **Onset:** usually in the **teens or early 20s**; may develop earlier
    3. **Stressful life events** have been associated with onset (e.g., postpartum period, illness) and exacerbation of symptoms.
    4. In adults, equally common in males and females
    5. **Course: chronic** and **fluctuating**
  B. Etiology
    1. **Neurobiologic factors:** neuroimaging studies point to **dysfunction** in the **frontal cortex** and **basal ganglia.**
    2. **Genetic factors**
      a. Greater concordance rates among **monozygotic twins** compared with dizygotic twins
      b. **Increased rates** among **first-degree relatives**
      c. First-degree relatives of individuals with **Tourette's disorder** have increased rates of OCD (see Chapter 22).
  C. Clinical presentation (Box 14-4)
    1. Patients often do not spontaneously report symptoms of OCD because of embarrassment or shame. At some point, patients usually are aware that their **symptoms are excessive and unreasonable.**
    2. Characterized by **obsessions or compulsions.** Functionally, **obsessions produce anxiety, compulsions decrease anxiety.**
      a. **Obsessions** are **repetitive thoughts**, impulses, or images that are experienced as senseless and intrusive and tend to focus on **certain themes** (e.g., **contamination**, pathologic doubt, religion, sex, aggression or harm, or order and asymmetry).
      b. **Compulsions** are **repetitive behaviors** or mental acts performed in response to an obsession and aimed at reducing distress, such as excessive hand washing, excessive checking (e.g., locks), and repetitive actions (e.g., turning light switches on and off 10 times).
    3. Compulsions may be maintained by their **reinforcing**

OCD: intrusive thoughts, images, or impulses; ritualistic behaviors.

properties (i.e., they result in a temporary reduction in distress).

4. **Signs:** may include red, chapped hands; repeated requests for medical tests (e.g., HIV) without indication; and concerns about cancer, AIDS, or poisoning

D. **Differential diagnosis**
   1. OCD-spectrum disorders (e.g., body dysmorphic disorder, trichotillomania)
   2. Obsessive-compulsive personality disorder
   3. Tourette's disorder

E. **Management**
   1. **Pharmacologic treatment** (see Table 14-3)
   2. **Cognitive-behavioral therapy:** such treatment involves "response prevention," in which patients are instructed not to engage in ritualistic behaviors following exposure to feared stimuli.
   3. **Surgical intervention** (e.g., cingulotomy) is considered an intervention of last resort; it continues to be used in severe cases that do not respond to medication to disrupt efferent pathways from the frontal cortex to the basal ganglia.

VI. **Posttraumatic Stress Disorder (PTSD) and Acute Stress Disorder (ASD)**

A. **Overview**
   1. **Symptoms of anxiety** develop **after direct or indirect exposure to a severe traumatic stressor** involving actual or threatened death or significant injury, and which involved feelings of intense fear or helplessness.
   2. **Traumatic stressors**
      a. Military combat
      b. Physical personal assault (e.g., mugging)
      c. Sexual abuse and/or sexual assault
      d. Natural or human catastrophic disasters
      e. Motor vehicle accidents
      f. Medical events (e.g., diagnosis of a life-threatening illness)
      g. Caregiving activities involving exposure to traumatic situations (e.g., rescue workers)

B. **Epidemiology and etiology**
   1. **PTSD**
      a. Symptoms usually develop within **3 months after the trauma**, although they may be **delayed for months or years.**
      b. **Course** is **variable**
      c. Twice as likely in **females** as in males
   2. **ASD:** symptoms develop within **4 weeks after the trauma** and last from 2 days to a **maximum of 4 weeks.**

C. **Clinical presentation**
   1. **Key features of PTSD and ASD**
      a. Reexperiencing the trauma

PTSD and ASD: the occurrence of anxiety symptoms after exposure to a traumatic stressor.

Example: An assault victim has distressing recollections and nightmares about the attack.
  b. **Persistent avoidance of situations that are reminders of the trauma**
   Example: An assault victim cannot go near the parking garage where the attack occurred.
  c. **Numbing of responsiveness** (PTSD)
   Example: An assault victim feels emotionally detached from other individuals.
  d. **Increased arousal**
   Example: On hearing the slightest noise, an assault victim is easily startled.
 2. **Other key features of ASD**
  a. Feeling **dazed**
  b. **Numbing of emotions**
  c. **Dissociative amnesia** (e.g., being unable to remember aspects of the event)
  d. **Derealization, depersonalization**
 3. **Associated features of PTSD**
  a. **Survivor guilt**
  b. Self-destructive behavior
  c. Impaired ability to modulate affect
  d. Increased health complaints; increased frequency of physician visits
  e. Comorbid conditions (e.g., major depression, other anxiety disorders, substance-related disorders)
D. **Differential diagnosis:** the type of stressor (e.g., traumatic) associated with PTSD distinguishes it from **adjustment disorder** (see Chapter 20).
E. Management
 1. **Pharmacologic agents** are used to alleviate the symptoms of PTSD and, in some cases, ASD (see Table 14-3).
 2. **Psychological interventions** for PTSD are aimed at helping patients confront the traumatic experience and integrate it intellectually and emotionally **in a supportive atmosphere** with:
  a. Individual therapy
  b. Support groups
  c. Coping skills training (e.g., relaxation skills)

15

Somatoform and Other Related Disorders

Target Topics

I. Overview

A. **Four related classes of disorders** are listed in the *Diagnostic and Statistical Manual of Mental Disorders,* 4th edition, text revision (DSM-IV-TR), and are discussed in this chapter: somatoform disorders, psychological factors affecting medical condition, factitious disorders, and malingering.

B. These four related classes of disorders all **share one common characteristic:** psychological influences play a prominent role in the expression of physical symptoms.

C. Characteristics

- Somatoform and related disorders may be distinguished using four characteristics (Table 15-1).

   1. **Symptom type:** physical or psychological

   2. **Symptom intentionality:** unintentional or deliberate production of symptoms

   3. **Physiologic basis:** presence or absence of a medical condition that can explain a patient's symptoms

   4. **Motivation:** presence or absence of known external incentives, such as financial gain

D. Etiology

   1. The following factors may play a role in causing these disorders:

TABLE 15-1   Characteristics of Somatoform-Related Disorders

Disorder	Symptom Type	Symptom Intentionality	Known Medical Condition	Known External Incentives
Somatoform disorders	Physical	Not deliberate	No	No
Psychological factors affecting a general medical condition	Physical	Not deliberate	Yes	No
Factitious disorder	Psychological and physical	Deliberate	No	No
Malingering	Psychological and physical	Deliberate	No	Yes

BOX 15-1   **DSM-IV-TR Classification of Somatoform Disorders**

Somatization disorder
Undifferentiated somatoform disorder
Hypochondriasis
Pain disorder
Conversion disorder
Body dysmorphic disorder
Somatoform disorder not otherwise specified

---

    a. **Psychosocial factors:** poor communication skills, intrapersonal conflict, expression of emotional distress through physical symptoms, and reinforcing properties of illness (e.g., avoiding obligations because one is ill)

    b. **Biological factors:** genetic predisposition, errors in sensory processing, and altered serotonin (neurotransmitter) levels

  2. **Psychiatric disorders** manifested by physical symptoms are **common in women** who have **experienced sexual abuse as children.**

II.   Somatoform Disorders

  A. **Overview**

    1. These disorders are characterized by the presence of physical symptoms that cannot be accounted for by a diagnosable medical condition.

    2. The DSM-IV-TR classification of somatoform disorders is listed in Box 15-1.

  B. **Epidemiology: prevalence** ranges from **5%** to **40%**, depending on the medical setting and medical specialty being surveyed.

    1. **Somatization disorder** occurs in less than 1% of the general population but may be found in 5–10% of outpatient primary care patients.

Somatoform disorders: physical symptoms that suggest a medical disorder but are inconsistent with its accepted presentation.

TABLE 15-2   Key Features of Somatoform Disorders

Disorder	Key Feature(s)	Patient Presentation
Somatization disorder	History of multiple physical complaints, beginning before age 30 and persisting for several years, that result in seeking of treatment or in functional impairment History of multiple symptoms: at least four pain, two gastrointestinal, one sexual, and one pseudoneurologic (see Box 15-2)	Numerous unsubstantiated symptoms
Undifferentiated somatoform disorder	One or more physical complaints grossly in excess of what would be expected based on physical findings Symptoms that cannot be explained by a known physical disorder or substance abuse and that have caused significant distress or impairment for at least 6 months	One or more unsubstantiated symptoms
Hypochondriasis	Preoccupying fear or belief that individual has serious disease; belief is not of delusional intensity Fear based on patient's interpretation of physical sensations as evidence of disease that persists despite medical reassurance and not of delusional intensity	Inappropriate belief that one has a serious disease
Pain disorder	Pain as focus of clinical presentation that causes clinically significant distress or functional impairment Pain that is not due to another psychiatric disorder and is not dyspareunia	Pain plus emotional and/or behavioral complications
Conversion disorder	Loss or change in voluntary motor or sensory functioning that suggests a general medical or neurologic disorder	Pseudoneurologic symptoms
Body dysmorphic disorder	Patient preoccupation with an imagined defect or grossly exaggerated defect in some aspect of individual's physical appearance	Inappropriate concern over physical appearance

    2. Pain symptoms are psychological in origin in as many as 40% of patients whose primary complaint is pain.

    3. Hypochondriasis may occur in as many as 10% of individuals in a primary care population.

    4. Conversion disorder and **body dysmorphic disorder** occur much less frequently than other somatoform disorders.

  C. Clinical presentation (Table 15-2)

    1. Patients with a possible somatoform disorder **believe** that they have a **physical disorder**, not a psychiatric illness, and are likely to strongly resist the idea that their symptoms relate more to emotional distress than to a physical condition.

    2. The types of somatoform disorders can be identified on the basis of their clinical features.

  D. Management

    1. Be alert for **coexisting psychiatric disorders** and **physical conditions** in the patient.

    2. Understand and **validate the patient's feelings of distress;** this involves empathic listening and considering that the patient's symptoms have a valid cause.

BOX 15-2	**The Patient With Somatization Disorder**

A 37-year-old woman sees her physician because of nausea and vomiting. The physician notices that the patient has an extensive history of medical problems not explained fully by findings, including sporadic neck, joint, chest, abdominal, and urinary tract pain; complaints of feeling bloated, nausea and vomiting, and diarrhea; transient diplopia; recurrent numbness in one foot; and irregular menses. She lives in a noisy, high-crime area with an abusive spouse, who is an alcoholic, and she has a demanding but low-paying job. The physician prescribes promethazine to control the nausea and vomiting, tells the patient how stress can exacerbate physical symptoms, and suggests options for stress management. The patient agrees to see a psychologist for help in coping with her stress, but she is skeptical that this type of treatment will be beneficial.

3. **Objective findings** serve as the basis for determining the need for various diagnostic and therapeutic procedures.
4. When the patient is undergoing psychotherapy, the **physician-patient interview focuses** primarily on **somatic** rather than on psychological problems.
5. Regardless of the clinical course of symptoms, **regular outpatient appointments** should be scheduled.
6. When chronic symptoms, severe psychosocial consequences, or morbid illness behavior are reported, **refer the patient for psychological treatment** (Box 15-2).

III. **Psychological Factors Affecting a General Medical Condition**
   A. Overview
      1. According to the DSM-IV-TR, **psychological factors** include mental disorders, psychological symptoms, personality traits or coping styles, maladaptive health behaviors, and stress-related physiologic responses.
      2. A diagnosis of "psychological factors affecting medical condition" should be considered when a specific **psychological** or **behavioral issue** (e.g., identifiable mental health concern) has a clinically significant adverse effect on the onset, course, outcome, or risk of a disease.
      3. This condition is more likely to **result** from the **cumulative effect** of day-to-day stressors than from a major crisis. The **disruption of a significant life event** is often more easily recognized (and thus dealt with) than stress that builds up as a result of coping with daily "hassles."
   B. **Clinical presentation:** patients complain of **physical symptoms** with **medically reasonable explanations** that may be exacerbated by an emotional or behavioral issue.
   C. Management
      1. **Patient education** about the **role of stress** in exacerbating physical symptoms helps patients recognize and begin managing their symptoms.
         a. Patients are often surprised by the suggestion that a

psychological issue is significantly **influencing their physical distress.**

    b. **Identifying psychological factors** may give patients the opportunity to consider the effect of psychological factors on a medical problem.

  2. Supportive, cognitive-behavioral, or insight-oriented **psychotherapy** may help patients understand the sources of emotional or behavioral stress or help them learn how to cope with stress effectively.

  3. **Stress management training** often involves biofeedback, relaxation skills, and assertiveness training.

IV. Factitious Disorders

  A. Overview

    1. These disorders involve the **intentional production of physical or psychological symptoms,** presumably to gain attention from health care providers. To minimize angry and rejecting behavior toward patients, physicians should help medical personnel understand a patient's disorder.

    2. Patients appear to have **no external incentives** for the production of symptoms (e.g., financial compensation).

    3. These disorders are relatively **rare.**

  B. Clinical presentation

    1. Patients present with **physical** or **psychological symptoms** that are **inconsistent with objective medical findings.**

      a. Many individuals with factitious disorder are **familiar with medical terminology** and the **health care system.**

      b. **Evidence,** often discovered by other health care personnel, may show that a particular patient is **intentionally producing symptoms.**

      c. Patients typically respond to evidence of their feigning of symptoms with **denial and anger** and are prone to **leave hospitals** or **clinics abruptly.**

    2. Inquiries among health care providers often indicate that a particular **patient** has **sought care for similar problems from many other physicians.**

    3. Factitious disorder with physical symptoms is also known as **Munchausen syndrome.**

    4. **Munchausen syndrome by proxy** is diagnosed when one individual, such as a parent or caretaker, intentionally produces symptoms in another individual, usually a child.

  C. Management

    1. **Avoid ordering unnecessary medical procedures.**

    2. Interpret the patient's behavior as a **"cry for help,"** and respond as if the patient were explicitly asking for help in alleviating emotional distress.

    3. **Notify child protective services** in cases of **Munchausen syndrome by proxy.**

Margin notes:

Factitious disorders: intentional production of symptoms of illness by patients, presumably to gain attention.

Munchausen syndrome by proxy: intentional production of symptoms in another person.

V. Malingering
  A. Overview
    1. Malingering involves the **deliberate production of feigned symptoms for specific gain** (e.g., seeking financial compensation, avoiding military duty, evading criminal prosecution, obtaining drugs).
    2. A **thorough medical evaluation** is necessary before a diagnosis of malingering can be made.
    3. Malingering is a relatively **rare** condition.
  B. Clinical presentation
    1. Patients present with **symptoms that cannot be adequately explained by objective medical findings.**
    2. **Presentation** often involves:
      a. **Medicolegal issues** associated with the symptoms (e.g., suing for injuries sustained in an automobile accident)
      b. Discrepancy between subjective distress and objective medical findings (e.g., pain grossly in excess of that experienced by most patients with such an injury)
      c. **Lack of compliance** with diagnostic and treatment procedures
  C. Management
    1. **Avoid angry confrontation** with malingering patients to maintain productive physician-patient relationships.
    2. **View medical symptoms as valid medical problems,** so that patients have an opportunity to "give in" in a face-saving manner.

> Malingering: conscious feigning of symptoms to achieve specific gain.

16

Substance Abuse and Dependence

Target Topics

▷ Commonly abused substances
▷ Neurobiology of substance abuse
▷ Symptoms of abuse and withdrawal
▷ Management of substance abuse

I. **Overview**
   A. Substance-related disorders are psychiatric disorders that involve **intoxication**, **withdrawal**, and **chronic use of drugs** and are considered **chronic, progressive** illnesses.
   B. **Commonly abused substances** are alcohol, sedative-hypnotics and anxiolytics, opiates, caffeine, nicotine, amphetamines, hallucinogens, marijuana, and inhalants.
   C. **Characteristics of substance use disorders** depend on the **substance used** and the **route of administration**. Substances that are injected, smoked, or snorted have a rapid onset and are more quickly addicting than substances that are ingested (Table 16-1).
   D. The *Diagnostic and Statistical Manual of Mental Disorders,* 4th edition, text revision (DSM-IV-TR), classification of substance-induced disorders is listed in Box 16-1.

Use of alcohol and some drugs can cause physiologic dependence.

II. **Terminology**
   A. **Substance abuse:** the continued maladaptive use of a substance despite physical endangerment, legal difficulties, interpersonal problems, impairment in major life activities, or related consequences
   B. **Substance dependence:** substance use that leads to social, oc-

BOX 16-1	DSM-IV-TR Classification of Substance-induced Disorders

Substance intoxication
Substance withdrawal
Substance-induced delirium
Substance-induced persisting dementia
Substance-induced persisting amnestic disorder
Substance-induced psychotic disorder
Substance-induced mood disorder
Substance-induced anxiety disorder
Substance-induced sexual dysfunction
Substance-induced sleep disorder

cupational, and often medical consequences involving **progressive use, tolerance**, and a **withdrawal syndrome** for many substances

   C. **Tolerance:** need for increasing amounts of a substance to obtain the same effect or a reduced effect than previously obtained from use of the same amount of the substance
   D. **Cross-tolerance:** common phenomenon in which addiction to one substance leads to addiction to another substance as a result of shared neurotransmitter pathways of addiction

III. **Epidemiology**
   A. **Incidence**
       1. In the United States, **15%** of individuals **over 18 years** of age have a **substance abuse** problem; about two thirds of these individuals abuse **alcohol.**
       2. Among patients receiving treatment for **alcohol abuse,** 80% use **one or more other drugs.**

About 25% of routine hospital admissions involve alcohol-related problems.

   B. **Substance abuse in the United States** has a broad social impact, manifested by:
       1. **Suicide rate:** 20% higher in the chemically dependent population than in the general population
       2. **Traffic accidents** and deaths
       3. **Impaired job performance** and increased likelihood of job loss
       4. **High mortality** and **high crime rates** related to substance use

Substance use disorders are associated with significant morbidity and mortality.

       5. **Fetal alcohol syndrome** and other drug-related neonatal conditions
       6. Domestic violence

IV. **Etiology**
   A. **Neurobiologic factors**
       1. **Alcohol and psychoactive drugs** act either directly or indirectly on **dopaminergic neurons** in the **mesolimbic dopamine pathway.**
           a. Neurons arising in the **ventral tegmental area** ascend through the **medial forebrain bundle** and

In the US, tobacco use is the leading cause of preventable illness and death.

TABLE 16-1 Effects of Substance Use

Substance	Effects of Use	Effects of Withdrawal	Medical Complications
Alcohol	Sense of well-being; ataxia, slurred speech; reduced consciousness; possible respiratory arrest	Hyperreflexia, weakness, vomiting, insomnia, tremors, hallucinations, agitation, anxiety, **elevated heart rate, elevated blood pressure, seizures, delirium tremens ("DTs")**	**Wernicke's encephalopathy, Korsakoff's syndrome, hepatic disease,** dementia, cerebellar degeneration, polyneuropathy, pancreatitis, ulcers, esophageal varices, vitamin deficiencies, **fetal alcohol syndrome**
Amphetamines Methylphenidate dextroamphetamine Methamphetamine Ephedrine Phenmetrazine	**Paranoia,** increased energy, restlessness, hypertension, tachycardia, pupil dilation, anorexia	**Postuse "crash":** depression, headache, lethargy, craving, hunger	Injected forms: **infectious diseases related to injection** (e.g., HIV, hepatitis B and C; endocarditis); skin abscess; tracks or tattoos Newborns: withdrawal syndromes
Caffeine	Alertness, insomnia, tachycardia, restlessness, anxiety	Mild headache, lethargy, dysphoria	None
Cocaine	Euphoria, sense of well-being and competence, paranoia, agitation, anorexia "High" is brief and immediate, lasting about 30 minutes	**Postuse "crash":** similar to withdrawal from amphetamines May last 1–2 weeks	**Sudden cardiac death,** areas of brain hypoperfusion similar to **small strokes** Perforated nasal septum, lip burns, "crack baby" syndrome
Hallucinogens "Ecstasy" (MDMA) Ketamine LSD Mescaline (in peyote) PCP Psilocybin (in mushrooms)	Sense of euphoria and well-being, perceptual disturbances, agitation, hypertension, tachycardia, **flashbacks** PCP: **violent and belligerent behavior**	**No physiologic withdrawal**	**MDMA: rhabdomyolysis, hyperthermia,** renal failure, "mini strokes" that may lead to permanent deficits PCP: convulsions Mushrooms: may be toxic or lethal

(Continued)

Substance	Intoxication	Withdrawal	Complications
Inhalants Gasoline Glue Nitrous oxide Paint	**Euphoria, confusion,** ataxia, delirium	No withdrawal symptoms	**Respiratory arrest or suffocation,** renal and liver failure Chronic use: dementia
Marijuana (cannabis)	Euphoria, confusion, disorientation, **psychosis in vulnerable individuals,** increased appetite Chronic use: **amotivational syndrome**	No withdrawal symptoms	Conjunctival injection, lung cancer
Nicotine*	Restlessness, insomnia, anxiety, arrhythmias	Craving, insomnia, irritability, increased appetite, decreased heart rate, anxiety, difficulty concentrating	Smoking: lung, pharyngeal, oral and bladder cancers; **emphysema; risk of cardiovascular symptoms** Low-birth-weight infants; premature delivery
Opiates Heroin Medically prescribed pain killers	Mood elevation, analgesia, central nervous system depression, **respiratory depression, miosis**	Tachycardia, hypertension, fever, restlessness, lacrimation, mydriasis, piloerection, nausea and vomiting, **diarrhea, intense craving** Uncomfortable but generally not lethal	Injected forms: **infectious diseases related to injection;** skin abscess; tracks or tattoos Newborns: withdrawal syndromes
Sedative-hypnotics, anxiolytics Barbiturates Benzodiazepines	Euphoria, reduced consciousness, disinhibition Sedatives: respiratory arrest	Anxiety, insomnia, tremors, **seizures,** psychosis, hallucinations, **cardiovascular collapse**	Usually none; frequently combined with other drugs, such as stimulants, to "come down" Benzodiazepines: high safety profile unless combined with other drugs or alcohol

LSD, lysergic acid diethylamide; *MDMA,* methylenedioxymethamphetamine; *PCP,* phencyclidine.
*About 23% of adults are smokers, and about 70% of smokers want to quit.

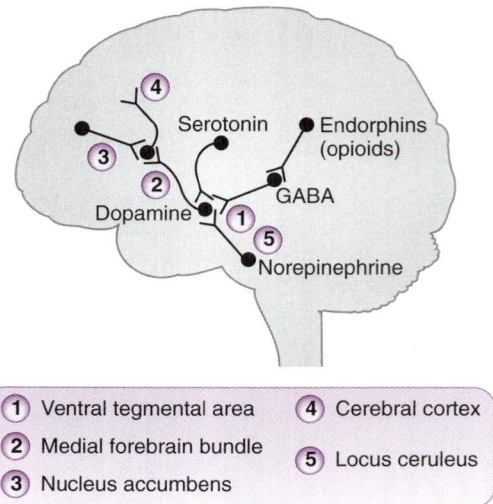

(1) Ventral tegmental area   (4) Cerebral cortex

(2) Medial forebrain bundle   (5) Locus ceruleus

(3) Nucleus accumbens

Figure 16-1 Schematic of receptor sites and pathways showing the areas of the brain and neurotransmitters identified with substance abuse. Dopamine release may be stimulated directly by substances of abuse or indirectly via other neurotransmitters, such as endorphins, norepinephrine, GABA, and serotonin.

Increased dopamine levels set up a reward system that leads to compulsive use.

---

distribute to the **nucleus accumbens** and **cerebral cortex** (Figure 16-1).

b. **Increased dopamine levels** are associated with gratification and pleasure and reduced stress.

c. **Chronic use** of **alcohol** and **psychoactive drugs** leads to genetic changes within the neurons via G proteins and second messengers, resulting in craving and withdrawal syndromes.

d. The resulting **reward pathway** may have priority over other drives, such as eating, drinking, and sex.

2. **Mechanisms of increased dopamine availability** vary for different substances.

a. **Alcohol:** may act directly on the dopamine pathway or indirectly through the opioid and GABA pathways

b. **Opiates**

(1) Act indirectly to stimulate the release of dopamine by **inhibiting GABA neurons**, which in turn normally inhibit dopaminergic release in the ventral tegmental area

(2) **Inhibit noradrenergic neurons of the locus ceruleus**, thereby reducing arousal of the entire central nervous system

c. **Nicotine:** increases dopamine release

d. **Amphetamines:** block reuptake of dopamine into presynaptic neurons and stimulate release of dopamine

e. **Cocaine:** blocks reuptake of dopamine into presynaptic neurons

TABLE 16-2   Common Findings in Substance Use Disorders

Behavioral Findings	Physical Findings	Laboratory Findings
Chronic anxiety, depression	Easy bruising	↑ Blood alcohol level or positive breath alcohol test
Insomnia	Sexually transmitted diseases	
Headaches	HIV, hepatitis B and C	↑ Mean corpuscular volume
"Blackouts"	Endocarditis	↑ Liver function tests
Sexual problems	Gastrointestinal symptoms (e.g., gastritis, ulcers)	↓ Levels of albumin, vitamin B_{12}, or folate
Single-vehicle automobile accidents, falls	Palpitations, tachycardia, hypertension	↑ Levels of uric acid and amylase
Irritability, belligerence, discharge against medical advice	Needle tracks, granulomas, abscesses, tattoos	Evidence of bone marrow suppression (e.g., low white blood cell or platelet count)
Poor hygiene	Perforated nasal septum, lip burns	
Absenteeism, missed appointments		Positive urine or serum drug screening
Family or work problems		

BOX 16-2   The Patient With Alcohol Withdrawal

A 45-year-old man is admitted to the hospital with acute appendicitis and undergoes uncomplicated emergency surgery. On the first postoperative day, the patient's blood pressure and heart rate are elevated, and he becomes belligerent and agitated, demanding to leave the hospital against medical advice. Although the patient stated on admission that he drinks alcohol only occasionally, his wife says that he regularly drinks as many as 12 cans of beer daily. The attending physician is able to obtain the patient's cooperation to begin a detoxification regimen using lorazepam, but the patient continues to deny that he has a problem with alcohol abuse.

---

      f. Hallucinogens: highly serotonergic; serotonin may be a modulator of the dopamine reward pathway

  B. Genetic factors: there is a genetic predisposition toward addiction.

      1. Adoption studies have shown that **sons of alcoholics** are **three to four times** more likely to **become alcoholics** than sons of nonalcoholics.

      2. There is a **60% concordance rate** between **monozygotic twins** and a 30% concordance rate between dizygotic twins for alcoholism.

> Substance use disorders have both psychosocial and genetic causes.

V. Clinical Presentation

  A. Screening: most patients *do not* see a physician with a complaint of substance abuse. The physician must screen for the disorder based on characteristic signs and symptoms and laboratory findings (Table 16-2; Box 16-2).

BOX 16-3	The Patient With Amphetamine Dependence

A 25-year-old woman has been using increasing amounts of intravenous amphetamines on a daily basis. She was terminated from her job 2 months ago and is using all of her savings to obtain drugs. She believes drug enforcement agents are following her and that her neighbors are part of a drug sting operation. She is barricaded within her home and will not allow her family to enter. Her husband calls the police, who recognize the woman's behavior as paranoid and transport her to a mental health facility for treatment. The patient agrees to begin chemical dependency treatment. She is withdrawn and lethargic for about 4 days, and during that time, the paranoia resolves. The patient begins to participate in a 12-step recovery group and demonstrates reality-based thought on the fourth day of hospitalization. After 10 days, she is transferred to a residential treatment facility for long-term follow-up care.

B. **CAGE questionnaire for alcohol abuse: three positive answers** correlate highly (95%) with alcohol abuse.
  1. Have you ever felt the need to <u>c</u>ut down on your drinking?
  2. Have you ever felt <u>a</u>nnoyed by criticism of your drinking?
  3. Have you ever had <u>g</u>uilty feelings about drinking?
  4. Have you ever taken a morning <u>e</u>ye opener?
C. **History taking:** the physician should obtain the following information from individuals with acknowledged substance use:
  1. **Usage history:** substance(s) used, age of first use, most recent use, frequency of use, route of use
  2. **Cessation history:** attempts to stop or periods of abstinence; withdrawal symptoms
  3. **Previous treatment:** inpatient or outpatient therapy; Alcoholics Anonymous (AA)
  4. **Psychosocial problems:** family history of chemical dependence; legal problems
  5. **Past medical history and review of systems:** detailed for substance-related medical conditions
D. **Dual diagnosis:** screening for **coexistence** of **substance use** and other **psychiatric disorders** is very important, because the risk of relapse is greatly increased if both types of disorders are not treated (e.g., a man with a dual diagnosis of cocaine abuse and bipolar disorder is much more likely to experience a relapse of the substance use if his mood swings are uncontrolled and untreated).

VI. **Management**
A. Substance use disorders are treated with both short-term and long-term medical and psychosocial **supportive interventions** (Box 16-3).

Always assess suicide risk in patients with chemical dependence.

Concurrent treatment of other psychiatric illnesses improves treatment outcomes.

TABLE 16-3   Pharmacologic Therapy for Substance Use Disorders

Substance	Therapy	Effect
Alcohol		
Dependence and abuse	Disulfiram (aversive prophylactic therapy)	Causes flushing, nausea, and hypertension when taken with alcohol
Withdrawal	Naltrexone	Reduces craving
	Benzodiazepines	Prevents and treats serious withdrawal symptoms and seizures
	Thiamine	Prevents Wernicke's encephalopathy and Korsakoff's syndrome
	Magnesium sulfate	Prevents hypomagnesemia and possible seizures
	Folic acid and multi-vitamins	Corrects deficiencies common in alcoholism
Cocaine		
Dependence	Desipramine or bromo-criptine	May reduce severity of postuse "crash" as well as craving and relapse
Nicotine		
Dependence and withdrawal	Nicotine gum, patch, inhaler spray	Reduces withdrawal symptoms and relapse
	Bupropion	Prevents withdrawal symptoms and relapse
Opiates		
Dependence	Methadone or LAMM (synthetic opioids with less sedation and euphoria)*	Reduces risk of heroin use; patient remains physically dependent
	Naltrexone	Reduces craving and drug effects if relapse occurs
Withdrawal	Clonidine	Reduces discomfort and withdrawal symptoms associated with adrenergic activity
Sedative-hypnotics, anxiolytics	Benzodiazepines or barbiturates in tapering doses	Prevents serious withdrawal symptoms such as seizures, anxiety, and elevated heart rate and blood pressure

LAMM, 1-α acetylmethadol.
*Drugs used in legally dispensed maintenance therapy.

1. Interventions are based on substance used, withdrawal syndrome, and level of dependence.
2. Intervention requires that the physician **be aware of the patient's stage of readiness for change** and **remain supportive** even when a high degree of resistance and denial is present (see Chapter 3, IV B).
3. **Inpatient or outpatient programs** are chosen based on the individual's ability to maintain abstinence, the presence of comorbid medical or psychiatric conditions, and the potential for serious withdrawal syndromes.

B. **Twelve-step programs** such as AA and other volunteer peer programs are the mainstay of long-term treatment and relapse prevention.

C. **Pharmacologic treatment** (Table 16-3)
   1. **Drug therapies** are useful in increasing safety and

Twelve-step recovery programs are the mainstay of treatment for substance use disorders.

comfort of **detoxification** and in **long-term prevention of relapse.**

2. **Substance-induced delirium** resulting from intoxication or withdrawal may require acute treatment with an antipsychotic drug (e.g., haloperidol) and a benzodiazepine (e.g., lorazepam) for agitation.

D. Behavioral counseling

1. Goals are to help the user develop **coping strategies** for dealing with urges and other precipitating causes of substance use and **skills for preventing relapse** (e.g., by identifying high-risk situations and making a plan to deal with them).

2. **Cognitive-behavioral therapy** also reduces the risk of relapse.

17

Eating Disorders and Obesity

Target Topics

▸ Epidemiology and etiology of eating disorders
▸ Symptoms of eating disorders
▸ Medical complications of eating disorders
▸ Management of eating disorders
▸ Characteristics and management of obesity

I. Overview

A. **Eating disorders** are severe disturbances in eating behavior that may involve one or more of the following:
   1. **Restricting food intake:** extremely limited diet, producing a physiologic state of semistarvation and weight that is significantly below normal
   2. **Purging:** use of inappropriate measures to prevent weight gain, such as self-induced vomiting; misuse of laxatives, diuretics, or enemas
   3. **Binge eating:** episodic consumption of a significantly larger-than-normal amount of food; associated with a feeling of lack of control

B. The *Diagnostic and Statistical Manual of Mental Disorders*, 4th edition, text revision (DSM-IV-TR), classification of eating disorders is listed in Box 17-1 and includes:
   1. **Anorexia nervosa** and **bulimia nervosa**
   2. **Eating disorder not otherwise specified (NOS):**
      a. A severe disturbance of eating behavior that does not meet the criteria for either anorexia nervosa or bulimia nervosa
      b. **Binge-eating disorder**, an eating disorder NOS,

Page 140 Behavioral Science

BOX 17-1	DSM-IV-TR Classification of Eating Disorders

Anorexia nervosa
Bulimia nervosa
Eating disorder not otherwise specified

involves repeated binge eating that is *not* associated with the use of inappropriate measures to prevent weight gain (e.g., purging, excessive exercise).

    C. **Obesity** is *not* associated consistently with a cluster of psychological or behavioral symptoms, and it is *not* considered a psychiatric disorder in the DSM-IV-TR (see section V).

II. **General Features of Eating Disorders**

    A. **Epidemiology**

        1. More than 90% of patients are **female.**

            a. **Anorexia:** 0.5% lifetime prevalence

            b. **Bulimia:** 1–3% lifetime prevalence

        2. **Eating disorder NOS: most prevalent** eating disorder, although precise statistics are not available

        3. **Onset:** typically in **adolescence** and **early adulthood**

        4. Occur in all socioeconomic classes and major ethnic groups in the United States

        5. Individuals who participate in **activities** in which **thinness is important for success** (e.g., modeling, acting, dancing, gymnastics) have an increased risk of being diagnosed with eating disorders.

    B. **Etiology**

        1. **Genetic factors,** as suggested by family and twin studies

        2. **Sociocultural factors,** as suggested by the increased prevalence of eating disorders in the United States and other industrialized societies, in which there is an emphasis on thinness as a perceived standard of beauty

        3. **Psychological factors**

            a. **Family-related factors,** such as strong emphasis on appearance and achievement

            b. **Factors associated with adolescent development,** such as fear of sexual development and separation from family

    C. **Clinical presentation** (Table 17-1)

    D. **Complications:** patients with eating disorders frequently seek treatment for **associated medical complications,** *not* the eating disorder itself (see Table 17-1).

    E. **Outcome**

        1. **Early detection** is associated with **improved prognosis.**

        2. **Adolescent and young adult females** are at **highest risk** for developing eating disorders and should be screened routinely for these disorders.

        3. Patients often are **resistant to treatment** because of intense **fear of gaining weight.**

Most individuals with eating disorders are adolescent or young adult females.

Depressive symptoms are frequently associated with eating disorders.

TABLE 17-1 Comparison of Anorexia Nervosa and Bulimia Nervosa

Disorder	Features	Comorbid Conditions	Complications*
Anorexia nervosa	Maintenance of **weight < 85% normal for age and height** **Distorted perceptions of own body size** Intense fear of gaining weight or becoming fat; self-esteem largely determined by weight **Amenorrhea:** absence of at least three consecutive menstrual cycles **Denial of serious health effects of very low body weight** Restricting type: obsessive-compulsive behavior, social withdrawal, restrained emotional expression, strong need for control	Depressive disorders Anxiety disorders Personality disorders	Hypotension Bradycardia Hypothermia Leukopenia, anemia Osteoporosis Dry skin, lanugo (fine, downy hair) Cardiac arrhythmias
Bulimia nervosa	Repeated **binge eating** Use of **inappropriate methods to prevent weight gain** Sense of lack of control during binge-eating episodes **Typically normal weight** Self-esteem largely determined by weight Restricted intake between binges Hiding binge eating and purging from others Impulsive behaviors (e.g., stealing, promiscuity, overspending)	Depressive disorders Anxiety disorders Substance use disorders Personality disorders (frequently borderline personality disorder)	Loss of dental enamel Fluid and electrolyte disturbances Cardiac arrhythmias Swollen parotid glands Calluses on back of hand from self-induced vomiting Esophageal tears or ruptures Dehydration

* Complications listed for bulimia nervosa also occur in patients who are diagnosed with the binge-eating/purging type of anorexia nervosa.

4. **Anorexia nervosa** is associated with a **mortality rate** of **5–20%**; death usually results from starvation, suicide, or cardiac arrhythmias.

III. Anorexia Nervosa (see Table 17-1)
- Although the word "anorexia" means loss of appetite, individuals with anorexia nervosa do *not* lose their appetite.

A. **Key feature:** intentional maintenance of body weight less than 85% of normal

B. **Types**
  1. **Restricting:** no regular binge eating or purging
  2. **Binge-eating/purging:** regular binge eating and/or purging

C. **Differential diagnosis**
  1. **Medical conditions that cause weight loss** (e.g., cancer, gastrointestinal disease, thyroid disease)
  2. **Major depressive disorder** (e.g., decreased appetite and/or weight loss)
  3. **Schizophrenia** (e.g., delusions about food)
  4. **Anxiety disorders** (e.g., fear of contamination)

Anorexia nervosa: body weight < 85% of normal.

| BOX 17-2 | The Patient With Bulimia Nervosa |

A 20-year-old college student has been binge eating and purging for the past 6 months. Although she is only 5 pounds over the normal-range weight for her height, she is extremely dissatisfied with her size and has recently started using amphetamines to lose weight. The woman visits the student health center because of a sore throat. The physician notices that her cheeks are puffy and that she has a callous on the back of her right hand, and he asks about symptoms of bulimia nervosa. The patient admits to occasional binge eating and vomiting but does not openly describe her eating history. The physician educates her about the health consequences of binge eating and purging, refers her to an eating disorders program for an evaluation, and asks her to return for a follow-up visit. The patient, tired of hiding her binging and purging, hesitantly agrees.

D. Management
   1. Treatment goals
      a. **Immediate** goal is reestablishing medical stability.
      b. **Long-term** goals include gaining weight at a recommended pace, learning healthy eating habits, and identifying and addressing relevant psychiatric and psychological issues.
   2. **Inpatient** or **outpatient** management depends on the patient's medical and psychiatric status, treatment history, and level of cooperation.
   3. **Treatment is multidisciplinary** and includes:
      a. **Medical intervention** to treat complications and monitor refeeding and weight restoration
      b. **Pharmacologic treatment** of comorbid psychiatric disorders, typically instituted after weight has been restored
      c. **Psychotherapy** (individual and family therapy)
      d. **Nutritional counseling**
      e. **Inpatient programs** involve monitoring food intake, attempts to purge, and exercise and providing privileges and positive feedback based on adherence to treatment goals.

> The mortality rate for anorexia nervosa is among the highest of all psychiatric disorders.

IV. **Bulimia Nervosa** (Box 17-2; see Table 17-1)
   A. **Key features:** repeated episodes of binge eating followed by inappropriate methods to prevent weight gain
   B. **Types**
      1. **Purging:** self-induced vomiting; misuse of laxatives, diuretics, or enemas
      2. **Nonpurging:** fasting and excessive exercise
   C. **Management**
      1. **Outpatient treatment** is most common.
      2. As with anorexia nervosa, **treatment is multidisciplinary** and includes:
         a. **Medical intervention:** treatment of complications

> Bulimia nervosa: recurrent binge eating and inappropriate methods to prevent weight gain.

> **b.** **Psychiatric interventions**
>> **(1)** Assessment and treatment of comorbid disorders
>> **(2)** **Antidepressant medication** to reduce bulimic symptoms
> **c.** **Psychotherapy:** cognitive-behavioral therapy; group and/or family therapy
> **d.** **Nutritional counseling**

V. Obesity

A. Definition

1. Obesity is defined as a weight that is **20% or more above ideal body weight** per standard height and weight tables.

   a. **Mild obesity:** 20–40% above ideal body weight
   b. **Moderate obesity:** 41–100% above ideal body weight
   c. **Morbid obesity:** >100% above ideal body weight

2. Obesity can also be measured using the **body mass index (BMI).**

$$BMI = \frac{\text{Weight (kg)}}{\text{Height (m)}^2}$$

   a. **Obesity:** BMI $\geq$ 30 kg/m^2
   b. **Overweight:** BMI of 25–29.9 kg/m^2

B. Prevalence

1. Obesity is **common.** In 1999, 61% of adults in the United States were overweight (34%) or obese (27%).

2. Obesity is more common in individuals of **lower socio-economic status,** particularly among **women,** and within **some ethnic groups** (e.g., African Americans, Mexican Americans).

C. Etiology

1. **Genetic factors**

   a. **Twin studies** show that body weight is more likely to be similar between **monozygotic** than dizygotic twins.
   b. **Adoptive studies** show that the adult weight of adoptees is closer to that of the biological parents than that of the adoptive parents.
   c. **Genetic studies** suggest that **leptin,** an obesity gene product found in adipose tissue, may play a role. Obesity may develop as the result of leptin resistance or reduced leptin release.

2. **Psychosocial and environmental factors**

   a. Increased caloric intake
   b. Reduced physical activity
   c. Food with high-fat content
   d. Increased accessibility of food

D. Effects of obesity on health

1. **Abdominal fat** is associated with **increased mortality** and **risk of disease.**

Antidepressants and cognitive behavioral therapy are effective treatments for bulimia nervosa.

Obesity affects > 25% of adults in the United States.

2. **Medical problems associated with obesity**
   a. Cardiovascular disease
   b. Hypertension
   c. Diabetes mellitus, type 2
   d. Hypercholesterolemia
   e. Osteoarthritis
   f. Sleep apnea
   g. Gallbladder disease

E. **Management:** Successful weight reduction is often followed by eventual regaining of weight.
   1. **Basic weight loss measures**
      a. **Diet**
      b. **Exercise:** aids in the maintenance of weight loss
      c. **Behavioral modification**
   2. **Additional measures**
      a. Weight loss medications (e.g., sibutramine, orlistat)
      b. **Surgical procedures** (e.g., gastric bypass)

Sleep and Sleep Disorders

Target Topics

▹ Sleep architecture
▹ Changes in sleep patterns with age
▹ Insomnia, sleep apnea, and narcolepsy
▹ Management of sleep disorders

I. Normal Sleep

A. Sleep architecture: the pattern of sleep through its progressive stages

1. Sleep consists of **rapid eye movement (REM)** and **non-REM** sleep.

2. **Non-REM** sleep is composed of **stages 1, 2, 3, and 4.** Sleep progresses through these stages before the initial REM period begins (Figure 18-1).

3. In the **young adult,** sleep stages are distributed (by percent) as follows: **75%** of sleep is **non-REM** (stage 1, 5%; stage 2, 45%; stages 3 and 4, 25%) and **25%** is **REM** sleep.

4. **Initial REM** sleep is **brief** (e.g., 10 minutes), but **subsequent REM** periods are **longer** (e.g., 15–40 minutes).

   a. Dreaming occurs during **REM** sleep.

   b. Four to six REM periods occur **each night,** at about **90-minute intervals.**

5. Sleep patterns are measured by a polysomnogram, which includes electroencephalographic (EEG), electro-oculographic, and electromyographic recordings (Table 18-1).

> The first REM period occurs about 90 minutes into the sleep cycle.

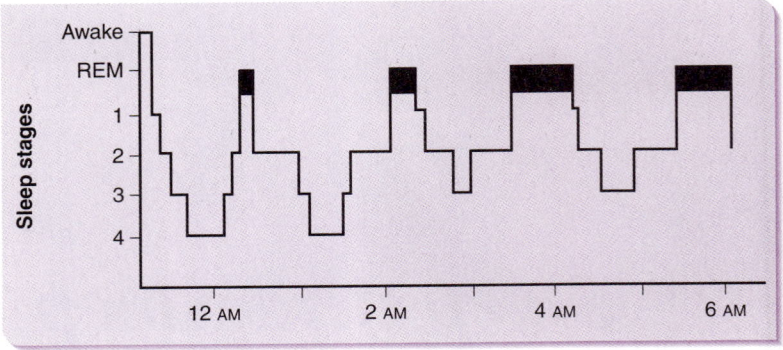

Figure 18-1 Conventional representation of a normal night sleep pattern. The first rapid eye movement (REM) period occurs about 90 minutes into the sleep cycle and lasts about 10 minutes. REM periods recur more frequently and are of longer duration later in the night. (From Kaufman DM. *Clinical Neurology for Psychiatrists.* 5th ed. Philadelphia: WB Saunders, an imprint of Elsevier Science, 2001, p. 414.)

B. Neurobiology of sleep
1. The suprachiasmatic nucleus of the hypothalamus acts as a "clock" that regulates the sleep-wake cycle. This cycle is influenced by environmental stimuli and the light-dark cycle and follows a **circadian pattern**.
2. The reticular activating system also plays a role in the regulation of the sleep-wake cycle.
3. **Neurotransmitters and sleep**
   a. **REM sleep** is associated with **increased acetylcholine** activity and **decreased dopamine, norepinephrine,** and **epinephrine** activity.
   b. **Non-REM sleep** is associated with **increased serotonin** activity.

C. Sleep requirements and sleep quality
1. **Newborns**
   a. Sleep an average of about **16 hours per day**
   b. REM sleep constitutes about **50%** of their sleep.
2. **Adults**
   a. Sleep an average of about **8 hours per day**
   b. REM sleep constitutes about **25%** of their sleep.
   c. **Changes in sleep patterns that occur with age** include:
      (1) Reduced delta sleep (stages 3 and 4 non-REM sleep)
      (2) Decreased REM sleep
      (3) Decreased total sleep time
      (4) Increased awakening

D. Sleep and health
1. An occasional night of sleep deprivation has a minimal effect on cognitive ability the following day; greater wakefulness leads to a **rebound of delta sleep** the following night.

Sleep becomes lighter and more fragmented with increasing age.

TABLE 18-1   Characteristics of Sleep Stages

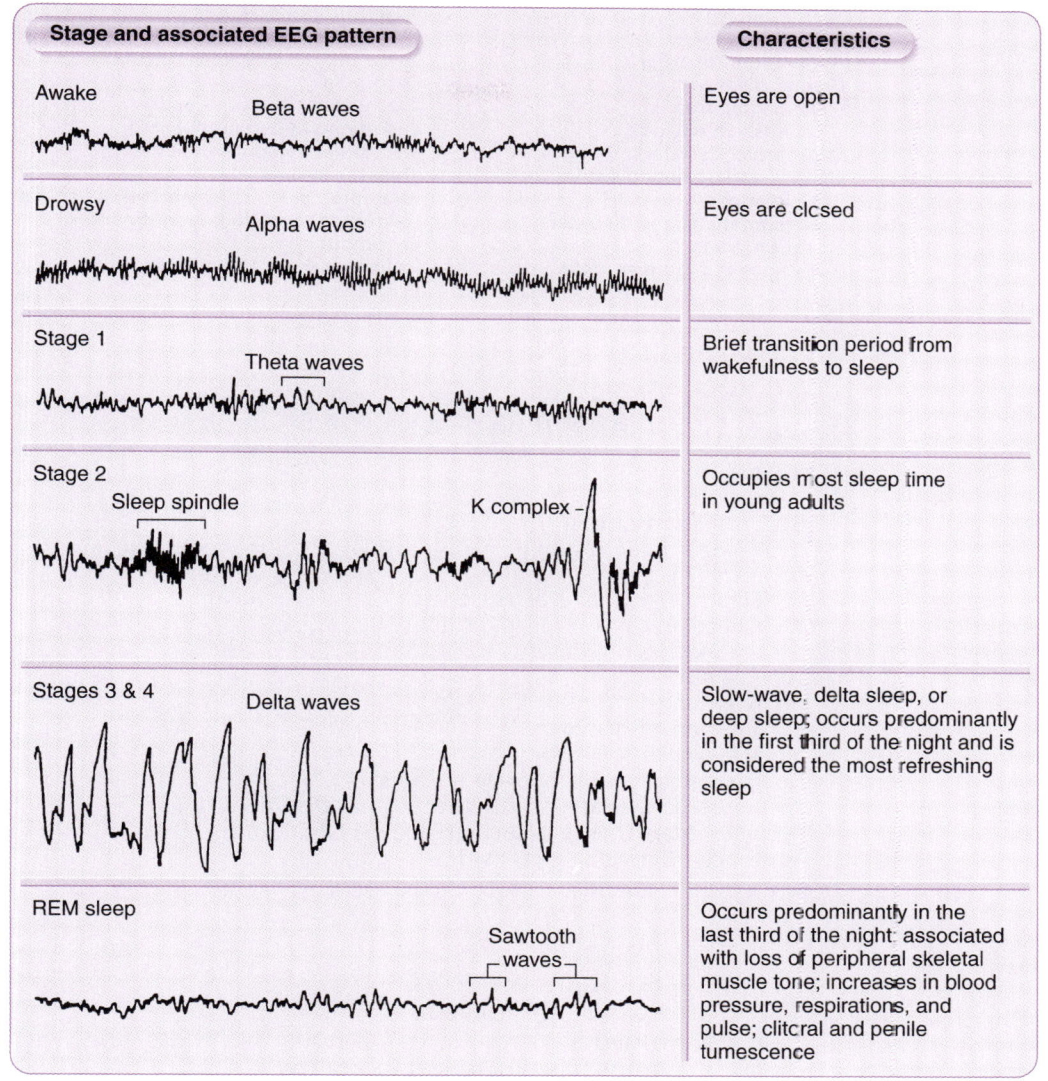

Stage and associated EEG pattern	Characteristics
Awake — Beta waves	Eyes are open
Drowsy — Alpha waves	Eyes are closed
Stage 1 — Theta waves	Brief transition period from wakefulness to sleep
Stage 2 — Sleep spindle, K complex	Occupies most sleep time in young adults
Stages 3 & 4 — Delta waves	Slow-wave, delta sleep, or deep sleep; occurs predominantly in the first third of the night and is considered the most refreshing sleep
REM sleep — Sawtooth waves	Occurs predominantly in the last third of the night; associated with loss of peripheral skeletal muscle tone; increases in blood pressure, respirations, and pulse; clitoral and penile tumescence

   2. Longer periods of sleep deprivation can lead to delusions and hallucinations.
   3. Individuals with **sleep problems** have an **increased risk** of:
      a. **Psychiatric disorders** (e.g., depression): sleep problems are associated with several psychiatric conditions (Table 18-2).
      b. Decreases in mental functioning

TABLE 18-2   Psychiatric Conditions Associated With Sleep Problems

Condition	Sleep Problem
Adjustment disorder	
Bipolar disorder	Insomnia
Mania/hypomania	Decreased need for sleep
Depressive episode	Insomnia, hypersomnolence
Depressive disorders	Insomnia, hypersomnolence
Generalized anxiety disorder	Initial insomnia
Panic disorder	Disrupted sleep (e.g., nocturnal panic attacks)
Posttraumatic stress disorder	Disrupted sleep (e.g., nightmares)
Schizophrenia	Insomnia
Substance-related disorders	Insomnia

BOX 18-1   **DSM-IV-TR Classification of Sleep Disorders**

Primary Sleep Disorders
  Dyssomnias
    Primary insomnia
    Primary hypersomnia
    Narcolepsy
    Breathing-related sleep disorder (e.g., sleep apnea)
    Circadian rhythm sleep disorder (e.g., jet lag)
    Dyssomnia not otherwise specified
  Parasomnias
    Nightmare disorder
    Sleep terror disorder
    Sleepwalking disorder
    Parasomnia not otherwise specified
Sleep Disorders Related to Another Mental Disorder
Sleep Disorders Due to a General Medical Condition
Substance-induced Sleep Disorders

    c. Traffic accidents
    d. Health problems
  4. Individuals who sleep ≤ 4 hours and those who sleep ≥ 10 hours have increased mortality.
  5. **Changes** in sleep architecture **seen in major depression**
    a. Shortened onset of REM sleep (REM latency)
    b. Predominance of REM earlier in sleep period
    c. Reduced delta sleep and total sleep time

II.   Classification of Sleep Disorders

  A. The *Diagnostic and Statistical Manual of Mental Disorders,* 4th edition, text revision (DSM-IV-TR), classification of sleep disorders is listed in Box 18-1.
  B. **Primary sleep disorders** may be classified in two categories:
    1. **Dyssomnias:** disorders involving difficulty initiating or maintaining sleep, or excessive sleepiness

2. **Parasomnias:** disorders involving abnormal behavioral or physiologic phenomena associated with sleep
C. **Clinical features and treatment** of some sleep disorders not discussed in the text are presented in Table 18-3.

III. **Insomnia**
  A. **Overview**
    1. Insomnia refers to **difficulty initiating** or **maintaining sleep** or experiencing nonrestorative sleep.
    2. Insomnia for **at least 1 month** that causes distress or impairment and is not due to another condition is one of the DSM-IV-TR criteria for **primary insomnia.**
  B. **Epidemiology**
    1. Occurs in **about 30%** of the general population
    2. More commonly reported by **females**
    3. Becomes more frequent with age
  C. **Etiology: causes and contributing factors** include:
    1. **Medical conditions** (e.g., pain)
    2. **Drugs** and **substance use** (e.g., amphetamines, caffeine)
    3. **Environmental factors** (e.g., noise, light) and **situational conditions** (e.g., stress, jet lag)
    4. **Poor sleep habits** (e.g., staying in bed for long periods despite being unable to fall asleep)
    5. **Psychiatric illness** (e.g., depression, anxiety)
  D. **Psychophysiologic insomnia:** the **presence of** a **sleep disturbance** that continues **after resolution of** the **precipitating factor**
    1. Patients with psychophysiologic insomnia have **poor conditioned sleep;** bedtime has become associated with increased arousal and anxiety about being unable to fall asleep.
    2. **Sleep** often **improves in novel environments** (e.g., hotels) that are not associated with the conditioned sleep response.
  E. **Consequences of chronic insomnia:** may include poor mood, decreased motivation, impaired attention and concentration
  F. **Management: early intervention** may prevent an acute sleep problem (e.g., transient insomnia) from becoming a chronic problem.
    1. **Underlying psychiatric** or **medical causes** should be addressed.
    2. **Behavioral methods** to promote sleep include sleep hygiene, stimulus control procedures, and relaxation skills (Table 18-4).
    3. **Sleep restriction therapy** curtails the amount of time initially allowed in bed to actual time asleep, with gradual increases as sleep time improves.
    4. **Pharmacologic treatment**
      a. **Benzodiazepines** (often reserved for short-term use because of their potential for abuse and tolerance) and nonbenzodiazepine hypnotics (see Table 10-6)

TABLE 18-3 Description and Treatment of Selected Sleep Disorders

Disorder	Epidemiology	Description	Treatment
Dyssomnias			
Circadian rhythm sleep disorder	May occur with shift work or jet lag	Circadian rhythm out of step with environmental schedule	Realignment of environmental schedule with circadian rhythm Exposure to light (in some cases)
Nocturnal myoclonus	Increased prevalence in older persons	Repetitive movements of leg during sleep, usually at 20- to 40-second intervals Associated with insomnia, awakening, and daytime sleepiness	Medication (e.g., benzodiazepines and levodopa)
Restless leg syndrome	More common with aging	Crawling sensations experienced in legs; accompanied by irresistible urge to move limb Associated with difficulty falling asleep, awakenings, and daytime sleepiness	Medication (e.g., benzodiazepines, levodopa, and carbamazepine)
Parasomnias			
Sleep terror disorder	Childhood onset	Repeated sudden displays of intense fear during **stage 3 and stage 4 sleep** Associated with scream and signs of autonomic arousal Individual is difficult to soothe and has no recall of event	Parental reassurance (usually resolves spontaneously during adolescence) Medication (in some cases)
Nightmare disorder	Nightmares common in **children**	Repeated dreams with frightening content during **REM sleep** Associated with increased stress Individual rapidly becomes alert on awakening and has full recall of event	Counseling for severe symptoms
Sleepwalking disorder (somnambulism)	Familial Sleepwalking episodes common in children: 10–30% Prevalence of disorder: 1–5%	Repeated occurrences in which individual walks during **stage 3 and stage 4 sleep** Individual has a blank gaze and is difficult to communicate with and awaken	Condition usually resolves spontaneously during adolescence Measures to ensure safety of individual (e.g., environmental changes to protect from harm) Medication (in some cases)

TABLE 18-4   Behavioral Methods for Treating Insomnia

Method	Comments
Sleep hygiene	Maintain regular bedtime and awakening schedule Avoid naps Restrict activities in bed (sleep and sexual relations only) "Wind down" prior to bedtime Maintain comfortable sleeping environment Exercise during daytime Avoid caffeinated products
Stimulus control	Retire to bed when sleepy If unable to fall asleep within 15–20 minutes, get out of bed and engage in relaxing, quiet activity Return to bed when sleepy Repeat as necessary

      b. **Antidepressants with sedating effects** (e.g., trazodone, mirtazapine, amitriptyline)

IV. **Narcolepsy**
- Narcolepsy is characterized by **daily, uncontrollable episodes of refreshing sleep** (e.g., about 10–20 minutes in duration) that occur for at least 3 months.

  A. **Epidemiology and etiology**
     1. Usually **begins during** the **teenage years** and is **lifelong**
     2. Rare; has a **familial** pattern

  B. **Clinical presentation**
- In narcolepsy, elements of REM sleep (e.g., sleep paralysis, hallucinations) intrude on the wakeful state.

     1. **Cataplexy** (~70% of cases): sudden muscle weakness occurring with strong emotion
     2. **Hypnagogic** hallucinations (perceptual disturbances on falling asleep) and **hypnopompic** hallucinations (perceptual disturbances on awakening)
     3. **Sleep paralysis:** transient inability to move upon awakening or falling asleep

  C. **Management**
     1. Scheduled **naps**
     2. **Pharmacologic treatment**
        a. **Stimulants** (e.g., methylphenidate and modafinil)
        b. **Antidepressant drugs** are used to treat cataplexy.

V. **Sleep Apnea**
  A. **Overview**
     1. Sleep apnea is a **breathing-related sleep disorder** involving frequent pauses in breathing that disrupt sleep and lead to excessive sleepiness (Box 18-2).
        a. **Obstructive sleep apnea:** intermittent obstruction of the upper airway
        b. **Central sleep apnea:** loss of respiratory effort

Narcolepsy: brief episodes of uncontrollable sleep.

Symptoms of sleep apnea: excessive sleepiness and loud snoring.

BOX 18-2	The Patient With Sleep Apnea

The wife of a 53-year-old obese man became concerned when she recently noticed that her husband had stopped breathing for brief periods while he was sleeping. She says that she has not slept with her husband for many months because of his loud snoring, and that she had been unaware of the problem until they recently shared a bed while on vacation. The man is unaware of these incidents, but he complains of feeling tired most of the day and of feeling unrefreshed when he awakens. The physician suspects sleep apnea and refers the patient to a sleep disorder clinic for evaluation and treatment.

   2. Respiratory abnormalities include **apneic episodes** (cessation of breathing ≥ 10 seconds) and **hypopnea** (abnormally slow or shallow respiration).
B. **Epidemiology and etiology**
   1. More common in **males**
   2. Associated with **obesity**
   3. Individuals with sleep apnea are at **increased risk for cardiovascular conditions,** such as cardiac arrhythmias, stroke, pulmonary and systemic hypertension, and sudden death.
C. **Clinical presentation: excessive sleepiness,** nonrefreshing sleep, loud **snoring,** frequent awakening, morning headache, and **erectile difficulty**
D. **Management of obstructive sleep apnea**
   1. Nasal continuous positive airway pressure
   2. **Weight loss** in obese individuals
   3. **Surgical procedures** (e.g., uvulopalatopharyngoplasty, tracheostomy)

19

Sexual Health and Sexual Disorders

Target Topics

▶ Sexual response cycle
▶ Sexual dysfunction and management
▶ Paraphilias
▶ Gender identity disorder
▶ Sexual activity and HIV

I. **Human Sexuality**
   A. **Masters and Johnson** described a four-stage model of human sexual response, which consists of **four phases**: excitement, plateau, orgasm, and resolution (Table 19-1).
   B. **Sexuality and aging**
      1. Sexual activity often **diminishes in the elderly** because of the **lack of a sexual partner.**
      2. **Changes in sexuality associated with aging**
         a. **Women**
            (1) Vaginal dryness
            (2) Thinning of vaginal lining
         b. **Men**
            (1) Longer time needed to achieve an erection; need for more direct stimulation to achieve erection
            (2) Decreased force of ejaculate
            (3) **Longer refractory period**
   C. **Sexual orientation**
      1. Sexual orientation may be **heterosexual, homosexual,** or **bisexual.**
      2. The specific determinants of homosexuality are not

Only males experience a refractory period.

Sexual desire does *not* diminish simply as a result of aging.

TABLE 19-1   Phases of the Sexual Response Cycle in Males and Females

Phase	Male Response	Female Response
Excitement	Penile erection Elevation of testes Increase in heart rate, blood pressure, and respiration	Vaginal lubrication Swelling of breasts; nipple erection Enlargement of the vagina Increase in heart rate, blood pressure, and respirations
Plateau	Increased size of testes	Significant vasocongestion of outer third of vagina
Orgasm	Ejaculation (semen first moves to urethra in emission stage and then is expelled during the ejaculation stage) Contraction of perineal muscles and anal sphincter	Contractions of uterus, outer third of vagina, and anal sphincter
Resolution	Return to baseline state Presence of refractory period,* which varies in length but generally becomes longer with increasing age	Return to baseline state Absence of refractory period; ability to achieve another orgasm shortly after initial climax

*The refractory period is the period following orgasm in which the male is unable to be restimulated to further orgasm.

BOX 19-1   DSM-IV-TR Classification of Sexual Dysfunction

Sexual Desire Disorders
  Hypoactive sexual desire disorder
  Sexual aversion disorder
Sexual Arousal Disorders
  Male erectile disorder
  Female sexual arousal disorder
Orgasmic Disorders
  Premature ejaculation
  Female orgasmic disorder
  Male orgasmic disorder
Sexual Pain Disorders
  Vaginismus (not due to medical condition)
  Dyspareunia (not due to medical condition)
Sexual Dysfunction Due to a General Medical Condition
Substance-induced Sexual Dysfunction
Sexual Dysfunction Not Otherwise Specified

---

known, but biological and genetic factors may play a role.

II.   Classification of Sexual Dysfunctions and Disorders

A.   The *Diagnostic and Statistical Manual of Mental Disorders,* 4th edition, text revision (DSM-IV-TR), classification of sexual dysfunction is listed in Box 19-1.

B.   The DSM-IV-TR also describes the paraphilias and gender identity disorders.

TABLE 19-2   Key Features of Sexual Dysfunctions

Dysfunction	Key Features
Hypoactive sexual desire disorder (desire phase)	Lack or deficiency of sexual fantasies and desire for sexual activity May be associated with problems with sexual arousal and orgasm
Sexual aversion disorder (desire phase)	Dislike and avoidance of sexual contact Lack of enjoyment of sexual activity May develop strong emotional reactions, such as extreme anxiety and panic, during sexual encounters May be associated with sexual trauma
Male erectile disorder (excitement phase) (see Box 19-2)	Inability to obtain or maintain erection Increased frequency of occurrence with advancing age (age is not a specific cause) Factors suggesting a psychological cause: presence of morning and nocturnal erections and erections with masturbation
Female sexual arousal disorder (excitement phase)	Inability to achieve or maintain adequate vaginal lubrication Arousal may be minimal or absent Possible painful intercourse or avoidance of sexual activity
Premature ejaculation (orgasm phase)	Occurrence of ejaculation before desired by male May be worse following periods during which individual has not had sexual relations Common in young males Occurs in about 30% of males
Female and male orgasmic disorder (orgasm phase)	Delay or failure in achieving orgasm following sexual excitement In males, orgasm often attained with sexual stimulation other than intercourse
Vaginismus	Reflexive, involuntary spasms of vaginal musculature that prohibit or interfere with intercourse May include difficulty with completing pelvic examination or inserting tampons May develop following sexual trauma Common in younger females with negative attitudes about sex
Dyspareunia	Genital pain with intercourse

III.   Sexual Dysfunctions

A.   **Overview** (Table 19-2)

1.   Sexual dysfunction involves a **disturbance in function** during the sexual response cycle or **pain associated with sexual intercourse.**

2.   It also involves **personal distress** or **relationship difficulties** resulting from a sexual problem.

B.   Etiology

1.   **Often multifactorial:** causes include psychological or behavioral factors, medical conditions, and drug or substance use (Table 19-3).

2.   Even when an organic factor is present, a **psychological response** (e.g., performance anxiety) often contributes to the sexual problem (Box 19-2).

Erectile disorder is one of most common sexual problems in males.

Approximately 50% of men with diabetes mellitus have erectile problems.

TABLE 19-3 Factors That May Affect Sexual Function

Psychological Factors	Medical Conditions	Prescription Drugs/ Substances Used
Lack of information about sexual issues Anxiety related to sexual activity Relationship problems History of traumatic sexual experiences High stress level	Endocrine disorders (e.g., diabetes mellitus, hypothyroidism) Vascular disorders (e.g., hypertension, atherosclerosis) Neurologic disorders (e.g., spinal cord injury, multiple sclerosis) Psychiatric disorders (e.g., depression, anxiety) Pelvic and genital surgery Genital diseases Trauma Renal and liver failure	Antihypertensives Antidepressants Antipsychotics Anxiolytics Sedatives Anticholinergics Lithium Hormones (e.g., estrogen) Opiates Tobacco Alcohol

BOX 19-2   The Man With Erectile Disorder

A 42-year-old man experienced erectile difficulties several weeks ago when he was unable to sustain an erection after consuming too much alcohol. Since then, his thoughts drift to his performance during lovemaking and he has been unable to remain aroused. He consults his physician and after completing a history and thorough physical examination, the physician finds the patient to be in good health. The patient admits to occasional social drinking, but there is no evidence of alcohol abuse. The physician educates the patient about the effect of alcohol on erectile functioning and explains that his anxiety about his performance is most likely interfering with his ability to enjoy sexual intimacy. The physician recommends the use of sensate focus exercises and schedules the patient for a return visit. At the follow-up visit, the man is pleased to report an improvement in his sexual functioning.

C. Management
   1. It is important to **evaluate** and **treat underlying medical conditions** and **related factors** (e.g., medication) that contribute to sexual symptoms.
   2. Treatment of sexual dysfunction may include **psychological, behavioral, medical,** or **pharmacologic interventions** or a combination of these treatments.
   3. **Behavioral techniques**
       a. **Sensate focus exercises:** goal is to **decrease the emphasis on performance** and to **increase the emphasis on pleasure,** a process likely to lead to improved sexual functioning.
       b. **Start-stop technique:** goal is to **increase familiarity with** and **control** over **arousal levels;** used in the treatment of **premature ejaculation.**

TABLE 19-4   Paraphilias

Disorder	Description
Exhibitionism	Displaying one's genitals to unsuspecting individuals
Fetishism	Having sexual urges or fantasies or engaging in sexual behavior using nonliving objects (e.g., female undergarments, shoes)
Frotteurism	Having sexual urges or fantasies or engaging in behaviors involving rubbing against or touching individuals without their consent
Pedophilia	Having sexual urges or fantasies about sexual activity with children or engaging in sexual acts with prepubescent children
Sexual masochism	Engaging in sexual urges, fantasies, or behaviors in which one is the recipient of acts that result in humiliation or physical distress (e.g., being intentionally hurt)
Sexual sadism	Having sexual urges or fantasies or engaging in behaviors in which one perpetrates acts involving psychological or physical harm or suffering to others (e.g., exerting dominance over another individual)
Voyeurism	Having sexual urges or fantasies or engaging in behavior that involves watching unsuspecting individuals while they are naked, undressing, or participating in sexual activity
Transvestic fetishism	Heterosexual males who have sexual urges or fantasies or engage in behaviors that involve dressing in female garments; must be differentiated from cross-dressing that occurs only as part of gender identity disorder

      c. **Squeeze technique:** goal is to **delay ejaculation;** used in the treatment of **premature ejaculation.**
   4. Pharmacotherapy
      a. **Sildenafil citrate:** for male erectile disorder
      b. Selective serotonin reuptake inhibitors (**SSRIs**): for premature ejaculation

> Premature ejaculation is the most common type of male sexual dysfunction.

IV. Paraphilias
  A. **Features** (Table 19-4)
    1. Paraphilias are disorders that involve sexual urges, fantasies, or behaviors that focus on **nonhuman objects,** involve **humiliation or suffering,** or involve **children** or other **nonconsenting individuals.** Many behaviors associated with paraphilias result in harm to others and are illegal.
    2. These features must be **recurrent; present** for **at least 6 months;** and involve impaired functioning, personal distress, or, in some cases, having acted on the sexual urges.
  B. Epidemiology
    1. More common in **males** and tend to be **chronic.**
    2. Most frequently seen paraphilias are **exhibitionism, voyeurism,** and **pedophilia.**
  C. **Management:** psychological intervention, antiandrogens

> Paraphilias are more common in males.

V. Gender Identity Disorder
  A. **Gender identity,** which is **established by 3 years** of age, refers to an individual's perception of being male or female.

B. Gender identity disorder is characterized by **persistent distress about** one's **gender** and a **strong, pervasive identification with** the **opposite sex.**

C. Individuals with this disorder may prefer to dress in attire and engage in activities typical of the opposite sex. Children with the disorder may assume the role of the opposite sex during playtime activities.

D. **Management:** may involve **hormone therapy** and **sex reassignment surgery**, which alter appearance and other physical sex characteristics.

VI. **HIV, AIDS, and Human Sexuality**

A. **Epidemiology**

1. **Number of individuals infected with HIV** in the United States: > 800,000; worldwide: estimated 40 million

2. **New cases of HIV infection in the United States annually**

   a. Majority of cases are **males**, particularly those who have **sex with other males.**

   b. The remainder of cases occur in both males and females who have been infected via **heterosexual contact** and via **injection drug use.**

B. **Transmission of HIV**

1. HIV is found in **blood, semen, vaginal fluid**, saliva, tears, and breast milk.

2. **Modes of transmission**

   a. **Sexual contact with an HIV-infected individual**

   b. **Contact with the blood of an HIV-infected individual:** via needle sharing, needle sticks, blood transfusions, and open sores on mucous membranes. Blood supplies are now tested; thus, the risk of HIV transmission via blood transfusions is extremely low.

   c. **Transmission from an HIV-positive mother to the fetus:** before birth, during birth, or through breastfeeding. Risk of perinatal HIV transmission is reduced when zidovudine **(AZT)** is **administered** to HIV-infected women from pregnancy through delivery and to **infants** after birth.

Receptive anal intercourse is associated with the highest risk of HIV transmission.

20

Other Psychiatric Disorders

Target Topics

▶ Etiology of cognitive disorders
▶ Dementia of the Alzheimer's type
▶ Management of cognitive disorders
▶ Clinical features and management of personality, adjustment, and dissociative disorders

I. Cognitive Disorders

A. Overview

1. Cognitive disorders are organic mental disorders that are characterized by symptoms such as confusion, agitation, and disorientation and include **delirium, dementia,** and **amnestic disorder.**

2. The *Diagnostic and Statistical Manual of Mental Disorders,* 4th edition, text revision (DSM-IV-TR), classification of cognitive disorders is based on etiology (Box 20-1).

3. **Major causes** include:
   a. **Substance use:** alcohol, toxins, medications
   b. **General medical conditions:** nutritional and metabolic disorders, liver disease
   c. **Neurologic conditions:** degenerative disorders, traumatic brain injuries, infections, tumors

4. **Distinguishing features** of delirium and dementia are presented in Table 20-1.

B. Delirium

• Delirium is a short-lived cognitive disorder that reflects an underlying medical condition.

1. **Epidemiology and etiology**
   a. **Risk factors**

Delirium is an acute, usually reversible cognitive disorder.

BOX 20-1	DSM-IV-TR Classification of Cognitive Disorders

Delirium
    Delirium due to a general medical condition
    Substance-induced delirium
    Delirium due to multiple etiologies
Dementia
    Dementia of the Alzheimer's type
    Vascular dementia
    Dementia due to other general medical conditions
    Substance-induced persisting dementia
    Dementia due to multiple etiologies
Amnestic Disorders
    Amnestic disorder due to a general medical condition
    Substance-induced persisting amnestic disorder

TABLE 20-1   Distinguishing Features of Delirium and Dementia

Feature	Delirium	Dementia
Onset	Acute, with prodrome	Slow
Course	Fluctuating	Steady decline
Memory	Impaired anterograde	Steady decline in short-term memory; then decline in long-term memory
Consciousness	Impaired; altered state of arousal	Unimpaired
Cognitive function	Distractibility	Aphasia, apraxia, or agnosia
Behavior	Periods of agitation	Depression, behavioral changes, agitation
Reversibility	Usually reversible	Reversible in only 15% of cases

The risk of delirium is greater if dementia is present.

    (1)   Very young or very advanced age
    (2)   Coexisting dementia
    (3)   History of previous delirium or brain injury
  b.   **Inpatient status:** delirium occurs in **10%** of **all patients in hospitals** and in **30%** of **patients in intensive care units.**
  c.   Development of delirium indicates the presence of a **potentially life-threatening medical condition.** Specific causes of delirium are presented in Table 20-2.
2.   **Clinical presentation** (see Table 20-1)
  a.   **Sleep-wake disturbances** ("sundowning")
  b.   **Delusions and hallucinations**
  c.   Autonomic dysfunction
  d.   Fluctuating states of arousal and confusion
3.   **Management**
  a.   **Identification** and **treatment** of the **underlying etiology** (Box 20-2)
  b.   **Antipsychotics** and/or **benzodiazepines** for agitation and psychosis

TABLE 20-2   Causes of Delirium

Cause	Example
Infection	HIV, encephalitis, sepsis
Withdrawal or intoxication disorders	Alcohol withdrawal, PCP intoxication
Metabolic or endocrine disturbances	Hyponatremia, hypoglycemia
Trauma	Head injury or surgery
Cardiovascular abnormalities	Cerebrovascular accident, hypertensive crisis
Organ system disease	Hepatic or renal dysfunction
Nutritional deficiencies	Thiamine
Medications	Steroids, digoxin, anticholinergics
Toxins	Heavy metals, poisons

PCP, phencyclidine.

BOX 20-2   **The Patient With Delirium Caused by a Medical Condition**

A previously healthy 62-year-old man is admitted to the hospital through the emergency department with a temperature of 39.4°C (102.9°F) and an oxygen saturation of 85% on 4 L of oxygen. A chest x-ray shows bilateral lower lobe pneumonia. After a few hours, the patient becomes confused and pulls out his intravenous line. During the night, he becomes more agitated and insists on going to the nurse's station "to catch the bus home." The physician prescribes haloperidol and lorazepam IV. After several hours of sleep and intravenous antibiotics, the patient's condition improves. As the pneumonia resolves, his confusion resolves, and no further pharmacologic treatment is necessary.

---

      c. **Reduction of environmental stimuli**, such as noise and unfamiliar visitors

C. **Dementia**

- Dementia is a **long-term illness of gradual onset** that involves **progressive cognitive decline.**

    1. **Epidemiology and etiology**

      a. The **prevalence** of dementia dramatically **increases** with advancing **age**, to between 16% and 25% in those individuals who are older than 85 years of age.

      b. **Types of dementia**

         (1) Dementia of the **Alzheimer's type:** the **most common** cause of dementia

         (2) **Vascular dementia:** accounts for 10–20% of dementias in the United States

         (3) **Parkinson's disease:** 20–60% of patients with Parkinson's disease develop dementia.

         (4) Other types of dementia are listed in Table 20-3.

      c. A patient may have more than one type of dementia.

    2. **Clinical presentation** (see Table 20-1)

      a. **Sleep-wake disturbances** ("sundowning"), **delusions** and **hallucinations**

> Two most common types of dementia: Alzheimer's type and vascular.

> Symptoms common to both delirium and dementia: sleep-wake disturbances, delusions, hallucinations.

TABLE 20-3 Features of Selected Non-Alzheimer's Dementias

Type of Dementia	Neurobiologic Findings	Features	Treatment
Vascular dementia	CT and MRI evidence of cerebro-vascular disease. History of hypertension, valvular heart disease, or arrhythmia	Stepwise decline in function Neurologic focal deficits and "soft" signs	Reduction of risk factors (e.g., smoking, hypertension, obesity, arrhythmia)
Dementia due to general conditions (e.g., head trauma)	Multifocal destruction; various locations and extent of injury	Neurologic, behavioral, and cognitive deficits, depending on injury	Address treatable etiologies Rehabilitation services
Parkinson's disease	Neuronal loss and Lewy bodies in substantia nigra	Shuffling, tremor, cogwheel rigidity	Treat Parkinson's symptoms pharmacologically; treat agitation and psychosis symptomatically
Huntington's disease	"Boxcar" ventricles seen in late disease, resulting from atrophy of striatum	Autosomal dominant trait Early onset of psychiatric symptoms, progressing to dementia and choreoathetosis in 30s and 40s	Behavioral and pharmacologic management of agitation and psychosis
Pick's disease	Pick bodies Frontal and temporal atrophy	Onset in 50s and 60s with personality changes, disinhibition, and progressive dementia	Behavioral and pharmacologic management of agitation and psychosis
Creutzfeldt-Jakob disease (mad cow disease)	Prion encephalopathy; spongiform neuropathologic changes	Myoclonus; periodic EEG activity Rapid progression	Behavioral and pharmacologic management of agitation and psychosis
Normal pressure hydrocephalus	MRI or CT of head showing enlarged ventricles	Triad of ataxia, dementia, urinary incontinence	Ventricular shunting
Vitamin B_{12} deficiency	Anemia, macrocytic anemia	Paresthesias, weakness, confusion	Vitamin B_{12} IM, for replacement and maintenance

CT, computed tomography; *EEG*, electroencephalogram; *IM*, intramuscularly; *MRI*, magnetic resonance imaging.

   b. Slow decline in cognitive function and memory

   c. Behavioral disturbances

  3. Differential diagnosis

   a. Amnestic disorder

    (1) Amnestic disorder, which is usually caused by **alcoholism** or **brain injury**, can be distinguished from dementia.

    (2) Key features include **memory loss**, with **preservation** of other **cognitive** and **social functions**.

   b. Pseudodementia

    (1) Pseudodementia occurs in **depressed patients** who appear to have cognitive decline but whose **symptoms resolve following treatment** of the depression (see Chapter 13).

    (2) Features that differentiate **pseudodementia** from dementia are **abrupt onset** and accompanying **depression** or irritability, lethargy, and recognition and distress about the cognitive symptoms.

> Dementia is often accompanied by depression.

  4. Management

   a. Workup for dementia should include the following basic laboratory and imaging studies, which help distinguish the type of dementia and its potential reversibility.

    (1) Blood studies: chemistry panel (electrolytes, glucose, liver, renal), complete blood count, thyroid-stimulating hormone level, vitamin B_{12} and folate levels, VDRL test, oxygen saturation, drug levels

    (2) Urinalysis

    (3) Imaging studies: electrocardiogram, chest radiograph; computed tomography (CT) or magnetic resonance imaging (MRI) of the head

    (4) Other studies, as indicated by physical examination or history

   b. Neuropsychological evaluation and sequential **Mini-Mental State Examination** help make the diagnosis of dementia and assess its progression (see Chapter 8).

   c. Treatment (see Table 20-3): About 15% of dementias can be reversed, or their progression can be arrested if the underlying cause is removed.

 D. **Dementia of the Alzheimer's type** (Box 20-3)

  • Characterized by progressive cognitive decline, with a survival of 8–10 years

  1. Epidemiology

   a. Women have a slightly **higher risk** than men.

   b. Patients with **Down syndrome** are at **high risk** of developing dementia by 40 years of age.

> Dementia of the Alzheimer's type constitutes 60% of dementias.

  2. Etiology

   a. Neuroanatomic changes

    (1) Atrophy with enlarged ventricles and sulci

| BOX 20-3 | **The Patient with Dementia of the Alzheimer's Type** |

An 85-year-old woman, who has been living independently, has become increasingly forgetful during the past several months and has forgotten to pay her bills. When her daughter tries to help her with business matters, the daughter finds that her mother cannot organize items properly or perform calculations correctly. Recently, the local police called the daughter when an officer found the woman wandering on a street when she became lost on the way to the grocery store. The woman's physician conducts a physical examination and orders laboratory studies and a CT scan of the head. The laboratory screening indicates no abnormalities, but the CT scan shows generalized atrophy, most prominently in the parietal lobes, with enlarged sulci and ventricles. The physician prescribes donepezil and helps arrange for the patient to be placed in an assisted-living facility.

        (2) β-**Amyloid deposits** in senile plaques
        (3) Neurofibrillary tangles
        (4) Loss of cholinergic neurons in the basal forebrain
    b. Genetic changes
        (1) Loci have been identified on **chromosomes 21, 14,** and **19.**
        (2) About 35–45% of patients with Alzheimer's disease have the apolipoprotein E4 gene on chromosome 19.
  3. Clinical presentation
    a. Features: slow, steady **decline in cognition, memory, and function**
    b. Course: **8–10 years;** death is often due to infection or another secondary process.
  4. Management
    a. Pharmacotherapy
        (1) Cholinesterase inhibitors (e.g., donepezil, rivastigmine, galantamine), which **slow** the progression of disease but *do not* reverse its course
        (2) Vitamin E, nonsteroidal anti-inflammatory drugs **(NSAIDs),** and **estrogen**
        (3) Symptomatic therapy with **antidepressants, antipsychotics,** and **mood stabilizers** as needed
    b. Psychotherapy: behavioral modalities (e.g., redirection; structured, safe environment with familiar caregivers)

II. Personality Disorders
  A. Overview
    1. "**Personality**" consists of one's habits, attitudes, and expectations that lie along a continuum from "trait" to "disorder."
      a. Personality traits are the ways in which individuals

Most individuals with personality disorders make others feel miserable.

TABLE 20-4   DSM-IV-TR Classification and Features of Personality Disorders

Personality Disorder	Descriptor	Features
Cluster A (odd)		
Paranoid	Suspicious	Distrust and suspiciousness to the extent that motives of others are interpreted as malevolent
Schizoid	Solitary	Detachment from social relationships and restricted range of emotional expression
Schizotypal	Peculiar	Acute discomfort in close relationships, cognitive or perceptual distortions, and eccentricities of behavior
Cluster B (dramatic, erratic, emotional)		
Antisocial	Unprincipled	Disregard for and violation of rights of others
Borderline	Volatile	Instability in interpersonal relationships, self-image, and affect; marked impulsivity
Histrionic	Attention seeking	Excessive emotionality and attention seeking
Narcissistic	Self-important	Grandiosity, need for adoration, and lack of empathy
Cluster C (anxious, fearful)		
Avoidant	Pathologically shy	Social inhibition, feelings of inadequacy, and hypersensitivity to negative evaluation
Dependent	Needy	Submissive and clinging behavior related to excessive need to be cared for
Obsessive-compulsive	Methodical	Preoccupation with orderliness, perfectionism, and control

perceive, think, and relate to their environment. Traits are the **normal characteristics** that make human beings distinct individuals.

  b. **Personality disorders** occur when these traits are used so rigidly and pervasively that they become maladaptive, leading to dysfunctional relationships (Table 20-4).

 2. **DSM-IV-TR classification** (Box 20-4)
  a. **Three clusters:** A, B, and C
  b. Recorded on axis II of the DSM-IV-TR multiaxial system (see Table 8-6)

B. **Epidemiology**
 1. Overall **prevalence: 10–14%**
 2. **Distribution between the sexes:** equal, although this pattern may vary considerably for specific disorders (e.g., antisocial personality disorder and paranoid personality disorder are more common in males).
 3. **Early onset:** beginning at least by **adolescence** or **early adulthood**

In the US, at least 1 in 10 individuals has a personality disorder.

Symptoms of personality disorders are usually evident by adolescence or early adulthood.

BOX 20-4 | **DSM-IV-TR Classification of Personality Disorders**

Cluster A
  Paranoid
  Schizoid
  Schizotypal
Cluster B
  Antisocial
  Borderline
  Histrionic
  Narcissistic
Cluster C
  Avoidant
  Dependent
  Obsessive-compulsive

BOX 20-5 | **The Patient With Borderline Personality Disorder**

A 23-year-old woman is brought to the emergency department by her parents after threatening to cut her wrists. When she is asked about the circumstances associated with her suicidal thoughts, she says that her boyfriend of 2 months ended their relationship earlier that day. She says that the emotional pain is unbearable, that she is "nothing" without him, and that she wishes she were dead. The woman's parents report that their daughter tried to commit suicide several months ago after an argument with a friend. They say that she has had many stormy relationships, eventually losing friends who grow weary of her unpredictable moods, her "idolizing" or "hateful" attitudes toward them, and her frequent suicidal threats. The suspected diagnosis is borderline personality disorder. The physician is concerned about acute suicide risk and arranges for the patient to be admitted to the psychiatric ward.

    C. Etiology
        1. Etiology is **multifactorial.**
        2. Personality development is the result of a complex interaction of biological, psychological, and social factors.
    D. Clinical presentation (see Table 20-4)
        1. Feelings of **unusual frustration, caution, rejection, detachment,** or **anger** by the physician toward a patient should alert the physician to the likely presence of a personality disorder.
        2. **Complaints by family members** about a patient's behavior may alert the physician to the presence of a personality disorder (Box 20-5).
        3. Most individuals with personality disorders believe that others are to blame for their difficulties and **see no reason to change their behavior.** A few individuals are motivated to **change to relieve the distress** caused by their interpersonal difficulties.

E.   Management
1.   **Establish well-defined limits** to the physician's availability.
2.   **Encourage patients to take responsibility** for change.
3.   Be **objective**, *not* judgmental, about a patient's behavior.
4.   **Psychotherapy:** the treatment of choice for patients who are motivated to change their behavior
5.   **Pharmacotherapy:** used to **manage specific symptoms** associated with the disorder (e.g., mood-stabilizing medication for mood instability) and to **treat coexisting conditions** (e.g., depression)

Consider personality disorders as problems to be managed, not cured.

III.   **Adjustment Disorders**
A.   Overview
1.   The key feature is the development of clinically significant **emotional** or **behavioral symptoms** that are a **reaction** to an **identifiable psychosocial stressor.**
2.   The **significance of the response** is indicated by either one of the following:
a.   **Marked emotional distress** exceeding that experienced by most individuals who encounter such a stressor
b.   **Significant impairment** in **performing** the individual's usual **social** or **occupational activities**
3.   The **DSM-IV-TR subtypes** are based primarily on clinical symptoms and include:
a.   With depressed mood
b.   With anxiety
c.   With mixed anxiety and depressed mood
d.   With disturbance of conduct
e.   With mixed disturbance of emotion and conduct
4.   **Adjustment disorder** may be **common**, with a **prevalence** in outpatient mental health settings of **5–20%.**

An adjustment disorder is a disruptive or distressful response to a discernible stressor.

B.   Clinical presentation
1.   **Symptoms** must **develop within 3 months** of the appearance of the stressor and **resolve within 6 months** of the disappearance of the stressor.
2.   **Stressors** may be single events (e.g., job loss); multiple events (e.g., divorce and relocation of residence); recurrent events (e.g., seasonal employment layoff); or continuous events (e.g., ongoing marital problems).
3.   Diagnosis of adjustment disorder is *not* **appropriate when the patient's distress is better accounted for by bereavement.**
C.   Management
1.   **Supportive psychotherapy:** the primary treatment of adjustment disorders
2.   **Pharmacologic therapy:** may be used to treat associated symptoms (e.g., hypnotics for sleep disturbance)

TABLE 20-5   Types and Features of Dissociative Disorders

Type of Disorder	Epidemiology	Features
Dissociative amnesia	Most common of the dissociative disorders More common in women and young adults	Inability to recall important personal information that is usually associated with trauma or stress and cannot be explained by ordinary forgetfulness
Dissociative fugue	Rare	Sudden, unexpected travel away from home or work, accompanied by an inability to recall one's personal history Confusion about one's identity or assumption of new identity
Dissociative identity disorder (formerly multiple personality disorder)	More common in women Often coexists with other mental disorders; up to two thirds of affected individuals commit suicide	Presence of two or more distinct personality states that alternately control behavior Varying extent of awareness of other personalities by others
Depersonalization disorder	More common in women than in men As many as 50% of adults have isolated experience of depersonalization at some point in life, usually associated with severe stress	Persistent or repeated feeling of being detached from one's body or one's mind, but with intact awareness of one's actual physical environment

IV.   **Dissociative Disorders**
    A.   **Overview**
        1.   The key feature is the **impaired integration** of an individual's **memories, consciousness,** and **perceptions,** resulting in the disruption of the individual's self-identity.
        2.   **Onset** may be **acute** or **gradual,** and the **course** may be **transient** or **chronic.**
        3.   Dissociative disorders described in the DSM-IV-TR include dissociative amnesia, dissociative fugue, dissociative identity disorder, and depersonalization disorder.
    B.   **Etiology**
        1.   Most individuals perceive themselves as having one basic personality, with their thoughts, emotions, and actions all interrelated in a consistent manner.
        2.   **Individuals** often **react to an event by dissociating from it;** that is, by automatically divorcing thoughts and memories of the event from those associated with other parts of their lives.
        3.   **Dissociation reactions** vary from **normal** "everyday" occurrences to **severe** responses that leave individuals distressed or impaired.
    C.   Types of dissociative disorders (Table 20-5)
    D.   Management
        1.   **Psychotherapy** is the treatment of choice.
        2.   **Pharmacotherapy**
            a.   Consider using **antidepressant** medications if coexisting depression is present.
            b.   **Avoid using benzodiazepines** to treat associated anxiety because of the risk of addiction.
        3.   Carefully assess **suicide risk.**

21

Abuse and Violence

Target Topics

▸ Physical and emotional problems associated with abuse and violence
▸ Types and signs of abuse and violence
▸ Role of the physician in managing the patient who is a victim of abuse

I. Overview

   A. Common responses to abuse and violence
   1. **Denial and blaming the victim** are common responses to episodes of abuse and violence by both victims and others. This is particularly true of victims of intrafamilial abuse and sexual assault.
   2. Abused individuals **often do not report** these **episodes to physicians** because of shame, guilt, embarrassment, fear of retaliation, or desire to protect their abusers.

   B. Associated physical and psychological health problems
   1. Individuals who experience abuse and violence have an **increased risk** of **long-term physical** and **psychological** health **problems**.
   2. Common immediate and long-term psychological sequelae
      a. Psychiatric disorders
         (1) Posttraumatic stress disorder and other anxiety disorders
         (2) Depression and increased risk of suicide
         (3) Substance use disorders
         (4) Dissociative disorders
         (5) Borderline personality disorder
         (6) Sexual dysfunction
      b. Difficulties with interpersonal relationships

> Victims of abuse often develop post-traumatic stress disorder, depression, and substance use disorders.

        c. Increased risk of being a victim of abuse or violence in the future

        d. Perpetration of abuse

  3. **Common long-term health-related outcomes**

        a. **Chronic pain**; increased physical complaints

        b. **Health-risk behaviors** (e.g., cigarette smoking, unprotected sex, poor diet, lack of exercise)

        c. Increased use of medical services

II. Child Maltreatment

A. Types of child maltreatment

  1. **Physical abuse:** any nonaccidental injury caused by a parent or caregiver

  2. **Sexual abuse:** engagement in a sexual encounter by an adult or significantly older child

  3. **Emotional abuse:** chronic emotional mistreatment (e.g., terrorizing, humiliating, rejecting, or isolating a child). These actions may involve **extreme forms of punishment** (e.g., locking a child in a closet, killing a child's pet).

  4. **Neglect:** chronic failure to provide basic physical, emotional, medical, and educational needs

  5. **Munchausen syndrome by proxy** (form of child maltreatment or abuse): parent or caregiver intentionally causes illness in a child or falsely reports symptoms (see Chapter 15)

B. Epidemiology

  1. The most frequently reported type of child maltreatment is neglect, followed by physical, sexual, and emotional abuse.

  2. The reported incidence is 13 per 1000; the actual incidence is unknown but is estimated to be 42 per 1000.

  3. Approximately 50% of abused children are 7 years of age or younger.

  4. Child abuse occurs equally in **boys and girls.**

  5. The majority of abusers are **parents** (77%), and some are other relatives (11%).

        a. Approximately **60%** of **abusers** are **women.**

        b. In **sexual abuse**, approximately **90%** of **abusers** are **men.**

  6. **Risk factors**

        a. **For abusers:** substance abuse, depression or other psychological disorders, lack of maturity, social isolation, high levels of stress, childhood history of abuse, poverty, concurrent partner abuse

        b. **For victims:** characteristics that make caregiving challenging (e.g., being disabled, having a difficult temperament); child of an unwanted pregnancy

C. Clinical presentation (Table 21-1)

  1. **Children** may show a decline in school performance, be reluctant to go home after school, have sleep problems and nightmares, secondary enuresis, or encopresis.

Neglect is the most frequently reported type of child maltreatment.

Adults who are abused as children are at increased risk of becoming abusers or victims of abuse.

Sexually transmitted disease in a child is a sign of sexual abuse.

TABLE 21-1   Physical and Behavioral Signs of Child Maltreatment

Type of Abuse	Physical Signs	Behavioral Signs
Physical abuse	**Injuries at various stages of healing,** bruises on uncommonly injured body surfaces **Bruises and welts** in shape of hand, belt, belt buckle, or teeth Immersion **burns** on feet (sock-like pattern), hands (glove-like pattern), or buttocks (circular pattern); rope burns on wrists or ankles; cigarette burns Fractures, including spiral fractures caused by twisting limbs; healed fractures on x-ray Internal abdominal injuries **"Shaken baby" syndrome** (subdural or subarachnoid hemorrhages, retinal hemorrhages, no evidence of external cranial trauma)	**Implausible explanations for injuries,** wearing long sleeves and pants to cover injuries **Aggressiveness toward other children** Destructiveness, cruelty to animals, setting fires
Sexual abuse	**Sexually transmitted disease,** repeated genitourinary infections Pregnancy Abrasions or bruises of inner thighs or external genitalia; anal trauma; rectal or genital bleeding, discharge, or pain	**Sexual knowledge or behavior beyond that expected for developmental level** Fear of undressing, unreasonable fear of physical examination, sudden fear of certain people or places, self-mutilation, secondary enuresis or encopresis, sleep disturbance
Emotional abuse	Abnormal weight gain or loss	**Anxious or depressed appearance,** difficulty with peer relationships, adult-like behavior or delays in physical or emotional development
Neglect	**Malnutrition,** failure to thrive Ingestion of toxic household substances Inadequately treated illness, severe diaper rash Frequent injuries Severe dental caries	**Attachment difficulties in infancy** Poor hygiene; inappropriate clothing for weather; frequent absence from school; begging or stealing food; lack of appropriate medical, dental, or vision care Developmental delays

  2.   **Adolescents** may become **runaways** and/or **substance abusers.**
 D.   Management (Box 21-1)
  1.   Be alert for **signs of abuse** (see Table 21-1).
  2.   Recognize **indicators of abusive parents,** who:
   a.   Provide a **history** of the child's **injuries** that is inconsistent with the medical evaluation

BOX 21-1	The Child With Evidence of Physical Abuse

A 5-year-old boy is brought to the pediatrician's office by his mother for his immunizations. While performing a physical examination, the pediatrician notices a clear impression of a belt buckle on the boy's back and several bruises on the buttocks. When asked about the boy's behavior, his mother responds that since his father left 1 year ago, her son rarely obeys her and often hits one of his siblings. She states that her husband is not providing financial support and that she is overwhelmed by caring for her three children on her own. When asked about the bruises in private interviews, the boy and his mother both report that he fell off his bicycle. The pediatrician says that the boy's injuries suggest that he has been hit with a belt and expresses concern for the boy's safety. He states that the law requires that the injuries be reported to child protective services. In addition, the pediatrician expresses concern for the boy's mother and gives her information about community programs that offer assistance to families who may need additional resources and support.

      b. Show **excessive concern** or a **lack of concern** for the child's injuries

      c. Make **statements** indicating that they have **unrealistic expectations for the child**

   3. Report child abuse

      a. **Physicians** have a **legal responsibility** to **report suspected child abuse** to the state child protective agency.

> All states require that physicians report suspected child maltreatment.

      b. It is generally recommended that parents be informed of the report, but it is *not required* if the physician believes that it will place the child in greater danger.

      c. A **physician** who makes a report in good faith is **immune from civil and criminal liability**.

III.   Intimate Partner Violence

   • Intimate partner violence (known as partner abuse, domestic violence, spousal abuse, or battering) is **physical, emotional,** or **sexual** intimidation or violation by a current or former intimate partner.

   A. Epidemiology

     1. In most cases, the abused individuals are **women** who are **abused by men.** Although men may be victims, women are more likely to be injured.

> Intimate partner violence is the most common cause of serious injury to women.

      a. **Injuries** from intimate partner violence account for approximately **one third** of all **emergency department visits** by women.

      b. Approximately **5% of pregnant women** are **battered.**

     2. **More than 50% of women** are **assaulted by a current or former partner** during their lifetime.

     3. Intimate partner violence frequently is associated with concurrent child abuse.

TABLE 21-2   Behavioral and Physical Signs of Intimate Partner Violence

Sign	Manifestation
Behavioral	
Patient-partner interaction	Partner who accompanies patient and dominates interview, reluctance of patient to speak or disagree with partner
Patient history	History that is inconsistent with injuries, delay in seeking treatment, minimization or denial of abuse
Adherence	Nonadherence with medical advice due to lack of access to transportation, money, or telephone
Physical	
Injury site	Head, neck, chest, breasts, and abdomen
Injury pattern	Multiple injuries at several sites, repeated injuries
Injury during pregnancy	Abdomen or breasts, in particular

   B. Risk factors (for both the abused and the abuser)
      1. Alcohol or **drug abuse**
      2. History of abuse as a child
      3. History of witnessing violent behavior in parents
      4. Low self-esteem
   C. Characteristics of an abusive relationship
      1. The principal issue is **control over the victim.**
      2. A repetitive **cycle of violence** involves the buildup of tension, violence, apologies, and promises of reform.
      3. Victims are afraid to leave abusers and must overcome barriers to leaving, which include fear of retaliation to self and children, lack of financial resources, lack of confidence in their ability to be independent, and emotional dependence on abusers.
      4. Abusers minimize their violent behavior and **blame their victims,** who often believe they deserve the abuse.
      5. Risk of harm is greatest when victims attempt to end the relationship.
   D. Clinical presentation (Table 21-2)
   E. Management
      1. Be alert for signs of abuse, and routinely **screen female patients** (see Table 21-2).
      2. If abuse is suspected, **interview patients** in the **absence of their partners.**
      3. Assess the degree of **immediate danger.**
      4. Provide information regarding community resources for shelter, counseling, and legal advocacy.
      5. Do *not* **refer partners** and **victims** for **joint counseling.**
      6. Reporting abuse
         a. Some states mandate the reporting of intimate partner violence.
         b. Mandatory reporting is controversial, because it may increase risk for further injury and deter victims from seeking medical care.
      7. Assess the safety of children in the home.

The severity of intimate partner violence escalates over time.

Couples counseling is contraindicated in situations of intimate partner violence.

IV. **Sexual Assault**
   A. **Definitions**
      1. Sexual assault is defined as any form of attempted or actual **nonconsenting sexual contact**, including a range of behaviors (e.g., kissing, fondling, rape) as well as verbal threats. It is a **crime of violence** in which sexual acts are used to control, overpower, degrade, or humiliate victims.
      2. **Rape**, the most common type of sexual assault, is attempted or actual oral, genital, or anal penetration by a part of the assailant's body or by an object.
   B. **Epidemiology**

Most victims of sexual assault know their assailant.

      1. **Most assailants are males** who are known to the victim.
      2. The **rate of** sexual assault **is highest** in **females younger than 19 years** of age.
      3. Approximately 18% of women and 3% of men report having experienced a rape or attempted rape in their lifetime.
   C. **Management**
      1. **Assess and treat physical injuries**, which are usually minor (e.g., lacerations, bruises).
      2. Obtain a **history** of the sexual assault in a compassionate manner that does not imply that the victim was at fault.
      3. **Collect evidence** following the protocol outlined in a standard rape kit.
      4. Provide **treatment** and **prophylaxis** for **sexually transmitted diseases** and for **pregnancy.**

Most victims of sexual assault do not report the crime to the police.

      5. If a rape crisis counselor is not present during the examination, **refer the patient to a rape crisis center** for guidance about reporting the crime, information about typical responses to sexual assault, and individual and/or group counseling.
      6. Formulate a plan with the patient for **follow-up medical care.**

V. **Elder Abuse and Neglect**
   A. **Types of elder abuse and neglect**, as defined by the National Center on Elder Abuse
      1. **Physical abuse:** use of physical force that may lead to physical injury, pain, or impairment, including the use of physical and chemical restraints
      2. **Sexual abuse:** any type of sexual involvement to which an elder does not or cannot give consent
      3. **Emotional abuse:** infliction of anguish, emotional pain, or distress by means such as threatening, humiliating, isolating, or treating the elder like an infant. Emotional abuse also involves the **violation of the elder's rights**, including denying an elder privacy or the right to make decisions about health care.
      4. **Financial or material exploitation:** inappropriate and often illegal use of the elder's money, property, or other resources

TABLE 21-3   Types and Signs of Elder Abuse

Type of Abuse	Signs
Physical abuse	Fractures, bruises, wounds, lacerations, burns (especially if injuries occur in a pattern, in a defined shape, in various stages of healing, or are inadequately explained) Laboratory evidence of overdosing or underdosing of prescribed medication
Sexual abuse	Bruises, lacerations, or bleeding Itching in genital or anal area; unexplained sexually transmitted disease; ripped, stained, or bloody underwear
Emotional abuse	Emotional upset or agitation; extreme withdrawal
Financial/material exploitation	Unauthorized appropriation of elder's financial assets or property; coercion to change deed, will, or bank account
Neglect	Dehydration or malnutrition Poor personal hygiene or inadequate clothing; unsanitary or unsafe living conditions Fecal impaction or urine burns Untreated health problems (e.g., bedsores) Lack of medical aids (e.g., glasses, dentures, hearing aids)
Abandonment	Desertion at institution (e.g., hospital) or public place (e.g., shopping mall)
Self-neglect	Same as for neglect

5. **Neglect:** failure or refusal of a caregiver to carry out the physical, emotional, and financial obligations required to meet the elder's care needs
6. **Abandonment:** deserting an elder for whom the caregiver is responsible, such as at a health institution or public place
7. **Self-neglect:** failure of an elder to provide for his or her own needs, resulting in threats to the elder's health and safety

B. Epidemiology
   1. **Self-neglect** is the **most common form of elder abuse,** followed by neglect by a caregiver.
   2. Elder abuse occurs in both **institutional** and **noninstitutional settings.** The most common abusers in noninstitutional settings are adult children, spouses, and other family members.
   3. The actual incidence is unknown; estimates range from 500,000 to 2 million cases per year, of which as few as 1 in 14 may be reported.
   4. **Victims** are **more likely** to be **women.**
   5. Possible risk factors
      a. **For abusers:** financial or emotional dependence on the elder, substance abuse, past or current psychiatric problems, family history of abuse, stress (e.g., financial problems, divorce, caregiver burden)
      b. **For victims:** advanced age, functional dependence on caregiver, living with others, social isolation, history of abuse, cognitive impairment

C. **Clinical presentation** (Table 21-3)
   1. **Signs of abuse and neglect in elders**

In noninstitutional settings, the most likely abusers of elders are adult children.

      a. Anxiety, **depression**, posttraumatic stress disorder
      b. Insomnia
      c. **Fear of caregiver**
      d. **Hesitating to speak freely**
      e. **Excessive hospitalizations** or **visits to emergency departments**

2. **Signs of elder abuse and neglect in caregivers**
      a. **Delay in seeking care for the elder**
      b. **Reluctance to answer questions,** vague and/or implausible answers about physical presentation, domination of the interview, unwillingness to allow the elder to be interviewed alone, tension or indifference between the elder and the caregiver
      c. Inadequate knowledge of the elder's medical problems
      d. Lack of visits to the elder in the hospital
      e. History of **physician or hospital "hopping"** with the elder
      f. Unwarranted concern about cost

D. **Management**
- **Physicians** play an important **role** in the **identification, treatment,** and **prevention** of **mistreatment of elders.** For some dependent elders, physicians may be the only contact the elders have except for their caregivers, who often are the abusers. **Management strategies for the physician** include:

1. Be alert for **signs of abuse** and **neglect** (see Table 21-3).
2. **Treat** physical **injuries** and other **medical problems.**
3. **Interview** the **elder** and the **caregiver individually** and avoid blame or confrontation.
4. **Develop plans to ensure the safety of the elder** (e.g., hospitalization, release to the care of a responsible family member or friend, referral to a shelter qualified to care for abused elders).
      a. **Educate the patient** about the escalating nature of the abuse.
      b. **Provide information about community resources** to maintain the security of patients in the least restrictive environment possible.
5. **Consider the patient's autonomy.** Elderly patients who have decision-making capacity may choose to remain in the abusive situation (see Chapter 25).
6. **Report suspected elder abuse,** if required. Most states mandate reporting of suspected elder abuse and offer immunity from criminal or civil liability if reports are made in good faith.

Childhood Psychiatric Disorders

22

Target Topics

▶ Attention-deficit/hyperactivity disorder
▶ Conduct disorder and oppositional defiant disorder
▶ Separation anxiety disorder
▶ Tourette's disorder
▶ Autistic disorder and other pervasive developmental disorders
▶ Mental retardation
▶ Learning disorders

I. Overview

A. Childhood psychiatric disorders are usually first diagnosed in infancy, childhood, or adolescence.

B. The estimated **prevalence** of all childhood psychiatric disorders is **15–20%**.

C. Childhood psychiatric disorders are generally **more common in boys**.

D. The *Diagnostic and Statistical Manual of Mental Disorders*, 4th edition, text revision (DSM-IV-TR), classification of childhood disorders is listed in Box 22-1.

> Almost all childhood psychiatric disorders are more prevalent in boys.

II. Attention-Deficit/Hyperactivity Disorder (ADHD)

A. Epidemiology and etiology

1. ADHD is one of the **most common childhood behavioral disorders.** The precise etiology is unknown; however, **genetic factors** play a role.
2. **Risk factors** include **prenatal maternal smoking** and

> Estimated prevalence of ADHD in school-age children is 3–5%.

BOX 22-1	**Some DSM-IV-TR Disorders Usually First Diagnosed in Infancy, Childhood, or Adolescence**

Attention-deficit and Disruptive Behavior Disorders
  Attention-deficit/hyperactivity disorder
  Conduct disorder
  Oppositional defiant disorder
Separation Anxiety Disorder
Tic Disorders
  Transient tic disorder
  Chronic tic disorder
  Tourette's disorder
Pervasive Development Disorders
  Autistic disorder
  Asperger's disorder
  Rett's disorder
Mental Retardation
Learning Disorders

alcohol abuse, perinatal exposure to toxins or infections, and history of abuse or neglect.

B. Clinical presentation

1. **Key features:** the following symptoms must be present **before 7 years** of age, must be **present for at least 6 months,** must occur to a degree that is **maladaptive** and **inconsistent** with **developmental** level, and must **occur in two or more settings.**

    a. **Inattention** (e.g., not completing tasks, being forgetful, or making careless mistakes)

    b. **Hyperactivity-impulsivity** (e.g., frequent interrupting or intruding on others, moving about inappropriately, or talking excessively)

2. **Associated features: academic underachievement,** difficulties in peer relationships, difficulty sleeping, poor handwriting, frequent accidents, low self-esteem, increased risk of **antisocial personality disorder** and **substance abuse**

3. **Comorbid conditions:** conduct disorder, oppositional defiant disorder, learning disorders, communication disorders, Tourette's disorder, mood disorder, anxiety disorder, and mental retardation.

4. **Most common course:** decrease in hyperactivity during adolescence, with a persistence of inattention and impulsivity in adulthood

C. Management

1. **Evaluation**

    a. Obtain **descriptions of the child's behavior** from teachers and parents, using standardized rating scales.

    b. Refer for **psychoeducational testing** to determine

ADHD involves inattention and/or hyperactivity-impulsivity.

TABLE 22-1   Comparison of Conduct Disorder and Oppositional Defiant Disorder

Disorder	Epidemiology	Clinical Features	Associated Features
Conduct disorder	Prevalence: 1–10% Better outcome if onset occurs in adolescence Predisposing factors: socio-economic deprivation, association with delinquent individuals; previous ADHD and/or ODD Prognosis: majority of cases resolve by adulthood	Aggression toward people and animals Destruction of property Deceitfulness or theft Serious violations of rules (e.g., truancy from school, running away from home)	Lack of appropriate feelings of remorse Sexual activity at early age Increased rate of suicidal ideation, suicide attempts and completions Increased risk of antisocial personality disorder and alcohol dependence in adulthood
Oppositional defiant disorder (ODD)	Prevalence: 2–16% Onset: usually before 8 years of age but no later than early adolescence Predisposing factors: difficult temperament, strong-willed personality; controlling, authoritarian, or permissive parents Prognosis: may develop into conduct disorder	Frequent refusal to comply with adult requests Deliberately annoying others; blaming others for misbehavior Vindictive, angry, argumentative Outbursts of temper	Verbal rather than physical expression of aggression Poor relationships with peers Symptoms more evident in contacts with familiar individuals

ADHD, attention-deficit/hyperactivity disorder.

whether learning disorders are contributing to school difficulties.

2. Pharmacotherapy: stimulants and atomoxetine (a selective norepinephrine reuptake inhibitor)

3. Behavioral therapy
 a. Teach parents **behavior management skills.**
 b. Work with teachers to **modify selected target behaviors.**
 c. Teach the child **self-control** and **social skills.**

Drugs most often involved in the treatment of ADHD are psychostimulants.

III. Disruptive Behavior Disorders: Conduct Disorder and Oppositional Defiant Disorder
 A. Clinical presentation
  1. Key features (Table 22-1)
   a. Conduct disorder: persistent pattern of behavior that **violates the rights of others** or societal rules
   b. Oppositional defiant disorder: pattern of negativistic, hostile, defiant behavior that **does *not* violate the rights of others** or societal rules (Box 22-2)
  2. Associated features: poor academic performance; use of tobacco, alcohol, or illicit drugs at a young age
  3. Predisposing family factors
   a. Increased incidence of **antisocial personality disorder,** ADHD, substance-related disorders, or mood disorders in parents

Conduct disorder may involve aggressive and illegal behavior.

BOX 22-2 | **The Boy With ADHD**

The teacher of a 6-year-old boy reports that the boy's behavior in his first-grade class is disruptive. He frequently leaves his seat, blurts out answers without raising his hand, and rarely finishes his assignments during class. His parents find it very difficult to get their son to do the simple chores that his older siblings did when they were the same age. Family members often are embarrassed by the boy's behavior at restaurants and at friends' homes; he seems unable to sit quietly and frequently breaks things. The parents seek assistance from a pediatrician, who asks them and the boy's teacher to evaluate the boy's behavior using standardized ADHD rating scales. Based on these results, the pediatrician prescribes methylphenidate, refers the family to a psychologist experienced in the treatment of ADHD, and arranges a follow-up visit to assess the boy's response to the drug.

---

        b. **Severe marital discord;** parenting practices that are abusive, neglectful, harsh, or inconsistent; frequent changes in caregivers

    4. **Comorbid conditions:** ADHD, learning disorders, depressive disorders, substance abuse

  B. **Management**

    1. **Parent training** (i.e., use of behavioral techniques to modify child's behavior) and **family therapy**

    2. **Individual psychotherapy**

    3. Treatment of comorbid conditions, using pharmacotherapy if indicated

    4. Additional **intervention for conduct disorder:** community programs, therapeutic foster homes, residential treatment programs, and efforts to decrease contact with delinquent peers

IV. **Separation Anxiety Disorder**

  • This condition involves developmentally **inappropriate** and **excessive anxiety** concerning separation from attachment figures (usually parents) (Box 22-3).

  A. **Clinical presentation**

    1. **Key features**

        a. **Persistent worry about harm** occurring to attachment figures

        b. **Reluctance to go to school** or to other places that require separation from attachment figures (school refusal or school phobia)

        c. **Reluctance to go to sleep** without being near attachment figures

        d. Repeated **nightmares** about separation

        e. Repeated **physical complaints** (e.g., headaches, stomachaches, vomiting)

BOX 22-3   The Girl With Separation Anxiety Disorder

An 8-year-old girl in the third grade has shown changes in her behavior since her grandfather, who lived with the girl's family, died a few months ago. The girl has frequent nightmares, and most nights she tries to get in bed with her parents. She no longer plays outdoors with friends and repeatedly asks her parents when they will die and what will happen to her when they do. She has complained of stomachaches in the mornings and has missed the past 6 days of school, although she denies having any recent negative experiences there. The girl's pediatrician acknowledges the significance of the loss of the grandfather and explains to the girl that she may be worried about losing her parents. The pediatrician describes how staying home from school intensifies the fear. He recommends an immediate return to school, refers her for cognitive-behavioral therapy, and arranges for a follow-up visit in 1 week.

      f. Withdrawal, sadness, and difficulty concentrating when separated from attachment figures
   2. **Onset:** often associated with **stressful life events**
  B. **Management**
    1. Parents should **praise and reinforce appropriate independent behavior** and avoid modeling anxiety.
    2. In school refusal, the immediate treatment goal is to **ensure that the child returns to school as soon as possible.** Each day away from school makes it more difficult to return.
      a. It is necessary to **identify** and **address factors** that contribute to the child's reluctance to go to school (e.g., bullying by a classmate).
      b. Psychological referral is recommended if the child does not return to school promptly.

V. **Tic Disorders: Tourette's Disorder**
  • Tourette's disorder is the **most severe tic disorder** and is characterized by several different types of motor tics and one or more vocal tics.
  A. **Epidemiology and etiology**
    1. **Prevalence** is low (< 1%).
    2. Precise etiology is unknown, but there is a strong genetic component.
  B. **Clinical presentation**
    1. **Key features**
      a. **Motor tics** (e.g., eye blinking, neck jerking, facial grimacing) typically precede **vocal tics** (e.g., throat clearing, grunting, sniffing).
      b. Vocal tics may include utterance of obscenities, a condition known as **coprolalia.**
    2. **Comorbid conditions:** ADHD, obsessive-compulsive disorder, and learning disorders.

> As many as 20% of children have tics at some time.

> Both motor and vocal tics occur in Tourette's disorder.

       3. Course: **fluctuating** with an **unpredictable prognosis**, although most affected patients show considerable improvement as adults.

   C. **Management**
       1. Patient **education**
       2. **Pharmacotherapy:** antipsychotic drugs
       3. **Supportive psychotherapy** for patients and families

VI. **Pervasive Developmental Disorders**
    • These **rare** disorders are characterized by **severe impairment** in several developmental areas.

   A. **Autistic disorder**
       1. **Epidemiology and etiology**
          a. **Onset:** before 3 years of age
          b. **Etiology:** strong **genetic** component
          c. **Associated conditions:** chromosomal abnormalities (e.g., fragile X syndrome), congenital infections (e.g., rubella)

       2. **Clinical presentation: key features**

> Autism is marked by significant deficits in social functioning and communication.

          a. **Impaired social interaction:** abnormal nonverbal behaviors (e.g., negative responses to cuddling in infants, lack of responsive smile and/or eye contact), lack of interest in others, inability to form peer relationships
          b. **Impaired communication:** delay in language development, absence of language, impaired use of language
          c. **Restricted and repetitive behaviors:** stereotypical movements, intense preoccupation with a particular area of interest, rigid adherence to routines
            • Some individuals with autism have extraordinary skills in a certain area (e.g., memory, music).

       3. **Associated features:** mental retardation, self-injurious behavior (e.g., headbanging, biting self), odd responses to sensory input (e.g., extreme sensitivity to touch or sound), hyperactivity, short attention span, impulsiveness, unusual eating or sleeping patterns, electroencephalographic abnormalities, seizures

       4. **Management**
          a. **Early identification** and **treatment** improves outcome, and development of language improves prognosis. Only a few individuals with autism can live independently as adults.
          b. **Treatment goals** include development of language and social and self-care skills and decreasing problem behaviors.
          c. **Treatment methods** include intensive **behavior modification** and **pharmacotherapy** to limit targeted symptoms such as self-injurious and aggressive behavior, hyperactivity, and repetitive behaviors.

B. Asperger's disorder
1. **Impairment in social abilities;** restricted interests and activities (somewhat **similar to autistic disorder)**
2. No significant delays in language and cognitive development

C. Rett's disorder
1. Occurs only in **girls**
2. Onset: **younger than 4 years of age,** after normal development
3. **Symptoms:** deceleration of head growth, stereotypical hand movements, loss of social interest, impaired language development

---

Rett's disorder occurs only in girls and begins by age 4.

VII. Mental Retardation
- Intellectual and adaptive functioning is significantly below average in individuals diagnosed with this disorder.
- Adaptive functioning is the degree to which individuals can effectively meet life demands appropriate to their age group and sociocultural background.

A. Epidemiology and etiology
1. **Prevalence:** approximately 1%
2. **Etiology:** often no specific cause can be identified, especially in cases of mild mental retardation.
   a. **Chromosomal abnormalities:** the two leading genetic causes of mental retardation are **Down syndrome** and **fragile X syndrome.**
   b. **Inherited metabolic conditions,** such as phenylketonuria (PKU) and **Tay-Sachs disease**
   c. **Prenatal factors,** such as maternal **use of alcohol and/or drugs** and **maternal rubella** and other infections
   d. **Perinatal factors,** such as prematurity and hypoxia
   e. **Acquired medical conditions,** such as trauma and poisoning
   f. **Environmental influences,** such as deprivation of stimulation

B. Clinical presentation
1. **Key features**
   a. Intelligence quotient **(IQ) approximately 70 or less**
   b. **Impaired adaptive functioning** in areas such as self-care, use of community resources, work, health, and safety
2. **Associated features: ADHD,** low self-esteem, stereotypical, repetitive movements (may be self-injurious)

Mental retardation: IQ ≤ 70 and significant deficits in adaptive functioning.

C. Degree of severity: most cases of mental retardation are mild (Table 22-2).

D. Management
- The severity of mental retardation and the existence of comorbid conditions influences the management approach.
1. Special **educational services** and **vocational training**

TABLE 22-2   Severity of Mental Retardation

Degree	Intelligence Quotient (IQ)	% of Total Cases	Need for Support
Mild	50–55 to ~ 70	85%	Intermittent*
Moderate	35–40 to 50–55	10%	Limited
Severe	20–25 to 35–40	3–4%	Extensive
Profound	< 20–25	1–2%	Constant

*In early years, affected children are often indistinguishable from those with normal intelligence.

2. **Behavioral therapy** aimed at increasing adaptive skills and reducing problem behaviors, such as aggression and self-injury
3. **Pharmacotherapy** for comorbid conditions (e.g., ADHD) and problem behaviors
4. **Supportive psychotherapy** for parents

VIII. Learning Disorders
A. **Epidemiology:** approximately 5% of students in public schools have a learning disorder.
B. **Etiology: genetic** predisposition, perinatal injury, and various medical conditions (e.g., fetal alcohol syndrome, lead poisoning) may play an etiologic role.
C. **Key feature:** performance on standardized achievement tests in reading, mathematics, or written expression that is substantially below expected levels for a child's IQ, age, and education
D. **Associated features:** low self-esteem, deficits in social skills, dropping out of school, difficulty in obtaining future employment
E. **Management**
   1. Treatment approaches include **remedial efforts** to improve specific skills, **compensatory strategies** to manage the skill deficits, and **psychotherapy** for associated emotional problems.
   2. Even with improvement, **some degree of impairment usually persists into adulthood.**

Medical Epidemiology

Target Topics

▶ Epidemiologic measurements
▶ Probability
▶ Risk
▶ Research study designs
▶ Sensitivity and specificity

I. Overview

A. **Epidemiology** is the study of **disease occurrence in populations** (groups).

B. Physicians apply epidemiologic knowledge to the **prevention, diagnosis,** and **treatment of disease in individuals.**

II. Epidemiologic Measurements

A. **Incidence** is the proportion of individuals initially free of a disorder who develop the disorder during a specific time period:

Incidence: new cases of a disease in a specific time period.

Incidence rate =

$$\frac{\text{Number of new cases of disorder}}{\text{Total number of individuals at risk for disorder}} \text{ per unit time}$$

Examples: During 12,000 person-years of observation, of 1200 individuals who were initially cancer-free, 30 were eventually diagnosed with cancer. One person-year of observation is equivalent to one person observed for 1 year. The **incidence rate** is 30 cases per 12,000 person-years × 1000 = 2.50 cases per 1000 person-years.

Of 15,000 children followed from birth to 7 years of age, 3000 were diagnosed with asthma. (The children were assumed to be asthma-free at birth.) The **cumulative incidence** for the 7-year period is 3000/15,000, or 20%.

Prevalence: all existing cases of a disease in a specific time period.

B. **Prevalence** is the proportion of a group with the disorder at a specific time (e.g., January 1, 2003) or during a specific time period (e.g., during the year 2003):

$$\text{Prevalence} = \frac{\text{Number of cases of disorder}}{\text{Total number of individuals at risk for disorder}}$$

Prevalence may be equivalent to incidence.

Example: Urine samples were collected from 30,000 randomly selected pregnant women prior to delivery and screened for toxins. Of these samples, 3000 women tested positive for alcohol. The prevalence of perinatal alcohol exposure is 3000 cases per 30,000 individuals, or 10%.

C. **Mortality rate** is the incidence of death in a group:

$$\text{Mortality rate} = \frac{\text{Total number of deaths}}{\text{Total number of individuals at risk for disorder}} \text{ per unit time}$$

1. **Crude mortality rate** refers to the total number of deaths in the population.
2. **Specific mortality rate** refers to the proportion of total deaths that occur in a subgroup of the population (e.g., among individuals in a specific age range, of a specific sex, or with a specific disorder).
3. **Adjusted mortality rate** adjusts or standardizes mortality rates to account for differences among groups in the distribution of specific characteristics, such as age, sex, or socioeconomic status.
   - **After adjustment** for a specific factor has been made, group **differences** in mortality rates **can no longer be attributed to that factor.**

Example: Crude mortality rates for the state of Florida (10.61 deaths per 1000 persons) are higher than for the state of Alaska (4.18 deaths per 1000 persons). Older individuals are more likely to die than younger individuals, and Florida has a greater proportion of older individuals than does Alaska. Is the difference in mortality rates between the two states a result of the higher proportion of older people in Florida when compared with Alaska? Or does an unknown factor cause the difference in mortality between these states?

Calculations show that, for each age group, **age-specific mortality rates** are similar between the states; therefore, individuals of the same age group die at the same rate in both states. In addition, the **age-adjusted mortality rates** for Florida (4.59 deaths per 1000 persons) and Alaska (4.42 deaths per 1000 persons) are similar. These similarities suggest that the older age of Florida's population, *not* some unknown factor that requires further investigation, accounts for the difference in crude mortality rates.

D. **Case fatality rate** is the proportion of individuals with a specific disorder who die of a particular disorder within a specific time period or during a given outbreak of the disorder.
    - This rate represents the **probability of death in diagnosed cases of the disorder.**

Example: The results of a study show that measles immunization decreases mortality among immunized patients who acquire the disease. Therefore, measles immunization decreases the measles **case fatality rate.**

E. **Some epidemiologic measurements are interrelated** (Figure 23-1).
    1. **Incidence and prevalence**
        a. In **acute conditions**, virtually every individual with the condition represents a new case; thus, **prevalence equals incidence.**
        b. In **chronic conditions**, new cases add to the number of existing cases; thus, **prevalence is greater than incidence.**
    2. **Case fatality rate and prevalence**
        a. An **increased case fatality rate** (i.e., a larger proportion of patients with a disorder dies) **decreases prevalence.**
        b. A **decreased case fatality rate without recovery** (i.e., patients live longer with the disorder) **increases prevalence.**

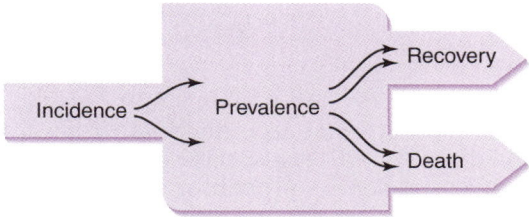

Figure 23-1   Diagram showing how incidence, recovery, and death affect prevalence.

III. Probability

- Probability *(p)* is a **measure of uncertainty or doubt.**
- The probability of an event is the **relative frequency of occurrence** (i.e., the number of times that the event does occur divided by the number of times that the event can occur).

A. Multiplication rule of probability

When combining probabilities, "and" = multiply.

1. The probability that **both** event A **and** event B occur **equals** the **probability of event A multiplied** by the **probability of event B.**
2. The probability that **neither** event A **nor** event B occurs **equals** the **probability** that event A does *not* occur **multiplied** by the **probability that event B does** *not* **occur.**
   - The probability that an event does *not* occur equals one minus the probability that it does occur $(1 - p)$.

B. Addition rule of probability

When combining probabilities, "or" = add.

1. **If event A and event B are mutually exclusive** (i.e., they cannot occur at the same time), the probability that either event A or event B occurs equals the sum of the probabilities of each event.
2. **If event A and event B can occur at the same time,** after adding the two individual probabilities, it is necessary to subtract the probability that the events both occur.

Example: Of 50 patients followed after a diagnosis of cancer, 10 patients survived for 5 years. Specific probabilities are calculated as follows:
Probability that patient A, a randomly selected patient, survived for 5 years:
$$10/50 = 0.20$$
Probability that patient A did *not* survive for 5 years:
$$1 - 0.20 = 0.80$$
Probability that *both* patient A *and* patient B survived for 5 years:
$$0.20 \times 0.20 = 0.04$$
Probability that *neither* patient A *nor* patient B survived for 5 years: probability that patient A did not survive multiplied by the probability that patient B did not survive, or
$$0.80 \times 0.80 = 0.64$$
Probability that *either* patient A *or* patient B survived for 5 years:
$$0.20 + 0.20 - 0.04 = 0.36$$

IV. Risk

- Risk is the probability that an individual without a disorder will acquire the disorder within a specific time period.
- Estimates of future disease probability in a specific patient (i.e., risk) are based on measurements of past disease frequency in a group of individuals similar to the patient (i.e., incidence).

Risk is based on past incidence and is an estimate of future probability.

BOX 23-1   Risk in a Cohort Study

Investigators study 2000 middle-aged women with no evidence of coronary heart disease (CHD) at study entry. Four hundred of the women are smokers. After 4 years of follow-up, 23 smokers and 77 nonsmokers develop CHD.

Risk Status	Develop CHD	Do Not Develop CHD	TOTALS
Exposed (smokers)	23	377	400
Unexposed (nonsmokers)	77	1523	1600
TOTALS	100	1900	2000

Exposed group
Risk = Incidence = 23/400, or 57.5 cases/1000 individuals

Unexposed group
Risk = Incidence = 77/1600, or 48.1 cases/1000 individuals

Relative risk
(risk ratio) = (incidence in exposed group)/(incidence in unexposed group)
= (57.5 cases/1000)/(48.1 cases/1000)
= 1.2
• Therefore, risk of CHD is 20% greater for the smokers than for the nonsmokers.

Attributable risk
(risk difference) = (incidence in exposed group) – (incidence in unexposed group)
= (57.5 cases/1000) – (48.1 cases/1000) = 9.4 cases/1000 or 3.8 cases/400

Attributable risk percent = (attributable risk)/(risk in exposed group) × 100%
= [(9.4 cases/1000)/(57.5 cases/1000)] × 100% = 16.3%
• Among the smokers, 3.8 of the 23 cases (16.3%) of CHD are attributable to smoking.

Population attributable risk = (incidence in population) – (incidence in unexposed group)
= (100 cases/2000) – (48.1 cases/1000)
= 1.9 cases/1000 or 3.8 cases/2000

Population attributable risk percent = [(population attributable risk)/(risk in population)] × 100%
= [(1.9 cases/1000)/(100 cases/2000)] × 100% = 3.8%
• In this population (cohort), 3.8 (3.8%) of the 100 cases of CHD are attributable to smoking.

   A. **Relative risk** (Box 23-1)
       • Relative risk is useful for **quantifying increased or decreased risk of a specific disorder** in a patient exposed to a certain factor.
     1. **Relative risk** (or **risk ratio**) is the ratio of the incidence

Relative risk indicates the strength of a risk factor.

of a disorder in two groups: **one exposed** to a certain factor (e.g., low-density lipoprotein cholesterol, LDL-C) and **one** *not* exposed to the factor.

2. If exposure to the factor increases risk, the exposed group is at greater risk than the unexposed group, yielding a risk ratio greater than 1.0. In this case, the factor is a **risk factor.**

> **Example:** The relative risk of coronary heart disease (CHD) among healthy, middle-aged adults with high levels of LDL-C is about 1.4. In these individuals, a high LDL-C level is a risk factor for CHD because it increases the risk of CHD; in this case, the risk is increased by about 40%.

3. If exposure to the factor decreases risk, the exposed group is at less risk than the unexposed group, yielding a risk ratio of less than 1.0. In this situation, the factor is a **protective factor.**

> **Example:** The relative risk of CHD among healthy, middle-aged adults with high levels of high-density lipoprotein cholesterol (HDL-C) is about 0.5. In these individuals, high HDL-C level is a protective factor for CHD because it decreases the risk of CHD by about 50%.

4. The **magnitude of a relative risk** indicates the **strength of a risk or protective factor.**
   a. **Larger relative risks** signify **stronger risk factors.**
   b. **Smaller relative risks** (i.e., closer to 0 than to 1.0) signify **stronger protective factors.**

> **Example:** High LDL-C is a stronger risk factor for CHD than is cigarette smoking. High LDL-C increases the risk of CHD by about 40% (relative risk = 1.4), whereas cigarette smoking increases the risk of CHD only by about 20% (relative risk = 1.2).

B. **Attributable risk** (see Box 23-1)

1. **Attributable risk** (or **risk difference**) is the difference in the risk of a disorder between a group exposed to a certain factor and a group *not* exposed to that factor.
   a. It is the **risk in the exposed group** that is **attributable to the risk factor.**
   b. It represents the **amount** that the risk would be **reduced in the exposed group if** the **risk factor were eliminated.**

2. **Attributable risk percent** is the attributable risk expressed as a percentage of the risk in the exposed group.

Attributable risk indicates the proportion of cases that can be prevented.

BOX 23-2   **Odds Ratio in a Case-Control Study**

Investigators study 100 adult women with coronary heart disease (CHD) (cases) and 100 adult women with no evidence of CHD (controls). The studies show that 75 of the cases and 10 of the controls are smokers.

	Cases	Controls
Exposed (smokers)	75	10
Unexposed (nonsmokers)	25	90
TOTALS	100	100

Odds that case is a smoker = 75/25 = 3/1
Odds that control is a smoker = 10/90 = 1/9

Odds ratio
Odds that case is a smoker/odds that control is a smoker = (3/1)/(1/9) = 27
Therefore, the odds that the cases are smokers, compared with the controls being smokers, are 27 to 1.

    C. **Population attributable risk** (see Box 23-1)
        1. **Population attributable risk** is the difference in risk between the entire population (i.e., exposed + unexposed) and a group *not* exposed to a certain factor.
            a. It is the risk **in the entire population** that is **attributable to the risk factor.**
            b. It represents the amount that the risk would be reduced in the entire population if the risk factor were eliminated.
        2. **Population attributable risk percent** is the population attributable risk expressed as a percentage of the risk in the population.
    D. **Odds ratio** (Box 23-2)
        1. The odds ratio is **used to estimate** the **risk ratio when risk cannot be calculated directly** (e.g., in a case-control study).
        2. If the incidence of a disorder is low (< 5%), the odds ratio is a good estimate of the risk ratio.

V. **Research Studies**
    A. **General design**
        1. **Experimental studies** deliberately control the exposure of participants to the factor of interest, usually a treatment, and include **clinical trials.**
        2. **Observational studies** detect differences between groups that are "naturally" exposed or unexposed to the factor in question, usually a risk factor or a prognostic factor, and include **cohort, case-control,** and **cross-sectional studies.**
    B. **Specific types**
        1. **Randomized controlled trials** (RCTs)
            a. **RCTs randomly allocate participants** who have the

disorder under investigation to either one of two groups:

(1) Experimental group receives the experimental intervention.

(2) Control group receives a **placebo** or usual treatment.

b. After following the participants to determine if the experimental group improves more than the control group, RCTs may **report results in the following terms:**

(1) Relative risk reduction (i.e., 1 – relative risk)

(2) Number needed to treat (i.e., number of patients needed to treat to achieve the observed effect in one patient)

c. Other terms used to report results of RCTs

(1) Efficacy (effect among those who actually receive the intervention and complete the protocol)

(2) Effectiveness (effect among all those originally assigned to receive the intervention regardless of whether they actually receive it or complete the protocol)

2. Cohort studies

Cohort studies group individuals according to exposure status and follow them to determine outcome incidence.

a. Cohort studies begin with a **group of individuals,** known as a **cohort,** who do *not* have the disorder under investigation (e.g., lung cancer), and classify them regarding their exposure (or lack of exposure) to the risk factor of interest (e.g., smoking).

b. After following cohort members to determine which members develop the disorder under investigation, cohort studies **compute relative risks** that compare incidence rates in the exposed group to incidence rates in the unexposed group.

3. Case-control studies

Case-control studies group individuals by outcome status and determine their exposure frequency by examining their history.

a. Case-control studies begin with a group of individuals **(cases)** who have the disorder under investigation and a comparison group **(controls)** who do *not* have the disorder.

b. After investigating the history of both groups to determine which participants had been exposed to the risk factor(s) of interest, case-control studies **compute odds ratios** that compare exposure frequency in cases to exposure frequency in controls.

4. Cross-sectional studies

a. Cross-sectional studies determine exposure and disorder status at **one specific point** in time, usually the present, to provide a "snapshot" in time.

b. These studies can be used to **survey prevalence** or to **identify associations** between potential **risk factors** and **disorders.**

5. Ecologic studies

a. Ecologic studies **compare average exposures and**

outcomes of groups rather than individuals (e.g., countries with higher average per capita wine consumption have lower average national cardiac mortality risk).

  b. Ecologic studies are useful for generating hypotheses to be tested in subsequent studies.

6. **Meta-analyses**

  a. Meta-analyses are **systematic overviews** that use explicitly stated methods to summarize the results of previous primary studies.

  - These studies can resolve uncertainty when the primary studies do not agree.

  b. **High-quality meta-analyses** can provide very strong evidence supporting the existence of an **association between exposure and outcome.**

  c. The **systematic method** involves:

  (1) Use of **explicit criteria** to decide which primary studies to include in the overview

  (2) **Comprehensive search** for primary studies that meet eligibility criteria

  (3) **Assessment of methodologic quality** of each eligible primary study

  (4) **Synthesis of primary study results** into one, appropriately weighted, summary result

C. Issues in study design

  - An investigator who shows that bias, chance, and confounding are not plausible explanations for an association between an exposure and an outcome may conclude that causation is the most convincing explanation for the association.

  - An association is **more likely to be causal** if it is **strong, consistent, and biologically plausible** and also shows the **correct temporal relationship.**

1. **Bias** is **systematic error,** which may occur at different stages of the research process.

  a. **Sampling bias** occurs when the individuals in a study (i.e., the sample) are *not* representative of the population being studied.

Bias is systematic error.

> **Example:** In a study purporting to examine memory function in patients with Alzheimer's disease, investigators include only institutionalized patients in the sample, thereby systematically excluding patients with better memory function (i.e., noninstitutionalized patients).

  b. **Selection bias** occurs when groups differ in ways other than the factor of interest.

> **Example:** In a study of the effects of exercise on obesity, investigators find that some of the obese

patients recruited to participate in the study do not want to participate in an exercise program. These patients are assigned to the nonexercise control group so that they do not leave the study. Thus, patients in the control group differ from patients in the exercise group in their willingness to exercise, which may reflect a difference in motivation to lose weight or some other factor that produces differential results.

c. **Measurement bias** occurs when either the exposure or the outcome is measured differently in different groups.

> **Example:** In a case-control study of analgesics as risk factors for end-stage renal disease, investigators question patients who have the disease (i.e., cases) more closely than those who do not have the disease (i.e., controls) about their use of acetaminophen and nonsteroidal anti-inflammatory drugs. The more intense questioning may elicit more analgesic use in the cases compared with the controls. In other words, the observed difference in exposure may result from differences in questioning techniques rather than a true difference in history of analgesic use.

2. **Confounding** occurs when an **extraneous factor** confuses, or confounds, understanding of the relationship between exposure and outcome.

> **Example:** Coffee drinkers are more likely than non–coffee drinkers to develop lung cancer, but *not* because ingestion of coffee causes lung cancer. Rather, coffee drinkers are more likely to smoke cigarettes, and smoking cigarettes causes cancer. In this example, **smoking is a confounding variable.**

3. **Methods for reducing bias and confounding**
   a. **Random sampling** of participants attempts to ensure that the sample is representative of the population of interest. This procedure **reduces sampling bias.**
   b. **Random allocation** of participants to groups attempts to ensure that the groups differ only in exposure to the experimental condition. This procedure **reduces selection bias and confounding.**
   c. **Matching** each participant in the exposed group with at least one comparison group participant with similar characteristics, except for the factor in question, helps ensure that the groups do not differ

on any of the matched characteristics, such as sex and age. This procedure **reduces selection bias and confounding.**

    d. **Masking** group allocation (synonymous with **blinding**) from participants and experimenters helps ensure that the actions of participants and experimenters are not affected by knowledge of group assignment.

        (1) This procedure **reduces measurement bias.**

        (2) Many RCTs give the control group a **placebo** to mask group assignment.

VI. Characteristics of Useful Medical Tests

  A. **Reliability** (or precision or reproducibility) is the extent to which the results of repeated measurements of a stable phenomenon are similar.

    1. Reliability is usually determined by **comparing repeated measurements of the same phenomenon.**

    2. A reliable measurement may or may not be valid, but an **unreliable measurement cannot be valid.**

> A reliable measure is reproducible and precise.

  B. **Validity** (or accuracy) is the extent to which a measurement or test **measures what it is intended to measure.**

    1. Validity of a new measure can be determined by **comparing results** using the new measure with results **using an established measure.**

    2. To be valid, a **measure must be reliable.**

> A valid measure or test is accurate and measures what it is intended to measure.

  C. **Sensitivity** is the ability of a test to correctly identify individuals who have a specific disorder (Box 23-3).

    1. The sensitivity of a test is the **proportion** of individuals with the disorder **who test positive.**

    2. A **sensitive (Sn) test** is **most useful** when it is **negative.**

    3. A **sensitive test** should be used when it is important to **minimize false-negative test results** (e.g., to avoid a missed diagnosis).

> A negative result on a sensitive test rules "out" disease (SnOUT).

  D. **Specificity** is the ability of a test to correctly identify individuals who do *not* have a specific disorder (see Box 23-3).

    1. The specificity of a test is the **proportion** of individuals without the disorder **who test negative.**

    2. A **specific (Sp) test** is **most useful** when it is **positive.**

    3. A **highly specific test** should be used when it is important to **minimize false-positive test results** (e.g., to avoid treating or testing people unnecessarily).

> A positive result on a specific test rules "in" disease (SpIN).

  E. **Accuracy** of a test is the **proportion of test results that are correct** (i.e., true) (see Box 23-3).

  F. **Predictive value of a test** (see Box 23-3)

    1. The predictive **value of a positive test** is the probability that a patient who tests positive has the disorder in question.

    2. The predictive **value of a negative test** is the probability that a patient who tests negative does *not* have the disorder in question.

    3. The predictive value of a test depends on the **prevalence**

> The predictive value of a test is the probability that a test result is correct.

BOX 23-3	Sensitivity, Specificity, Accuracy, and Predictive Value

As part of a program to determine whether a newly developed diagnostic test for diabetes mellitus can correctly identify patients with and without diabetes, investigators use the test on 100 patients; 50 have diabetes and 50 do not have diabetes. The investigators obtain the following results:

- 45 of 50 patients with diabetes test positive for the disease (**true-positive** result, or TP)
- 5 of 50 patients with diabetes test negative (**false-negative** result, or FN)
- 40 of 50 patients without diabetes test negative for the disease (**true-negative** result, or TN)
- 10 of 50 patients without diabetes test positive (**false-positive** result, or FP)

Disorder Status

Test Result	Negative	Positive	TOTALS
Positive	45 (TP)	10 (FP)	55
Negative	5 (FN)	40 (TN)	45
TOTALS	50	50	100

Sensitivity = TP/total number of patients with the disorder = 45/50 = 0.90
- The test correctly identifies 90% of patients with diabetes.
- The test misclassifies 10% of patients with diabetes, who may not receive the necessary treatment.

Specificity = TN/total number of patients without the disorder = 40/50 = 0.80
- The test correctly identifies 80% of patients without diabetes.
- The test misclassifies 20% of patients without diabetes, who may undergo unnecessary tests and procedures.

- Knowledge of sensitivity and specificity is most useful in deciding whether to use a certain test in a specific clinical context.

Accuracy = (TP + TN)/total number of patients tested = (45 + 40)/100 = 0.85

Positive predictive value = TP/total number of positive tests = 45/55 = 0.82

Negative predictive value = TN/total number of negative tests = 40/45 = 0.89

- Knowledge of predictive values is most useful in estimating the probability that a particular test result is accurate. Physicians are able to use this information to help decide whether to rely on a particular result.

---

of the disorder in a group with characteristics similar to those of the patient.

  a. **Positive test results** are more likely to be correct in a group with higher prevalence of the disorder.

  Example: A positive breast self-examination, in which a patient detects a lump in her breast, is

> more likely to be correct in an older woman than in a younger woman, because the older woman is a member of a group with a higher prevalence of breast cancer.

    b. **Negative test results** are more likely to be correct in a group with a lower prevalence of the disorder.

> **Example:** A negative breast self-examination is more likely to be correct in a younger woman than in an older woman, because the younger woman is a member of a group with a lower prevalence of breast cancer.

VII. Levels of Prevention

A. **Primary prevention procedures**, such as immunizations, counseling to adopt healthy lifestyles, and chlorination and fluoridation of the water supply, are aimed at preventing disease in healthy individuals.

B. **Secondary prevention procedures**, such as most screening tests, are aimed at preventing symptomatic disease in asymptomatic individuals (i.e., people with a disease in its early stages).

C. **Tertiary prevention procedures**, such as physical rehabilitation and the use of a beta-blocker to reduce mortality in patients with acute myocardial infarction, are aimed at preventing further complications or reoccurrence in patients with clinically evident disease.

Biostatistics

Target Topics

▷ Frequency distributions
▷ Hypothesis testing and probability values
▷ Interval estimation and confidence intervals
▷ Specific statistical tests

I. Frequency Distributions

- Frequency distributions represent the **frequency of occurrence** of all values of a variable in a data set.
- These distributions are used to determine the **probability of occurrence** of a specific data value or range of values.

A. Characteristics of a frequency distribution

1. **Central tendency**
   - **Mean, median,** and **mode** are measures of central tendency that describe typical data in different ways.
   a. The **mean** (or average) is the geometric center of the distribution.
      - The mean is the **sum of all data values divided by the number of data values**.
   b. The **median** is the **middle data value** (i.e., 50th percentile).
      - The median is the value below which, and above which, half of all data values occur.
   c. The **mode** is the **most frequently occurring data value.**

2. **Dispersion** (or **variability**)
   - **Standard deviation (SD)** and **standard error (SE)** are measures of dispersion around the central tendency that describes the spread of data values.
   a. The **SD** represents the average distance of all data values from the mean.

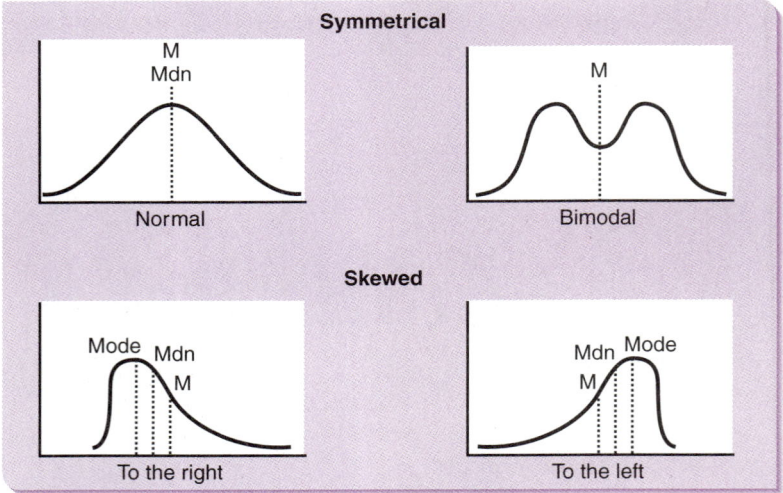

Figure 24-1 Frequency of various types of distributions, with the relative positions of the mean (M) and the median (Mdn). When the shape is skewed to the right, the tail of the curve points to the right; when the shape is skewed to the left, the tail of the curve points to the left.

- A **larger SD** indicates that the data values are dispersed more widely about the mean.
  b. The **SE** estimates the **magnitude of error** in the sample statistic.
    (1) A **larger SE** indicates that the range within which the population statistic lies (i.e., **confidence interval**) is wider.
    (2) **As sample size increases, SE decreases.**
3. **Shape**
  - Different frequency distributions have different shapes (Figure 24-1).
  a. In a **symmetrical distribution**, one side of the distribution is the mirror image of the other.
    - The **mean and median are equal.**
  b. In a **skewed distribution**, the peak (mode) of the distribution is closer to one side.
    - The **mean and median are *not* equal.**
    (1) If the **mean is greater than the median**, the distribution is **skewed** to the **right (positive).**
    (2) If the **mean is less than the median**, the distribution is **skewed** to the **left (negative).**
B. **Normal distribution** (also known as a **gaussian** or **bell-shaped distribution**) (Figure 24-2)
  1. A normal distribution is a **theoretical distribution** (i.e., defined by an equation rather than by data) in which the **mean, median, and mode are equal.**
  2. In a normal distribution, approximately 68% of data values fall within ± one SD of the mean, **approximately 95% of data values fall within ± two SDs of the**

A normal distribution is symmetrical and has the same mean, median, and mode.

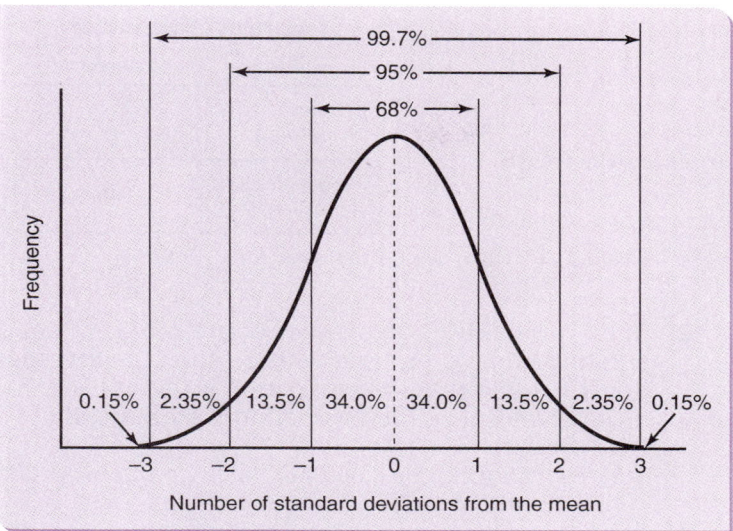

Figure 24-2   Normal distribution, showing the area under the curve for ±1, ±2, and ±3 deviations from the mean.

mean, and 99.7% of data values fall within ± three SDs of the mean.

3. One method for determining the **normal limits** of a measurement is to consider that **95%** of individuals who fall **within the mean ± two SDs are normal.**

> **Example:** To determine whether long-term intense conditioning in elite athletes produces abnormal cardiac dimensions, investigators compared cardiac dimensions in the athletes with the normal limits of these dimensions, as defined by the mean ± two SDs in a large group of healthy adults.

Normal limits can be considered as the mean ± two SDs, which includes 95% of individuals.

II. **Hypothesis Testing**
   - The goal of hypothesis testing is to determine whether the association between exposure to the supposed risk factor, cause, or intervention and clinical outcome is too large to be explained by random variation (i.e., chance), which would make it statistically significant.
   A. **Logic of hypothesis testing**
      1. The **null hypothesis (H_0)** states that there is **no association** between the exposure and outcome of interest.
         a. The null hypothesis is a "**straw horse**" set up to be **discredited** or **nullified** by the **data** obtained from the study.
         b. **To reject the null hypothesis** (i.e., to reject "no association") is to **conclude** that **there is an association.**

Hypothesis test result		True status of association: Present	True status of association: Absent
	Significant	Correct (1-β) (power)	Type I error (α) (false-positive)
	Not significant	Type II error (β) (false-negative)	Correct

Figure 24-3 Two types of error in hypothesis testing.

A statistically significant result is unlikely to occur as the result of chance.

2. If the **probability** (*p*) of an association is less than a preestablished level (α; usually 0.05), then the investigator concludes that the association is too unlikely to result from chance (i.e., the association is **statistically significant).**
   - The *p* value can be calculated using an appropriate statistical procedure.
3. If an association is statistically significant (i.e., does *not* occur on the basis of chance), and if bias and confounding are *not* viable explanations for the association, then the association may reflect a **causal relationship between exposure and outcome.**

> **Example:** In a study relating patient characteristics to serum creatine levels in patients recovering from myocardial infarction, investigators tested the **null hypothesis** that serum creatine levels are equal in men and women. They found that mean (±SD) serum creatine levels are 1.13 mg/dL (±0.16) in men and 0.92 mg/dL (±0.13) in women ($p < 0.05$). Because *p* is less than 0.05, the investigators rejected the null hypothesis and concluded that serum creatine levels in men are significantly different from those in women.

B. Types of error in hypothesis testing (Figure 24-3)

1. **Type I error (α),** which is usually set at **0.05,** is the probability of concluding incorrectly that the association found in the study is statistically significant (i.e., of rejecting a true null hypothesis).

> **Example:** The interpretation of the previously described study of serum creatine levels after a myocardial infarction could be incorrect. The probability of the occurrence of a **type I error** (i.e., outcome is the result of chance rather than an actual difference between men and women) is α (0.05 or 5%).

2. **Type II error (β)** is the probability of concluding incorrectly that the association found in the study is *not* statis-

ically significant (i.e., of *not* rejecting a false null hypothesis).

> **Example:** In the previously described study of serum creatine levels after a myocardial infarction, if *p* had been greater than 0.05, the investigators would have retained the null hypothesis (i.e., decided that the serum creatine difference between men and women was small enough to have occurred by chance), thus concluding that the study result is *not* statistically significant. The probability of the occurrence of a **type II error** (i.e., outcome is *not* the result of chance but it is statistically significant) is β.

3. **Statistical power** $(1 - \beta)$ is the probability of concluding correctly that the association found in the study is statistically significant (i.e., of rejecting a false null hypothesis).
   - **As sample size increases, statistical power also increases.**

> **Example:** In a randomized, double-blind, placebo-controlled primary prevention trial of 29,133 male smokers, investigators examined whether dietary supplementation with vitamin E reduced the risk of lung cancer. After 5–8 years of follow-up, investigators found no significant difference in the incidence of lung cancer between men who received vitamin E and men who received a placebo.
>
> Did the study fail to find an association because (1) there is no association to be found, or (2) there is an association, but this study lacked the power to find it? The well-designed and well-executed study had an extremely large sample size. Thus, investigators could argue convincingly that the study had sufficient statistical power and would have found the association had there been one.

C. **Clinical significance or meaningfulness**
   1. Although an association between an exposure and a clinical outcome may be statistically significant, it may *not* be clinically meaningful.
   2. Decisions about clinical meaningfulness are based on clinical judgment, *not* on statistical analyses.

> Clinical judgment may determine that a statistically significant association is *not* clinically meaningful.

III. **Interval Estimation**
   - The goal of interval estimation is to show that the interval, or range, within which a statistic is most likely to be located does *not* include the value that would indicate "no difference."
A. **Logic of interval estimation** (Box 24-1)
   1. A statistic computed from a sample is the best estimate of

---

BOX 24-1 | **Interpretation of Confidence Intervals (CIs)**

In a study of the association between analgesic use and risk of Alzheimer's disease, investigators followed a cohort of 1686 participants from 1980 to 1995. About 80% of the participants were followed for 5 or more years.

The relative risk of Alzheimer's disease associated with reported use of nonsteroidal anti-inflammatory drugs (NSAIDs) is 0.50 (95% CI: 0.30–0.85). Although this result indicates that the best point estimate of relative risk of Alzheimer's disease in NSAID users is 0.50, the CI suggests that the real relative risk may be as low as 0.30 or as high as 0.85. If risk in users were equal to risk in nonusers, the ratio of the two risks (i.e., the relative risk) would equal 1.0. Because the CI does *not* include 1.0, the possibility that the risk in NSAID users equals the risk in NSAID nonusers can be excluded with 95% confidence. The result supports the hypothesis that NSAID use is associated with decreased risk for Alzheimer's disease.

The relative risk of Alzheimer's disease with reported use of aspirin is 0.81 (95% CI: 0.52–1.28). Although this result indicates that the best point estimate of relative risk of Alzheimer's disease in aspirin users is 0.81, the CI suggests that the real relative risk may be as low as 0.52 or as high as 1.28. Because the CI includes 1.0, the possibility that the risk in aspirin users equals the risk in aspirin nonusers cannot be excluded with 95% confidence. Therefore, this result does *not* support the hypothesis that aspirin use is associated with decreased risk of Alzheimer's disease.

> It may be concluded with 95% confidence that the true value of a statistic falls within the 95% CI.

> Wide CIs reflect imprecise measurements.

that statistic in the target population, but the **sample statistic is likely to contain some error.**

2. The **95% confidence interval (CI) quantifies this error** by indicating an interval surrounding the sample statistic that has a 95% probability of containing the population statistic.

3. If the 95% CI does *not* include the value that indicates "no association," then it can be concluded with 95% confidence that there is an association between exposure and outcome and that it did *not* occur by chance.

4. If the 95% CI includes the value that would indicate "no association," then it cannot be concluded with 95% confidence that there is an association between exposure and outcome.

B. The **width of CIs varies directly with the precision of the measurement** (i.e., more precise measurements result in narrower CIs).

IV. Specific Statistical Tests

- Tests of statistical significance compute the probability of the observed association, assuming that the observed association is determined by chance.
- If this probability is small (i.e., < 5%), the result is considered statistically significant.

A. The **chi-square (χ^2) test** determines whether proportions obtained in a study are different from proportions expected by chance.

B. **Analysis of variance and the *t*-test** determine whether differences between sample means are greater than would be expected by chance.
  1. The *t*-test compares differences between means from two groups.
  2. **Analysis of variance** compares differences among means from more than two groups.
C. **Correlation analysis** yields a **correlation coefficient (*r*)**, which quantifies the strength and direction of an association between two variables.
  1. The **magnitude of *r*** can vary from 0 to ±1.0, with larger absolute values indicating greater strength of association.
  2. The **sign of *r*** indicates the direction of the association between the two variables: a **positive coefficient** indicates a **direct relationship**, and a **negative coefficient** indicates an **inverse relationship.**
  3. **Correlation** indicates **magnitude of association,** *not* causation.

> **Example:** A study of 700 patients with obstructive sleep apnea syndrome found a significant correlation between number of apneic episodes per hour of sleep and body mass index ($r = 0.35$, $p < 0.001$).
>
> The correlation coefficient *r* indicates a statistical association between body mass and respiratory disturbance during sleep (i.e., as body mass increases, frequency of respiratory disturbance during sleep also increases). The correlation does *not* prove that greater body mass causes respiratory disturbance during sleep, or vice versa.

D. **Multivariate analysis** shows the relationship between a set of predictor or exposure variables (e.g., hypertension, smoking, lipid levels) and a clinical outcome variable (e.g., coronary heart disease).

> Multivariate analysis adjusts for, or controls the influence of, confounding variables.

  1. **Different types of data require different multivariate procedures.**
    a. **Multiple regression analysis** is used when the outcome variable is **quantitative** (e.g., blood pressure in mm Hg, lipid levels in mg/dL).
    b. **Logistic regression analysis** is used when the outcome variable is **categorical** (e.g., dead or alive, does or does not have a disease).
    c. **Survival analysis** is used when the outcome variable is **time** (e.g., survival time in months).
  2. Despite procedural differences, **all multivariate approaches answer the same two questions:**
    a. What is the association between a predictor variable and the outcome variable after adjusting for the other predictor variables?

b. What is the total association between the set of predictor variables and the outcome variable?

Example: The **Framingham Heart Study** used multivariate analysis to answer these two questions. This study showed that smoking, serum lipid levels, and hypertension (predictors) were independent risk factors for coronary heart disease (CHD) occurrence (outcome). Each factor predicted future occurrence of CHD independently of the other two factors (e.g., associations between smoking and CHD and between serum lipid levels and CHD did *not* account for the association between hypertension and CHD risk). All three predictors together explained less than 50% of the new cases of CHD.

Medical Practice and the Health Care System

25

Ethical and Legal Issues in Medicine

Target Topics

▶ Medical ethics
▶ Jurisprudence
▶ Professional behavior

I. Overview
- Ethics is a system of moral principles holding physicians to certain rules of conduct.
- Medical licensing boards and medical societies formulate codes of professional conduct.

II. Fundamentals of Ethics in the Physician-Patient Relationship
A. Beneficence: physicians should act in the best interest of their patients.
B. Nonmaleficence: physicians should "**do no harm.**"
C. Patient autonomy: patients have a right to make decisions about their own medical care.
   1. Self-determination means that **patients can refuse treatment**, even if lack of treatment may lead to a negative outcome.
   2. This right may **conflict with the physician's desire** to act in the best interest of his or her patients.

D. Honesty: the physician should tell the patient the truth about the patient's medical condition.
1. This act is a fundamental aspect of **building trust** in the physician-patient relationship (see Chapter 1).
2. When a physician believes that the truth about a patient's diagnosis or medical care may harm the patient, the **physician** is still **ethically responsible** for conveying such information to the patient.
3. The physician may wait briefly to inform the patient until concerns about harm to the patient have subsided or an appropriate method for the delivery of such information is determined.

III. Competence
A. Competence to make decisions about one's health care requires that the individual understand the **benefits and risks of care, treatment alternatives**, and **consequences of lack of treatment.**
B. Determining competence
1. Competence is determined by the **court.**
2. **Physician-conducted assessments** may help the court to determine if a patient is competent or incompetent.
3. A patient may be found **competent in one area** (e.g., medical treatment) but **not competent in another** (e.g., decisions about finances).
C. Who is competent?
1. Individuals **18 years of age and older**
2. **Emancipated minors:** individuals **younger than 18** years of age who satisfy one or more of the following criteria:
   a. **Live independently** and are **self-supporting**
   b. Are **married**
   c. Have **served** or are **currently serving in the military**
   d. **Have dependent children**

IV. Informed Consent
• Informed consent refers to the process by which patients give their consent for medical procedures.
A. Requirements for informed consent
1. **Patients must be given information** about their **diagnosis, recommended treatment, risks** and **benefits** of treatment, treatment **alternatives**, and the likely **outcome without treatment.**
2. Patients should make a choice in the **absence of coercion** and **undue influence.**
3. Patients must be **competent.**
   a. **Minors** require the **consent** of their **parent** or **legal guardian** for medical care.
   b. In many states, **minors may give informed consent for certain types of care**, such as prenatal visits, treatment for substance abuse or sexually transmitted diseases, and contraception.

TABLE 25-1 Examples of Informed Consent and Confidentiality: Physician's Response to Clinical Situations

Situation	Physician's Response
The parents of a minor child who has a life-threatening medical emergency cannot be located.	Provide emergency care.
The parents of a 5-year-old girl refuse, on religious grounds, to give permission for their daughter to receive chemotherapy for a type of cancer that has a 95% survival rate with treatment.	Seek court assistance to obtain consent for the child to undergo chemotherapy.
A 55-year-old man is injured in a motor vehicle accident and is unconscious and in need of surgery to repair a ruptured spleen.	If next-of-kin is available, discuss care options. If kin is not available and there is no reason to assume that the patient does not want medical care, provide emergency surgery.
The parents of a 19-year-old man contact their son's physician, asking to be given information about the results of their son's recent HIV test. Their son does not authorize the release of this information to his parents.	Do not release the test results to the parents.
A 14-year-old girl admits that she is being sexually abused by her uncle. Her mother asks that this information not be disclosed to social services.	Report suspicions of child abuse to the appropriate state protective agency.

4. **Psychiatric illness** does *not* mean that an individual cannot make an informed decision or be competent; however, psychiatric illness (e.g., delusions) **may compromise and interfere with the individual's decision-making capacity.**

B. **Exceptions to obtaining informed consent** (Table 25-1)
   1. **Therapeutic privilege:** the physician, believing that telling a patient about treatment might have a harmful effect, can decide to forgo obtaining informed consent.
   2. **Implied consent:** permission to treat is assumed in **medical emergencies** in which a patient cannot give consent (e.g., a patient is in a coma). This type of consent is based on the idea that reasonable individuals would wish to receive care in an emergency.
   3. **Patient is a minor**
      a. **Emergency medical care** can be given if attempts to contact a parent or legal guardian are unsuccessful and delaying treatment could endanger the patient's life or health.
      b. When parents refuse treatment for their child for a life-threatening condition (e.g., parents who are Jehovah's Witnesses refuse to give permission for a blood transfusion for their child based on religious grounds), a request can be made for **court-authorized treatment.**
      c. When parents refuse medical care for their child,

notification of child protective agencies is sometimes indicated.

4. **Waiver of consent:** a patient has relinquished his or her right to be further informed.

V. **Confidentiality**
   A. **Communications between physicians and patients** are **privileged** and **confidential.**
   B. **Physicians** (as well as those working with physicians, such as nurses) **cannot release information** about a patient's care **without** the express **consent of the patient.**
   C. **Exceptions to confidentiality** (see Table 25-1)
      1. **Intent to harm or kill another individual;** threat is credible
         • The **Tarasoff decision** led to statutes requiring that physicians have a **duty to warn** intended victims about a patient's threat and a **duty to protect** these victims. This may necessitate arranging voluntary or involuntary hospitalization of a patient.
      2. **Imminent danger of suicide**
         a. To **protect** a patient **from self-harm,** the physician may contact the patient's family, friends, and/or the police.
         b. **Involuntary psychiatric hospitalization** may be necessary.
      3. **Inability to provide basic self-care** or to protect from self-harm
      4. **Suspected child or elder abuse**
         a. In all states, physicians are mandated by law to report **suspected child abuse** to the appropriate social service agency.
         b. Most states also mandate reporting of suspected elder abuse.
         c. It is not necessary to confirm abuse to submit a report (see Chapter 21).
      5. **Court order**
         a. A physician may receive a **subpoena,** which orders the physician to appear in court and/or produce medical records.
         b. If the contents of the medical record are a concern, the physician may ask the judge to consider the issue.
      6. **Reportable diseases**
         a. States require that physicians report specific illnesses to the state health department, including **AIDS** and **syphilis.**
         b. Some states may also require or permit **physicians** to **breach confidentiality** in specific circumstances, such as notifying:
            (1) The **division of motor vehicles** about a patient with a seizure disorder who drives a motor vehicle

Significant risk of suicide is a reason to suspend confidentiality.

Physicians are required by law to report suspected child abuse.

(2) The **partner of an HIV-positive patient** when the patient is putting the partner at significant risk of HIV infection.

VI. **Involuntary and Voluntary Psychiatric Hospitalization**
   A. Patients in **inpatient psychiatric facilities** who have entered voluntarily or involuntarily have the **right to receive treatment.**
   B. **Involuntary psychiatric hospitalization** is necessary for:
      1. Patients who are deemed to be an **imminent threat to their own safety** or the **safety of others** and who **refuse voluntary admission**
      2. Patients who are **unable to care for their basic needs** because of mental illness
   C. **Involuntary admission procedures may vary** from state to state but generally involve a court request for detention.
   D. **Patient evaluation** must occur within a short period (e.g., often 72 hours), at which time a determination is usually made either to release or to retain the patient for treatment.
      1. Patients hospitalized involuntarily have the **right to refuse treatment.**
      2. **Exceptions** include:
         a. When a **court order for commitment** is accompanied by a **court order to treat**
         b. When **emergency treatment** is deemed necessary to **protect** the patient or others **from harm**

VII. **Advance Directives**
   A. Advance directives are means by which **competent individuals** express their **wishes for** their **future health care** in the event that they no longer can make such decisions for themselves.
      1. To make an advance directive, individuals must have **decision-making capacity** and must be able to:
         a. **Understand** the medical problem and its significance
         b. Rationally **evaluate** treatment options
         c. **Communicate** choices
      2. **Types of advance directives**
         a. **Living will:** document that gives instructions about the medical care a patient wants at the end of life
         b. **Health care proxy** (durable power of attorney for health care): an individual appointed by a patient to make medical decisions for the patient if the patient is unable to do so.

         A health care proxy should make decisions based on the patient's wishes, *not* those of the proxy or the physician.

      3. **Laws** regulating the contents and use of advance directives **vary by state.** Facilities funded by Medicare or Medicaid are required to provide written information to patients about state laws regarding their right to accept or refuse treatment and to create advance directives.
   B. **Surrogate decision-making laws**
      1. This system allows **relatives,** and **sometimes close**

BOX 25-1	A Solution to Practicing Within the Scope of Professional Boundaries

A young mother with three small children is seen by a physician in a clinic. She tells the physician that she has no transportation or food and asks him if he can spare $15 so that she can buy food for an evening meal for her family. The physician shows concern for her circumstances. Realizing that it is inappropriate to offer the patient cash, he introduces her to the clinic social worker, who arranges a taxi voucher to a community food pantry and helps the patient fill out the application for additional financial assistance.

BOX 25-2	A Physician's Response to an Unethical Patient Request

A 24-year-old woman comes to the physician's office with a temperature of 39.4°C (103°F). The physician diagnoses acute bacterial pharyngitis and prescribes cefaclor. The patient says that she does not have enough money to pay for the medication, but her husband's health insurance covers prescriptions for him. She asks the physician to write the prescription in her husband's name. The physician, who prefers to prescribe a higher-priced antibiotic less susceptible to resistance, explains that he cannot do this but provides the patient with a prescription for a generic medication that she can afford. He instructs her to call within 24–48 hours if her symptoms do not improve.

friends, to **make medical decisions for patients who do not have advance directives.**
2. A surrogate decision-maker is supposed to act according to the wishes of the patient, or if those wishes are unknown, in the best interest of the patient.
3. **Statutes vary by state** in terms of the:
   a. **Individuals who can serve as surrogates** (e.g., patient's spouse, adult child, parent)
   b. Extent of the surrogate's decision-making authority
4. In **states that do not have surrogacy laws,** physicians often continue to rely on a **next-of-kin** hierarchy.

VIII. **Violating Professional Boundaries in the Physician-Patient Relationship** (Boxes 25-1 and 25-2)
   A. Violating professional boundaries may be intentional or unintentional.
   B. **Ethical codes** prohibit physicians from having sexual relations with current patients.
      1. **Sexual relationships with patients** are grounds for **disciplinary action** by licensing boards, medical societies, and peer review committees.
      2. Although feelings of sexual attraction toward patients may develop during the course of a professional relation-

Ethical codes prohibit sexual relations with current patients.

ship, **acting on these feelings** is unprofessional, can harm the patient, and **may put physicians at risk for malpractice claims** and **criminal prosecution.**

IX. **Medical Malpractice**
- Medical malpractice is the performance of **medical duties** by a physician at a level below or in conflict with the community standard of care that **results in patient harm.**
  A. **Four criteria of malpractice**
    1. **Dereliction:** negligence
    2. **Duty:** establishment of a patient-physician relationship, with a physician's duty to care for the patient
    3. **Direct causation:** act of omission or commission that directly led to the negative outcome
    4. **Damage:** harm to patient
  B. **Medical malpractice** is a tort or civil wrong, **not** a crime.

X. **Physician-assisted Suicide**
  A. **Physician-assisted suicide:** a physician provides a patient with the means (e.g., medication) and/or information necessary to commit suicide, and the patient commits the act.
  B. **Euthanasia:** a physician administers medication or another intervention to a patient to cause death.
  C. **Double effect:** a physician provides **palliative treatment** to relieve pain and suffering, which **hastens death** as a side effect. This action is *not* physician-assisted suicide or euthanasia.

XI. **Impaired Physicians**
- Ethically, physicians must protect patients from harm and intervene with physicians who are impaired in their ability to practice medicine.
- **Reporting** of impaired physicians is **required in some states.**
  A. **Common reasons for physician impairment** include:
    1. **Drug and alcohol use**
    2. Psychiatric illness
    3. Medical illness
  B. Depending on the circumstances, **interventions may include:**
    1. Directly **discussing the problem with the impaired colleague**
    2. **Notifying a superior** (e.g., attending physician, department head)
    3. **Notifying** the **medical licensing board**
  C. **Confidential rehabilitation services** are aimed at **physician recovery** and restoring the physician's ability to continue and/or resume medical practice.

"4 Ds" of malpractice:

Dereliction
Duty
Direct causation
Damage

A physician who withholds life-sustaining treatment is not committing physician-assisted suicide.

26

Health Care Delivery Systems

Target Topics

▶ Health care delivery structure and providers
▶ Trends in health care costs
▶ Programs for financing health care

I. Health Care Delivery Structure

A. Overview

1. Hospital care is expensive, and efforts have been made over the past 20 years to decrease hospital utilization.
2. There has been a **shift** in provision of care **from inpatient settings to ambulatory care settings** and to patients' homes.
3. The **need for long-term care** is **increasing**.

B. Hospitals

1. The **decrease in hospital utilization** is due to factors such as:
   a. **Cost-containment measures** (e.g., increase in managed care)
   b. New and **improved technologies** and **drug therapies**
2. In **2001**, the United States had 5801 hospitals with approximately 987,000 beds; a **67% occupancy rate** indicates there is a **surplus of hospital beds.**

C. Ambulatory care

   • Services provided to patients in settings such as:
1. Physicians' offices
2. Ambulatory surgery centers

The average length of stay for hospital inpatients decreased from 7.5 days in 1980 to 4.9 days in 2000.

TABLE 26-1   Types of Long-term Care Programs and Facilities

Type of Care	Services Provided	Comments
Home health	In-home care for individuals who have recently been discharged from the hospital or who are homebound and unable to get to a physician's office May include nursing, personal care, and social services, as well as physical, speech, and occupational therapy	Eligibility: the patient must require care from a nurse, physical therapist, occupational therapist, or speech therapist Providers include for-profit and not-for-profit organizations (e.g., visiting nurse associations)
Respite	Provides a break (respite) for family caregivers of persons unable to stay alone safely Services range from sitting with the person to providing total care	May last from hours to weeks; provided by health care professionals or volunteers Settings include the home, adult day care centers, and nursing homes
Rehabilitation	Treatment for patients disabled by neuromuscular conditions (e.g., stroke, spinal cord injury), substance abuse, or psychiatric disorders focuses on optimizing the individual's physical, emotional, and social abilities to perform expected roles May include medical, nursing, psychological, pastoral counseling, and social services, as well as physical, occupational, and recreational therapy	Programs are conducted in hospitals and outpatient clinics
Nursing home	Provides 24-hour care for patients with significant physical problems, functional disabilities, or cognitive impairment May include nursing, personal care, social, recreational, and other therapeutic services	Average cost is > $3800 per month Medicaid pays about 50% of nursing home costs; patients and families, about 27%
Hospice	Palliative care, including pain management, and supportive services for terminally ill patients (life expectancy less than 6 months) and their families Similar to home health care services, plus respite care, counseling, spiritual care, and bereavement services	Most hospice care is provided in the home Use of these services is increasing

      3. Urgent care centers
      4. Hospital-based outpatient centers
   D. **Long-term care** (Table 26-1)
      1. Facilities and programs that provide **services for people with chronic conditions and functional limitations,** including:
         a. Home health care
         b. Respite care
         c. Rehabilitation programs

BOX 26-1	The Patient Who Is Recommended for Hospice Care

An 85-year-old woman with pancreatic cancer is not expected to live more than 4 months and will require more care as her illness progresses. The woman, who has been living with her daughter for the past 3 years, wants to die at home, and her daughter expresses the same wish. The physician suggests that they consider hospice care, which will provide palliative care to maintain the woman's dignity, control her pain, and manage her symptoms. Hospice care will allow her to stay at home and receive help from a variety of providers, including nurses, home health aides, and counselors. The woman's daughter also will have services available, such as respite care during her mother's illness and bereavement care for 1 year after her mother dies. Medicare Part A will pay for most of these services. The woman and her daughter agree that hospice care would be the best alternative, and the physician refers them to a program in their area.

       d. Nursing homes
       e. Hospice (Box 26-1)
  2. Includes a range of **health care, personal care, social,** and **housing services** provided in institutional, home, and community-based settings
  3. **Nursing homes** are identified most closely with long-term care.
       a. In **2000,** there were approximately 17,000 nursing homes in the United States, with about **1.8 million beds** and an **82% occupancy rate.**
       b. The trend is toward fewer but larger facilities.
       c. **Types of facilities**
          (1) **Skilled nursing facilities:** provide short-term, inpatient, skilled nursing care and rehabilitative services at a level below that provided in a hospital (some coverage by Medicare after a 3-day hospital stay)
          (2) **Nursing homes:** provide long-term room and board, nursing and personal care, and some therapies to patients unable to live alone because of physical, functional, or cognitive impairment (paid for by resident, some long-term care insurance plans, and Medicaid)
          (3) Many facilities offer both levels of care.
  4. The **need for long-term care** is **expected to continue to rise** because of an increase in the number of people who:
       a. Are older than 65 years of age
       b. Are living longer with chronic diseases
       c. Have survived previously fatal conditions
E. Federal facilities and programs
  1. **Veterans Administration** (VA)
       a. **Eligibility: veterans** who have served in the military and who have been **honorably discharged**
       b. **Services: acute care** and some long-term care ser-

vices; **long-term care** services often are available only to veterans who have **service-connected disabilities.**

2. **Indian Health Service** (IHS)
   a. **Eligibility: Native Americans** who are members of federally recognized tribes (or their descendants) and who live in an area served by IHS
   b. **Services: personal health care** and **public health services** provided either directly through IHS facilities or through tribal services funded by IHS
3. **Public health system**
   a. Includes **public health agencies** (e.g., state and local health departments) and other agencies (e.g., Environmental Protection Agency) concerned with the **health of communities** and **population groups**
   b. **Services**
      (1) **Assessing the health and disease status** of the community
      (2) **Formulating policies** to deal with community health problems
      (3) **Treating these problems** through environmental, behavioral, and medical services
   c. As part of the public health system's **disease surveillance** function, physicians are required to report certain diseases (e.g., chlamydia) to the health department (see Chapter 25).

II. Health Care Providers
A. Physicians
1. In the United States, there are approximately 772,000 practicing physicians: 727,000 medical doctors (MDs) and 45,000 doctors of osteopathic medicine (DOs).
2. About **34% of MDs** and **64% of DOs** practice in the **primary care specialties** of family practice, internal medicine, obstetrics/gynecology, and pediatrics.
   • In 2001, the specialties with the highest number of physicians were internal medicine, family practice, pediatrics, obstetrics/gynecology, psychiatry, and general surgery.

Inner cities and rural areas have a shortage of physicians.

3. In the United States, **89%** of physicians **practice in metropolitan areas,** with only 14% serving nonmetropolitan areas.
4. Over the past 35 years, the **physician-to-patient ratio has increased;** in 2001, the ratio was 286 physicians per 100,000 population.
5. The **role of the physician is changing,** with reliance on physician extenders (e.g., nurse practitioners, physician assistants), an increase in managed care, and more integrated health care delivery systems requiring greater collaboration and cooperation.
B. Other health care providers include:
1. Nurses, such as registered nurses (RNs), licensed practical

nurses (LPNs), certified nursing assistants (CNAs), and specialty nurses (e.g., nurse practitioners)
2. Physician assistants (PAs)
3. Physical, occupational, respiratory, and speech therapists
4. Pharmacists
5. Psychologists
6. Skilled technologists and technicians (e.g., clinical laboratory technologists, phlebotomists)

III. **Costs of Health Care**
A. In **2000, national health expenditures** were **$1.3 trillion,** comprising 13.2% of the gross domestic product (GDP). Since 1992, this percentage has been fairly stable, but it is expected to increase to about 17% by 2011.
B. Although health care expenditures are higher in the United States than in any other industrialized country, the **United States lags behind many other countries** in health status indicators such as **infant mortality** and **life expectancy.**
C. **Hospital care and physician care** account for **more than 50% of health care spending,** followed by **prescription drugs** (the **fastest rising component**), nursing home care, and program administration.
    • To improve cost-effectiveness, lower paid workers are often substituted for higher paid workers if they can provide the same quality of care.

> More than 50% of health care costs represent hospital and physician care.

D. Sources of payment for health care expenses
    1. **Private insurance:** 34%
    2. **Medicare:** 17%
    3. **Medicaid** and State Children's Health Insurance Program (**SCHIP**): 16%
    4. **Out-of-pocket:** 15%
    5. Other public programs (e.g., VA and IHS): 12%
    6. Other private sources: 6%

IV. **Financing Health Care**
A. Overview
    1. In 2001, about **83%** of the United States population **younger than 65 years of age** were **covered by health insurance.**
    2. Most health **insurance** plans include some **cost-sharing responsibilities** for the patient through mechanisms such as:
        a. **Deductibles:** a set amount the patient must pay for health services before the insurance plan begins to pay
        b. **Coinsurance:** a percentage of the approved cost for each health care service, paid by the patient after the deductible is met
        c. **Copayments:** a set fee paid by the patient for a service (e.g., $10 per physician visit)

> In 2001, approximately 42 million people in the United States did *not* have health insurance.

B. **Private health insurance**
    1. Most people under 65 years of age obtain health care cov-

| BOX 26-2 | The HMO Patient Who Is Referred to a Specialist |

A 76-year-old woman with chronic knee problems learns that she will need knee-replacement surgery. The orthopedic surgeon she previously saw is not in her current HMO network, and if she uses him, she will be responsible for the cost of the operation. Her primary care physician recommends an in-network surgeon, and the woman reluctantly agrees to see him.

erage through private, **employer-sponsored, group health insurance.**

2. **Blue Cross/Blue Shield:** The Blue Cross (hospital coverage) and Blue Shield (physician coverage) system is the largest insurer in the United States.

C. Fee-for-service plans

1. In these plans, the insurance carrier **pays the provider for each covered service** the patient receives. The health care **provider sets** the **price** for each service.

2. There is **no restriction on choice of provider.**

3. Care by a **specialist does** *not* **require a referral.**

4. Patients must pay **deductibles** and **coinsurance.**

D. Managed care organizations (MCOs)

1. MCOs integrate health insurance, financing, and delivery of health care to enrollees. Attempts are made to control costs by:

a. **Contracting with a network of providers** to supply services, usually at a predetermined cost

b. Requiring **patients who use providers outside the network** to **pay more** for these services out-of-pocket

c. **Monitoring medical resources** through utilization review and quality assurance programs

2. Health maintenance organizations (HMOs)

a. An HMO is a managed care plan that is **prepaid a certain amount per enrollee** and provides all of the health care needed by the enrollee for this **capitated payment.**

b. To improve the cost-effectiveness of services provided, **patient care is managed** and **prevention is emphasized.**

c. Patients are usually assigned or required to choose a **primary care physician** from within the HMO network who has "**gatekeeper**" functions (e.g., deciding on referrals to specialists within the network) (Box 26-2).

d. Patients are **less likely to have deductibles and coinsurance** and usually have **lower copayments** than those enrolled in other insurance plans.

In 2001, about 28% of the US population were enrolled in HMOs.

   e. **Types of HMOs**
      (1) **Staff model:** physicians are salaried employees of the HMO.
      (2) **Group model:** the HMO contracts with an independent multispeciality medical group practice, which provides care to HMO enrollees.
      (3) **Independent practice association (IPA) model:** the HMO contracts with an association of independent physicians and independent multispeciality medical group practices, which provides care to HMO enrollees as well as patients with other forms of insurance.
      (4) **Network model:** the HMO contracts with two or more independent multispeciality medical group practices, and the enrollee chooses one of these groups as his or her main source of health care.
   f. Some HMOs have a **point of service** (POS) option in which the patient may choose a provider not in the HMO's network, but the **patient pays a portion of the fee** for this service.

3. **Preferred provider organizations** (PPOs)
   a. A PPO is a managed care plan that is **paid a premium for each patient.** In-network physicians are paid for each covered service, but at a **discounted rate** that is lower than their fee for non-PPO patients.
   b. Patients usually pay deductibles, coinsurance, and copayments and are able to **choose a health care provider either in or out of the network;** however, patients pay less if the provider is in-network.
   c. There usually are **no gatekeepers** for referrals to specialists.

E. **Federal and state-funded programs**
   1. **Medicare**
      a. This **federally funded program**, established in 1965, provides health care coverage for individuals who:
         (1) Are **65** years of age **and older**
         (2) Are **disabled** and **younger than 65** years of age
         (3) Have **end-stage renal disease**
      b. Table 26-2 summarizes eligibility requirements and benefits provided under **Medicare Part A** (hospital insurance) and **Part B** (physician and outpatient medical insurance).
      c. **Supplemental insurance**
         (1) **Medigap** policies: sold by private insurance companies to provide coverage for some **services *not* covered** in the original Medicare plan, such as outpatient prescription drugs and additional preventive screenings
         (2) **Long-term care insurance:** sold by private insurance companies to provide medical and personal care services, such as bathing and

TABLE 26-2   Medicare and Medicaid

Program	Eligibility	Coverage	Comments
Medicare	65 years of age or older Disabled and younger than age 65 End-stage renal disease	Part A: Deductible is paid for hospitalizations; copayments may be paid by the insured Benefits include: Inpatient hospital care Skilled nursing facility care Home health care Hospice care Part B: Insured is responsible for monthly premiums, deductible, and coinsurance (about 20% of approved charges) Benefits include (some or all): Outpatient hospital services Physician services Physical therapy Clinical laboratory services Durable medical equipment Dialysis Ambulance Preventive services (e.g., colorectal cancer screening)	Hospital payments are based on diagnosis-related groups (DRGs), in which a payment amount is set for each diagnosis Medicare does *not* cover prescription drugs, eyeglasses, hearing aids, and nursing home care In 2001, there were 40 million enrollees
Medicaid	Some individuals and families with limited income and resources	Benefits may include: Inpatient and outpatient hospital care Physician services Home health care Nursing home care Clinical laboratory services Hospice care Durable medical equipment Dialysis Ambulance services Family planning services Some prescriptions Early and periodic screening, diagnosis, and treatment services for children	In 2001, there were 34 million enrollees, but only about 40% of the poor were covered by Medicaid

dressing, when a person needs assistance with activities of daily living

2. **Medicaid**
   a. This joint **federal** and **state-funded** program helps pay for medical services for some people with **limited income** and **resources**, including:
      (1) **Families with children**
      (2) **Pregnant** women
      (3) **Aged, blind,** or **disabled** individuals
   b. **Eligibility requirements and benefits** vary from state to state (see Table 26-2).

c.   **State Children's Health Insurance Program (SCHIP)**

   (1)   This program was established by the federal government in 1997 to encourage states to provide **health care coverage for children of low-income families** whose parents' income was too high to be eligible for Medicaid coverage but too low to enable them to purchase private health insurance.

   (2)   States can expand their Medicaid program to include this coverage or develop a separate child health program.

In 2001, approximately 4.6 million children received assistance from SCHIP.

Tests

COMMON LABORATORY VALUES

Test	Conventional Units	SI Units
Blood, Plasma, Serum		
Alanine aminotransferase (ALT, GPT at 30°C)	8-20 U/L	8-20 U/L
Amylase, serum	25-125 U/L	25-125 U/L
Aspartate aminotransferase (AST, GOT at 30°C)	8-20 U/L	8-20 U/L
Bilirubin, serum (adult) Total // Direct	0.1-1.0 mg/dL // 0.0-0.3 mg/dL	2-17 μmol/L // 0-5 μmol/L
Calcium, serum (Ca^{2+})	8.4-10.2 mg/dL	2.1-2.8 mmol/L
Cholesterol, serum	Rec: < 200 mg/dL	< 5.2 mmol/L
Cortisol, serum	8:00 AM: 6-23 μg/dL // 4:00 PM: 3-15 μg/dL 8:00 PM: ≤ 50% of 8:00 AM	170-630 nmol/L // 80-410 nmol/L Fraction of 8:00 AM: ≤ 0.50
Creatine kinase, serum	Male: 25-90 U/L Female: 10-70 U/L	25-90 U/L 10-70 U/L
Creatinine, serum	0.6-1.2 mg/dL	53-106 μmol/L
Electrolytes, serum		
Sodium (Na^+)	136-145 mEq/L	135-145 mmol/L
Chloride (Cl^-)	95-105 mEq/L	95-105 mmol/L
Potassium (K^+)	3.5-5.0 mEq/L	3.5-5.0 mmol/L
Bicarbonate (HCO_3^-)	22-28 mEq/L	22-28 mmol/L
Magnesium (Mg^{2+})	1.5-2.0 mEq/L	1.5-2.0 mmol/L
Estriol, total, serum (in pregnancy)		
24-28 wk // 32-36 wk	30-170 ng/mL // 60-280 ng/mL	104-590 // 208-970 nmol/L
28-32 wk // 36-40 wk	40-220 ng/mL // 80-350 ng/mL	140-760 // 280-1210 nmol/L
Ferritin, serum	Male: 15-200 ng/mL Female: 12-150 ng/mL	15-200 μg/L 12-150 μg/L
Follicle-stimulating hormone, serum/ plasma (FSH)	Male: 4-25 mIU/mL Female: premenopause 4-30 mIU/mL midcycle peak 10-90 mIU/mL postmenopause 40-250 mIU/mL	4-25 U/L 4-30 U/L 10-90 U/L 40-250 U/L
Gases, arterial blood (room air)		
pH	7.35-7.45	[H^+] 36-44 nmol/L
P_{CO_2}	33-45 mm Hg	4.4-5.9 kPa
P_{O_2}	75-105 mm Hg	10.0-14.0 kPa
Glucose, serum	Fasting: 70-110 mg/dL 2 hr postprandial: < 120 mg/dL	3.8-6.1 mmol/L < 6.6 mmol/L
Growth hormone–arginine stimulation	Fasting: < 5 ng/mL provocative stimuli: > 7 ng/mL	< 5 μg/L > 7 μg/L
Immunoglobulins, serum		
IgA	76-390 mg/dL	0.76-3.90 g/L
IgE	0-380 IU/mL	0-380 kIU/L
IgG	650-1500 mg/dL	6.5-15 g/L
IgM	40-345 mg/dL	0.4-3.45 g/L

COMMON LABORATORY VALUES—cont'd

Test	Conventional Units	SI Units
Blood, Plasma, Serum—cont'd		
Iron	50-170 µg/dL	9-30 µmol/L
Lactate dehydrogenase, serum (LDH)	45-90 U/L	45-90 U/L
Luteinizing hormone, serum/plasma (LH)	Male: 6-23 mIU/mL	6-23 U/L
	Female: follicular phase	
	5-30 mIU/mL	5-30 U/L
	midcycle 75-150 mIU/mL	75-150 U/L
	postmenopause	
	30-200 mIU/mL	30-200 U/L
Osmolality, serum	275-295 mOsm/kg	275-295 mOsm/kg
Parathyroid hormone, serum, N-terminal	230-630 pg/mL	230-630 ng/L
Phosphatase (alkaline), serum (p-NPP at 30°C)	20-70 U/L	20-70 U/L
Phosphorus (inorganic), serum	3.0-4.5 mg/dL	1.0-1.5 mmol/L
Prolactin, serum (hPRL)	< 20 ng/mL	< 20 µg/L
Proteins, serum		
Total (recumbent)	6.0-8.0 g/dL	60-80 g/L
Albumin	3.5-5.5 g/dL	35-55 g/L
Globulin	2.3-3.5 g/dL	23-35 g/L
Thyroid-stimulating hormone, serum or plasma (TSH)	0.5-5.0 µU/mL	0.5-5.0 mU/L
Thyroidal iodine (^{123}I) uptake	8%-30% of administered dose/24 hr	0.08-0.30/24 hr
Thyroxine (T_4), serum	4.5-12 µg/dL	58-154 nmol/L
Triglycerides, serum	35-160 mg/dL	0.4-1.81 mmol/L
Triiodothyronine (T_3), serum (RIA)	115-190 ng/dL	1.8-2.9 nmol/L
Triiodothyronine (T_3) resin uptake	25%-38%	0.25-0.38
Urea nitrogen, serum (BUN)	7-18 mg/dL	1.2-3.0 mmol urea/L
Uric acid, serum	3.0-8.2 mg/dL	0.18-0.48 mmol/L
Cerebrospinal Fluid (CSF)		
Cell count	0-5 cells/mm^3	0-5 × 10^6/L
Chloride	118-132 mEq/L	118-132 mmol/L
Gamma globulin	3%-12% total proteins	0.03-0.12
Glucose	50-75 mg/dL	2.8-4.2 mmol/L
Pressure	70-180 mm H$_2$O	70-180 mm H$_2$O
Proteins, total	< 40 mg/dL	< 0.40 g/L
Hematology		
Bleeding time (template)	2-7 min	2-7 min
Erythrocyte count	Male: 4.3-5.9 million/mm^3	4.3-5.9 × 10^{12}/L
	Female: 3.5-5.5 million/mm^3	3.5-5.5 × 10^{12}/L
Erythrocyte sedimentation rate (Westergren)	Male: 0-15 mm/hr	0-15 mm/hr
	Female: 0-20 mm/hr	0-20 mm/hr

Continued

COMMON LABORATORY VALUES—cont'd

Test	Conventional Units	SI Units
Hematology—cont'd		
Hematocrit (Hct)	Male: 40%-54%	0.40-0.54
	Female: 37%-47%	0.37-0.47
Hemoglobin A_{IC}	≤ 6%	≤ 0.06%
Hemoglobin, blood (Hb)	Male: 13.5-17.5 g/dL	2.09-2.71 mmol/L
	Female: 12.0-16.0 g/dL	1.86-2.48 mmol/L
Hemoglobin, plasma	1-4 mg/dL	0.16-0.62 mmol/L
Leukocyte count and differential		
Leukocyte count	4500-11,000/mm³	$4.5\text{-}11.0 \times 10^9/L$
Segmented neutrophils	54%-62%	0.54-0.62
Bands	3%-5%	0.03-0.05
Eosinophils	1%-3%	0.01-0.03
Basophils	0%-0.75%	0-0.0075
Lymphocytes	25%-33%	0.25-0.33
Monocytes	3%-7%	0.03-0.07
Mean corpuscular hemoglobin (MCH)	25.4-34.6 pg/cell	0.39-0.54 fmol/cell
Mean corpuscular hemoglobin concentration (MCHC)	31%-37% Hb/cell	4.81-5.74 mmol Hb/L
Mean corpuscular volume (MCV)	80-100 μm³	80-100 fl
Partial thromboplastin time (activated) (aPTT)	25-40 sec	25-40 sec
Platelet count	150,000-400,000/mm³	$150\text{-}400 \times 10^9/L$
Prothrombin time (PT)	12-14 sec	12-14 sec
Reticulocyte count	0.5%-1.5% of red cells	0.005-0.015
Thrombin time	< 2 sec deviation from control	< 2 sec deviation from control
Volume		
Plasma	Male: 25-43 mL/kg	0.025-0.043 L/kg
	Female: 28-45 mL/kg	0.028-0.045 L/kg
Red cell	Male: 20-36 mL/kg	0.020-0.036 L/kg
	Female: 19-31 mL/kg	0.019-0.031 L/kg
Sweat		
Chloride	0-35 mmol/L	0-35 mmol/L
Urine		
Calcium	100-300 mg/24 hr	2.5-7.5 mmol/24 hr
Creatinine clearance	Male: 97-137 mL/min	
	Female: 88-128 mL/min	
Estriol, total (in pregnancy)		
30 wk	6-18 mg/24 hr	21-62 μmol/24 hr
35 wk	9-28 mg/24 hr	31-97 μmol/24 hr
40 wk	13-42 mg/24 hr	45-146 μmol/24 hr
17-Hydroxycorticosteroids	Male: 3.0-9.0 mg/24 hr	8.2-25.0 μmol/24 hr
	Female: 2.0-8.0 mg/24 hr	5.5-22.0 μmol/24 hr
17-Ketosteroids, total	Male: 8-22 mg/24 hr	28-76 μmol/24 hr
	Female: 6-15 mg/24 hr	21-52 μmol/24 hr
Osmolality	50-1400 mOsm/kg	
Oxalate	8-40 μg/mL	90-445 μmol/L
Proteins, total	< 150 mg/24 hr	< 0.15 g/24 hr

TEST 1

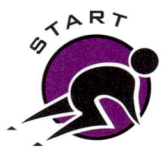

DIRECTIONS: Each numbered item or incomplete statement is followed by options arranged in alphabetical or logical order. Select the best answer to each question. Some options may be partially correct, but there is only **ONE BEST** answer.

1. A 25-year-old woman is taken to the emergency department because of shortness of breath. She is diagnosed with endocarditis and admitted to the hospital. Track marks are noted on both arms. Within 12 hours after admission, pupillary dilation and lacrimation are noted. She is restless and experiencing abdominal cramping and diarrhea. Which of the following substances is most likely to be found in this patient's urine drug screen?

- A. Alcohol
- B. Alprazolam
- C. Cannabis
- D. Cocaine
- E. Heroin

2. The parents of a 2-year-old girl who has frequent tantrums first try to soothe her but then decide to ignore her. The tantrums decrease and eventually stop. Eliminating the tantrums by ignoring them is an example of

- A. extinction
- B. negative reinforcement
- C. shaping
- D. stimulus generalization

3. A 19-year-old man begins experiencing auditory and visual hallucinations a few weeks after going away to college. His urine drug screen is negative. Which of the following studies would be the best choice to rule out pathologic anatomic changes in this patient?

- A. Electroencephalography (EEG)
- B. Magnetic resonance imaging (MRI)
- C. Magnetic resonance spectroscopy (MRS)
- D. Positron emission tomography (PET)
- E. Single-photon emission computed tomography (SPECT)

4. A 16-year-old boy with diabetes recently has not been adhering to his daily medical regimen. Which of the following approaches would be best for the physician to use in encouraging this patient to adhere to his regimen?

- A. Describe health problems that may develop over the next 10–20 years if he does not adhere to his regimen
- B. Reprimand the boy's parents for not taking responsibility for their son's health
- C. Try to involve the boy's friends in supporting his adherence
- D. Work with the boy's parents to develop punishments for nonadherence

229

5. A 67-year-old patient has multiple sclerosis and recently has become confined to a wheelchair. He receives both Medicare and Medicaid benefits. His wife is planning to have a ramp built up to the front door to accommodate his wheelchair. Which of the following will be the primary payer for the ramp?

○ A. Medicaid
○ B. Medicare Part A
○ C. Medicare Part B
○ D. Out-of-pocket payments

6. An 18-year-old woman has daily headaches that are so severe that she is unable to go to school. When the physician asks her about recent stressors, she says that the headaches began about a month ago when her parents began pressuring her to go to college. The physician, who is concerned because his own daughter refuses to go to college, begins to feel angry with the patient. The physician's anger is an example of

○ A. countertransference
○ B. displacement
○ C. regression
○ D. sublimation
○ E. transference

7. A physician finds it difficult to keep the office visit of a patient on schedule because she rambles on about numerous things and tells stories unrelated to her medical complaint. She shows no signs of cognitive problems. Which of the following approaches could the physician use to keep this patient focused during the interview?

○ A. Set a timer to indicate how many minutes remain for the visit
○ B. Redirect the conversation with paraphrased statements
○ C. Use facilitating remarks
○ D. Use mainly open-ended questions

8. Total cholesterol values in a random sample of 400 healthy men are assumed to follow a normal distribution, with mean equal to 160 mg/dL and standard deviation (SD) equal to 20 mg/dL. Which of the following best represents the normal limits for total cholesterol values in this population?

○ A. 100–220 mg/dL
○ B. 120–200 mg/dL
○ C. 140–180 mg/dL
○ D. 158–162 mg/dL
○ E. 159–161 mg/dL

9. Which of the following findings is most likely to be seen in a 21-year-old woman diagnosed with anorexia nervosa, restricting type?

○ A. Bradycardia
○ B. Dental enamel erosion
○ C. Electrolyte disturbance
○ D. Esophageal tears
○ E. Swollen salivary glands

10. A 33-year-old executive complains of headaches, difficulty concentrating, sleep problems, and fatigue. She says that although things are going well in her life, she worries all the time about "little things," such as getting her work done. Her symptoms have been present most days over the past year. Which of the following is the most likely diagnosis?

○ A. Adjustment disorder
○ B. Agoraphobia
○ C. Generalized anxiety disorder
○ D. Panic disorder
○ E. Posttraumatic stress disorder (PTSD)

11. A physician is concerned about the quality of attachment between a 13-month-old infant and her caregivers. Which of the following signs is the strongest indicator of poor attachment?

○ A. Failure to thrive
○ B. Persistence of newborn reflexes
○ C. Presence of colic
○ D. Separation anxiety
○ E. Stranger anxiety

12. Which of the following features is most likely to be present in a 19-year-old woman with anorexia nervosa, restricting type?

○ A. Impulsive behavior
○ B. Loss of appetite
○ C. Obsessions and compulsions
○ D. Purging
○ E. Substance abuse

13. The daughter of a 71-year-old woman reports to the physician that her mother has been unable to maintain her checkbook lately and has been misplacing items in the home. The patient explains that the items are mislaid because men from the gas company have been coming into her home at night while she sleeps and have been moving things around. Her response demonstrates

○ A. delusional thinking
○ B. disorientation
○ C. hallucinations
○ D. poor judgment
○ E. thought blocking

14. A hospitalized patient is angry and frustrated because she feels that her physician is always rushed, does not listen well, and does not keep her informed of treatment plans. A medical student is responsive to her needs, but she accuses him of being abrupt and insensitive. Which of the following defense mechanisms is this patient using?

○ A. Displacement
○ B. Identification
○ C. Projection
○ D. Rationalization
○ E. Reaction formation

15. The teacher of a 7-year-old boy complains that the boy interferes with other students' learning, makes careless mistakes in his work, and earns grades that are much lower than his ability. His parents say that he acts before he thinks, has frequent accidents, and has trouble falling asleep at night. Which of the following is the most likely diagnosis?

○ A. Attention-deficit/hyperactivity disorder (ADHD)
○ B. Conduct disorder
○ C. Learning disorder
○ D. Mental retardation
○ E. Oppositional defiant disorder

16. A 14-year-old boy believes that he is being observed by aliens. In which section of the psychiatric evaluation would the physician record information about the presence and content of delusions?

○ A. Family history
○ B. Global assessment of functioning
○ C. Identifying information
○ D. Mental status examination
○ E. Strengths and weaknesses

17. The parents of a 5-year-old boy tell him that each day he puts away his toys he will be able to play 15 minutes longer with one of his parents. Which of the following reinforcement schedules is being used with this child?

❍ A. Continuous
❍ B. Fixed-interval
❍ C. Fixed-ratio
❍ D. Variable-interval
❍ E. Variable-ratio

18. Which of the following recommendations would best help a 5-year-old child cope with hospitalization and surgery?

❍ A. Encourage the parents to be present at the hospital as much as possible
❍ B. Instruct the parents to offer rewards for good behavior in the hospital
❍ C. Recommend that the parents read information about hospitals to the child before admission
❍ D. Suggest that the child bring favorite toys from home

19. The cerebrospinal fluid (CSF) of a 50-year-old suicide victim is examined at autopsy. The victim has no history of mental illness other than recent depression. Which of the following is most likely to be found in this CSF sample?

❍ A. Decreased choline and acetic acid
❍ B. Decreased 5-hydroxyindoleacetic acid (5-HIAA)
❍ C. Increased homovanillic acid (HVA)
❍ D. Increased 3-methoxy-4-hydroxyphenylglycol (MHPG)
❍ E. Increased norepinephrine

20. An 18-year-old pregnant woman who has received no prenatal care comes to the hospital in labor and delivers a low-birth-weight infant with a flattened nasal bridge, a relatively small cranium, small nail beds, and small and curved fingers. Which of the following substances is the most likely cause of the developmental defects in this infant?

❍ A. Alcohol
❍ B. Cocaine
❍ C. Marijuana
❍ D. Methamphetamine
❍ E. Nicotine

21. A 61-year-old man sees his physician because he is having trouble sleeping. The man says, "I'm having a hard time since my wife died 3 weeks ago. We were married for 40 years, and I just can't get used to her not being here. Nights are the worst. It takes me a couple of hours to get to sleep." Which of the following responses by the physician would be the most empathic?

❍ A. "Have you thought about starting a new hobby? Staying busy helps."
❍ B. "I know how you feel. My mother died when I was a kid, and it was really hard for me."
❍ C. "I'll give you a prescription that will help you get to sleep and sleep well through the night."
❍ D. "It sounds like you miss your wife very much. Losing her has had an enormous impact on your life."
❍ E. "You still have many good years to look forward to. You'll feel better soon."

22. A 49-year-old accountant with depression is administered a formal Mini-Mental State Examination. She makes five errors when subtracting by serial 7s. Based on her performance, in which cognitive area is this patient most likely to have a deficit?

○ A. Concentration
○ B. Immediate recall
○ C. Intelligence
○ D. Judgment
○ E. Long-term memory

23. A 23-year-old woman has a severe cough and a sore throat and is accompanied to the physician's office by her mother. The patient responds pleasantly and factually as her medical history is being taken. When the physician asks her about the scars on her wrists, she becomes angry and curses and tells the physician that he is incompetent and storms out of the room. The patient's mother says that her daughter's social life is marked by a pattern of unstable and intense relationships, impulsive buying sprees, and several suicide attempts and that she has not been able to keep a job or friends because of her behavior. Which of the following is the most appropriate diagnosis?

○ A. Antisocial personality disorder
○ B. Borderline personality disorder
○ C. Histrionic personality disorder
○ D. Narcissistic personality disorder

24. A 5-year-old girl is taken to the pediatrician by her mother for her annual checkup. The child is a victim of sexual abuse, although her mother is unaware of it. Which of the following is the most likely concern expressed by the mother to the pediatrician?

○ A. The child has been enacting sexual behavior with her dolls
○ B. The child has been stealing food
○ C. The child has no friends
○ D. The child has physical developmental delays
○ E. The child has recently developed a tic

25. A 35-year-old married woman was diagnosed with liver cancer 10 months ago and has been receiving hospice care for the past 2 months. The patient tells her physician that she is planning a trip to Europe next year and that she would like to have a child "when she gets better." According to Elisabeth Kübler-Ross, this patient is in which stage of dying?

○ A. Denial
○ B. Anger
○ C. Bargaining
○ D. Depression
○ E. Acceptance

26. Patients taking medication that causes side effects, such as headaches and nausea, are less likely to continue taking the medication. Conversely, patients taking medication that produces immediate benefits are more likely to continue taking the medication. These basic principles pertain to which of the following theories?

○ A. Cognitive
○ B. Learning
○ C. Psychoanalytic
○ D. Social cognitive

27. A 92-year-old man is brought to the emergency department by his daughter, who cares for him. He has a broken arm and multiple bruises on his back, which are in various stages of healing. If his daughter has caused these injuries, which of the following behaviors might she exhibit?

- ○ A. She brought her father to the emergency department immediately after he broke his arm
- ○ B. She is attentive to her father
- ○ C. She is unwilling to allow her father to be interviewed alone
- ○ D. She provides information that indicates that she is knowledgeable about her father's medical condition
- ○ E. She provides specific details about her father's injuries

28. The son of a 72-year-old woman worries that his mother should not be living independently because of her difficulty in remembering things. She has a history of a progressive decline in memory but otherwise is in good health. The physician suspects dementia due to Alzheimer's disease. Which of the following would be the best test to evaluate this patient?

- ○ A. Mini-Mental State Examination (MMSE)
- ○ B. Minnesota Multiphasic Personality Inventory (MMPI)
- ○ C. Rorschach test
- ○ D. Thematic Apperception Test

29. Diastolic blood pressure values in a random sample of 100 men are assumed to follow a normal distribution, with mean equal to 85 mm Hg and standard deviation (SD) equal to 10 mm Hg. What is the probability that a patient randomly selected from this sample has a diastolic blood pressure value of 105 mm Hg or greater?

- ○ A. 2.35%
- ○ B. 2.50%
- ○ C. 5.0%
- ○ D. 16%
- ○ E. 32%

30. A 60-year-old woman decides to prepare a living will. Which of the following instructions would be included in this document?

- ○ A. How she wants her property and assets to be disposed of when she dies
- ○ B. What kind of funeral she wants when she dies
- ○ C. What medical care she wants to receive at the end of her life if she is no longer able to make decisions for herself
- ○ D. Whether she wants the physician to perform euthanasia if she becomes terminally ill
- ○ E. Who should be appointed to make medical decisions for her in the event that she loses decisional capacity

31. A 61-year-old man complains of memory loss and says that he is afraid he has Alzheimer's disease. A diagnostic interview shows that the patient's only symptom is a memory lapse of events that occurred while he was shopping at a supermarket and was threatened by an armed robber during a holdup of the store. Which of the following is the most appropriate diagnosis?

- ○ A. Depersonalization disorder
- ○ B. Dissociative amnesia
- ○ C. Dissociative fugue
- ○ D. Dissociative identity disorder

32. The wife of a man with bipolar I disorder asks the physician about the likelihood that their 17-year-old daughter or their 15-year-old son will develop a mood disorder. Which of the following statements accurately describes the risk in these children?

○ A. The daughter has a greater risk of developing a bipolar disorder during the next 10 years than at any other time in her life
○ B. The daughter has a greater risk of developing bipolar I disorder than bipolar II disorder
○ C. The daughter has a greater risk of developing a cyclothymic disorder than does the son
○ D. The son has a greater risk of developing a depressive disorder than does the daughter
○ E. The husband's diagnosis has no bearing on his children's risk of developing a mood disorder

33. A 61-year-old woman, whose mother died of cervical cancer, sees her physician because of vaginal bleeding that began 6 months earlier. The patient's menstrual periods stopped when she was age 50. Which of the following defense mechanisms best explains the 6-month delay in this patient seeking treatment?

○ A. Denial
○ B. Isolation
○ C. Reaction formation
○ D. Regression
○ E. Suppression

34. Which of the following features is rated by an Apgar score?

○ A. Developmental milestones in children younger than 6 years of age
○ B. Health status of a newborn infant immediately after birth
○ C. Quality of attachment between an infant and its caregiver
○ D. Stage of development of secondary sex characteristics

35. A 40-year-old woman bursts into tears as she tells her physician that she has been "in a black hole" for the past 3 weeks. She says that she has been feeling "incredibly fatigued" and is unable to remember details most of the time. She falls asleep as soon as she gets into bed each night, but then awakens at about 3:00 AM and remains awake until morning. She has no appetite. Which of the following is the most likely diagnosis?

○ A. Adjustment disorder with depressed mood
○ B. Bipolar I disorder
○ C. Bipolar II disorder
○ D. Dysthymic disorder
○ E. Major depressive disorder

36. The parents of a 17-year-old girl bring their daughter to the physician's office because they think she is underweight and is not eating enough. The girl thinks that her parents are overreacting and says that she needs to lose more weight because her thighs are fat. Her weight is significantly below normal for her height. The girl started menstruating when she was 13 years old but has not had a menstrual period for the past 5 months. Which of the following is the most likely diagnosis?

○ A. Anorexia nervosa
○ B. Bulimia nervosa
○ C. Eating disorder not otherwise specified
○ D. Major depressive disorder
○ E. Obsessive-compulsive disorder

37. A 60-year-old man is diagnosed with a disorder involving repetitive movements of his legs that occur at 20- to 40-second intervals during sleep. He also has insomnia and feels sleepy during the day. Which of the following is the most likely diagnosis?

○ A. Narcolepsy
○ B. Nocturnal myoclonus
○ C. Obstructive sleep apnea
○ D. Restless leg syndrome

38. A man who is a recovering alcoholic with a 3-year period of abstinence is visiting friends who are drinking alcohol. He has an urge to have a glass of wine. After considering the potential consequences, he decides not to drink. The decision to resist the urge to drink is a function of which of the following psychological domains?

○ A. Ego
○ B. Id
○ C. Superego
○ D. Unconscious mind

39. A 35-year-old physically healthy woman sees her physician because she feels depressed, has trouble sleeping, and thinks she is a "hopelessly incompetent woman." She has experienced these symptoms on more days than not since her late teens, and has never been free of symptoms for more than a few days at a time. Which of the following is the most likely diagnosis?

○ A. Adjustment disorder with depressed mood
○ B. Bipolar II disorder
○ C. Cyclothymic disorder
○ D. Dysthymic disorder
○ E. Major depressive disorder

40. In a study examining the association of serum cholesterol levels with mortality in persons older than age 70, the investigators find significantly higher mortality in a group with high serum cholesterol levels compared with a group with low serum cholesterol levels. The investigators conclude that serum cholesterol level is a risk factor for mortality in persons older than age 70. This conclusion may be faulty because

○ A. bias and confounding have not been excluded as likely explanations of the results
○ B. the result does not focus on mortality associated with a specific medical disorder
○ C. the result may not be clinically important
○ D. the sample size is too small

41. At a routine checkup, the physician checks the reflexes of a 1-month-old infant. He strokes the sole of the infant's foot to see if she responds by extending her big toe and fanning her other toes. Which of the following newborn reflexes is the physician testing?

○ A. Babinski reflex
○ B. Grasp reflex
○ C. Moro reflex
○ D. Rooting reflex
○ E. Stepping reflex

42. A 70-year-old man with dementia is to be scheduled for hip replacement surgery. The physician questions whether the patient has the cognitive ability to provide informed consent for the surgery. Which of the following is the physician's best course of action?

○ A. Arrange to have a psychiatric consultation to assess the patient's decisional capacity
○ B. Declare the patient legally incompetent to make health care decisions
○ C. Determine whether there is family consensus to proceed with surgery
○ D. Proceed with surgery without the patient's express consent

43. A 48-year-old woman sees her physician with complaints of falling and being "clumsy." The physician notices an ataxic gait. A CT scan of her head shows cerebellar degenerative changes. The physician should screen for which of the following substances of abuse?

○ A. Alcohol
○ B. Amphetamines
○ C. Benzodiazepines
○ D. Cocaine
○ E. Opiates

44. A patient with social phobia experiences tachycardia before making public presentations. Which neurotransmitter, working in which system, is most likely responsible for these symptoms?

○ A. Acetylcholine in the parasympathetic system
○ B. Acetylcholine in the sympathetic system
○ C. Dopamine in the reticular activating system
○ D. Norepinephrine in the sympathetic system
○ E. Serotonin in the limbic system

45. With advancing age, sleep is characterized by which of the following changes?

○ A. Decrease in nighttime awakenings
○ B. Increase in delta sleep
○ C. Increase in rapid eye movement (REM) sleep
○ D. Increase in sleep stages 1 and 2

46. A 14-year-old girl was practicing a leap during a dance class when she fell and hit her head. She is brought to the emergency room, unconscious, by her dance instructor. The physician wants to perform an emergency craniotomy because of a possible brain hemorrhage. Repeated attempts to locate the girl's parents for their consent are unsuccessful. Which of the following is an appropriate action by the physician?

○ A. Ask the dance instructor to provide consent in lieu of the parents
○ B. Keep the patient comfortable until the parents can be reached
○ C. Proceed with surgery while continuing efforts are made to contact the parents for consent
○ D. Seek emergency authorization from the court to proceed with surgery

47. A 74-year-old woman is brought to the physician by her daughter, who is concerned about her mother's driving safety. The physician conducts a mental status examination by asking the patient to repeat three words immediately after he says them. Five minutes later, he asks the patient to repeat the same three words. Which of the patient's abilities is being tested?

○ A. Abstract thought
○ B. Concentration
○ C. Fund of knowledge
○ D. Judgment
○ E. Memory

48. A 40-year-old man with schizophrenia is being treated with fluphenazine. The physician notices that the patient paces and is restless after each dose of the drug. In an effort to reduce the patient's agitation, the physician increases the dose of fluphenazine, which worsens his symptoms. This patient is experiencing which of the following conditions?

○ A. Akathisia
○ B. Akinesia
○ C. Dystonia
○ D. Neuroleptic malignant syndrome (NMS)
○ E. Tardive dyskinesia

49. A 41-year-old man sees his physician because of an abrupt onset of erectile difficulties. During the examination, the physician asks about the patient's marital relationship, his job, and his level of stress. The man admits that he and his wife have recently been experiencing marital tension because of the long hours that he works at a stressful job, but he says that he has experienced this level of stress on his job for several years. The physical examination is unremarkable. Which of the following is most likely the primary factor contributing to this patient's erectile difficulties?

○ A. Age
○ B. Long work hours
○ C. Marital relationship
○ D. Stress level

50. Suicide occurs more often in which of the following cultural groups?

○ A. African Americans
○ B. Asian Americans
○ C. Hispanic Americans
○ D. Native Americans

ANSWERS AND DISCUSSIONS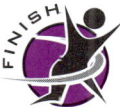

1. E (heroin) is correct. Endocarditis is a medical complication of intravenous substance abuse. The withdrawal symptoms described are characteristic of opiate withdrawal, such as occurs in heroin addiction. Opiate withdrawal is uncomfortable but usually not life-threatening.

   A   (alcohol) is incorrect. Alcohol withdrawal can be life-threatening. Symptoms can range from elevated blood pressure, elevated heart rate, and tremors to seizures and delirium tremens accompanied by hallucinations and metabolic and cardiovascular instability. They do not include endocarditis.

   B   (alprazolam) is incorrect. Alprazolam is a benzodiazepine. Withdrawal from benzodiazepines may cause seizures and is associated with anxiety, insomnia, and other activating symptoms, such as elevated heart rate. Although alprazolam can be injected, it is more likely to be ingested.

   C   (cannabis) is incorrect. Cannabis use is not associated with physiologic tolerance or a particular withdrawal syndrome other than craving.

   D   (cocaine) is incorrect. Cocaine can be injected, but usually is snorted or smoked. Intense craving, lethargy, and depression characterize withdrawal.

2. A (extinction) is correct. Extinction occurs when reinforcement is discontinued, resulting in cessation of the previous response. In this case, when the parents try to soothe their daughter when she is having tantrums, their attention serves as positive reinforcement for the behavior (tantrums). When the parents withdraw their attention (i.e., positive reinforcement), the tantrums eventually stop.

   B   (negative reinforcement) is incorrect. In negative reinforcement, an unpleasant stimulus is removed. The removal strengthens the behavior that caused the unpleasant stimulus to cease. For example, a child is throwing a tantrum because he wants a toy, and his parents agree to buy it so that he will stop crying. The parents' response of giving in to the child's demands now has been negatively reinforced. The next time the child throws a tantrum, the parents will be more likely to give in because the aversive event (i.e., crying) ceased with this behavior.

   C   (shaping) is incorrect. Shaping is the reinforcement of behaviors as they become more and more similar to a desired behavior. For example, a man is encouraged to begin walking 10 minutes a day, 3 days a week. Upon reaching this initial goal, his physician praises him and recommends that he increase his walking time to 30 minutes, 5 days a week.

D (stimulus generalization) is incorrect. Stimulus generalization occurs in a classical conditioning paradigm when stimuli similar to a conditioned stimulus produce the same response as the conditioned response. For example, chemotherapy produces nausea in many people. After several treatment sessions in which chemotherapy (unconditioned stimulus) and nausea (unconditioned response) repeatedly are paired, the patient may experience nausea (conditioned response) when exposed to stimuli associated with the treatment environment (e.g., the waiting room).

3. B (magnetic resonance imaging) is correct. MRI provides the most definitive picture of anatomic structures in the brain. It is important to rule out tumors or other anomalies with any new onset of mental status changes.

A (electroencephalography) is incorrect. The EEG does not give an anatomic image of the brain. Rather, it measures electrical brain activity.

C (magnetic resonance spectroscopy) is incorrect. MRS can determine the use of organic substances in the brain, but an MRI provides a clearer anatomic picture than does an MRS.

D (positron emission tomography) is incorrect. The PET scan is a functional (not an anatomic) test used to monitor tumor activity.

E (single-photon emission computed tomography) is incorrect. The SPECT scan is a functional study and is appropriate for patients with dementia, but not for patients experiencing psychotic symptoms. The SPECT scan provides information about brain function by monitoring blood flow and receptor binding.

4. C (try to involve the boy's friends in supporting his adherence) is correct. Normal adolescent development involves asserting independence, questioning authority, and feeling invincible. As a result, adolescents frequently do not adhere to medical recommendations. Peer relationships are very important to adolescents. If friends of a teenage patient support and encourage the patient to adhere to medical recommendations, the likelihood of adherence is increased.

A (describe health problems that may develop over the next 10–20 years if he does not adhere to his regimen) is incorrect. Most teens in middle adolescence have not developed the cognitive capacity to foresee the long-term consequences of their behavior. Focusing on short-term positive consequences is a better strategy.

B (reprimand the boy's parents for not taking responsibility for their son's health) is incorrect. The responsibility for daily self-care should be progressively transferred to chronically ill teens as they grow older.

D (work with the boy's parents to develop punishments for non-adherence) is incorrect. The emphasis should be on working with the adolescent to maximize adherence. Reinforcement of desired behavior is generally preferred to the use of punishment.

5. D (out-of-pocket payments) is correct. Medicare and Medicaid pay for many hospital and medical expenses but do not pay for making a home more accessible to a wheelchair patient.

A (Medicaid) is incorrect. Medicaid helps pay for medical care for some individuals with low income and limited resources. Benefits vary from state to state but commonly include inpatient and outpatient hospital care, physician services, home health care, and durable medical equipment.

B (Medicare Part A) is incorrect. Medicare Part A covers such benefits as inpatient hospital services, skilled nursing facility care, home health care, and hospice care.

C (Medicare Part B) is incorrect. Medicare Part B includes such benefits as outpatient hospital services, physician services, physical therapy, clinical laboratory services, durable medical equipment, dialysis, ambulance service, and some preventive services.

6. A (countertransference) is correct. Countertransference refers to an unconscious process in which the physician brings feelings and attitudes from previous experiences and applies those feelings to the patient. In this case, the patient has not said or done anything that could cause the physician to become angry with her. The physician's anger can best be explained as a reflection of his feelings toward his daughter.

B (displacement) is incorrect. Displacement is a defense mechanism in which a person redirects feelings toward a person or thing other than the object that originally elicited the feelings. For example, if the physician had an argument with his daughter and then yelled at his nurse, he would be displacing his anger at his daughter to his nurse.

C (regression) is incorrect. Regression is a defense mechanism in which a person resorts to earlier behaviors as a way of dealing with emotional conflict.

D (sublimation) is incorrect. Sublimation is a defense mechanism in which a person expresses a feeling that is unacceptable to him or her in a constructive or adaptive way.

E (transference) is incorrect. Transference occurs when the patient brings feelings or attitudes from previous relationships and applies those feelings to the physician. In this case, a transference reaction might involve the patient feeling angry with the physician when he asks about her plans for college, because it reminds her of being pressured by her parents to attend college.

---

7. B (redirect the conversation with paraphrased statements) is correct. Paraphrasing what the patient has said politely redirects the discussion to the medical complaint. Another helpful strategy is the use of close-ended questions, which can narrow the focus of the conversation.

A (set a timer to indicate how many minutes remain for the visit) is incorrect. Setting a timer that indicates the number of remaining minutes for a visit is not an appropriate interviewing strategy and is most likely to offend a patient.

C (use facilitating remarks) is incorrect. Facilitating remarks (e.g., "and then what happened?") help when a physician is interviewing a patient who is shy or reluctant to talk about a problem.

D (use mainly open-ended questions) is incorrect. Open-ended questions elicit less structured responses. They are effective early in the interview and allow patients to freely describe symptoms and concerns. However, use of open-ended questions when interviewing a rambling patient may lead to a loss of focus, and thus it may become necessary to limit their use during the interview.

---

8. B (120–200 mg/dL) is correct. The normal limits are usually set to include 95% of the population. In a normal distribution, 95% of the values fall within the mean ± 2SD. In this example:

$$160 \text{ mg/dL} + (2 \cdot 20 \text{ mg/dL}) = 200 \text{ mg/dL}$$
$$160 \text{ mg/dL} - (2 \cdot 20 \text{ mg/dL}) = 120 \text{ mg/dL}$$

A (100–220 mg/dL) is incorrect. These limits are equal to the mean ± 3SD. In a normal distribution, 99.7% of the values fall within ± 3SD of the mean.

C (140–180 mg/dL) is incorrect. These limits are equal to the mean ± 1SD. In a normal distribution, 68% of the values fall within ± 1SD of the mean.

D (158–162 mg/dL) is incorrect. These limits are equal to the mean ± 2 standard error of the mean (SEM). In the same way that the SD of a mean represents the average dispersion of data values around the population mean, the SEM represents the average dispersal of sample means around the population mean. The 95% confidence interval of a mean is equal to the mean ± 2SEM. Therefore, these limits indicate the 95% confidence interval around the mean.

$$\text{SEM} = \text{SD}/\sqrt{n} = 20 \text{ mg/dL} / \sqrt{400 \text{ mg/dL}} = 1 \text{ mg/dL}$$

E (159–161 mg/dL) is incorrect. These limits are equal to the mean ± 1SEM.

9. A (bradycardia) is correct. A slow heart rate is common in individuals with anorexia nervosa, and it is a medical complication associated with significant weight loss. Other complications of anorexia nervosa, restricting type, include hypotension, hypothermia, leukopenia, anemia, osteoporosis, dry skin, and lanugo (fine, downy hair on the body).

B (dental enamel erosion) is incorrect. This is a complication of bulimia nervosa, purging type, and of anorexia nervosa, binge-eating/purging type. It occurs particularly on the front teeth, is accompanied by decay, and is caused by repeated vomiting.

C (electrolyte disturbance) is incorrect. Electrolyte disturbance is a complication of bulimia nervosa, purging type, and anorexia nervosa, binge-eating/purging type. It is caused by repeated vomiting or laxative abuse. Patients with eating disorders who engage in purging should have regular assessment of their electrolytes.

D (esophageal tears) is incorrect. Esophageal tears are a rare complication of bulimia nervosa, purging type, and anorexia nervosa, binge-eating/purging type. They are related to repeated vomiting.

E (swollen salivary glands) is incorrect. Swollen parotid or salivary glands are a complication of bulimia nervosa, purging type, and anorexia nervosa, binge-eating/purging type. The swollen glands produce a "chipmunk-like" appearance in patients who engage in purging.

10. C (generalized anxiety disorder) is correct. Generalized anxiety disorder is characterized by the presence of excessive worry and associated symptoms (in this patient, sleep problems, concentration difficulties, and fatigue) that persist most days for at least 6 months.

A (adjustment disorder) is incorrect. Adjustment disorder involves the development of symptoms in response to an identified psychosocial stressor. This patient states that her life is going well, suggesting the absence of any specific stressor.

B (agoraphobia) is incorrect. Agoraphobia is anxiety about being in places where escape would be difficult or embarrassing or where help might not be accessible if panic symptoms developed. This patient is not complaining about such symptoms.

D (panic disorder) is incorrect. Panic disorder involves recurrent unexpected panic attacks. This patient complains of chronic anxiety and other complaints that persist most of the time. This chronic pattern is in contrast to the episodic surge of anxiety associated with discrete panic attacks.

E (posttraumatic stress disorder) is incorrect. Although some of the complaints described may occur in PTSD (e.g., sleep disturbance, concentration difficulties), there is no mention of exposure to a traumatic stressor. Further screening to rule out a history of traumatic experiences or PTSD symptoms (e.g., recurrent nightmares) would be appropriate in an individual who presents with a high level of anxiety.

11. A (failure to thrive) is correct. Infants who fail to thrive have reduced growth and delayed development. These signs may be caused by factors other than poor attachment, but their presence is a red flag signaling that a physician should evaluate the infant for possible attachment problems.

B (persistence of newborn reflexes) is incorrect. Persistence of newborn reflexes beyond the age when they would normally disappear is an indicator of central nervous system dysfunction.

C (presence of colic) is incorrect. Colic, or prolonged crying, is common in infants up to age 3 months. It is sometimes associated with poor attachment to caregivers. However, colic usually occurs in healthy, well-fed infants.

D (separation anxiety) is incorrect. Infants with separation anxiety are fearful when they are separated from their caregivers. This behavior is normal in infants between 10 and 18 months of age.

E (stranger anxiety) is incorrect. Stranger anxiety is fearfulness in infants when they are approached by a stranger. This normal reaction occurs at about 8 months of age.

12. C (obsessions and compulsions) is correct. Obsessions and compulsions commonly occur in anorexia nervosa. They may be related to food or other themes such as checking or counting. Common features of obsessive-compulsive personality include perfectionism and an increased need for control. When the obsessions and compulsions are not related to food, body shape, or weight, a diagnosis of obsessive-compulsive disorder may be indicated.

A (impulsive behavior) is incorrect. Impulsive behaviors such as stealing, promiscuity, and overspending are commonly associated with bulimia nervosa and anorexia nervosa, binge-eating/purging type.

B (loss of appetite) is incorrect. Although the general medical definition of anorexia is "loss of appetite," an individual with anorexia nervosa does not lose his or her appetite.

D (purging) is incorrect. Purging is characteristic of most cases of bulimia nervosa and many cases of anorexia nervosa, binge-eating/purging type. It is not consistently a feature of anorexia nervosa, restricting type.

E   (substance abuse) is incorrect. Substance abuse is common in patients with bulimia nervosa or anorexia nervosa, binge-eating/purging type.

13. A   (delusional thinking) is correct. A delusion is a fixed, false belief. Trying to convince this patient about the falsity of a delusion is most likely to have the opposite result (i.e., this patient will be more convinced than ever that her belief is true).

B   (disorientation) is incorrect. Orientation is assessed in three spheres: person, place, and time. A person is oriented when she (or he) knows who she is (person), where she is (place), and the current time (day/month/year). Disorientation is the absence of being oriented in one or more of these spheres.

C   (hallucinations) is incorrect. The patient believes that the men from the gas company come into her home at night, but she has not mentioned actually seeing them or hearing them during these visits.

D   (poor judgment) is incorrect. Poor judgment involves poor self-care or engaging in harmful or impulsive behavior. A patient with delusional thinking may exhibit poor judgment; this patient has not been described as having self-care deficits or as having engaged in harmful or impulsive acts.

E   (thought blocking) is incorrect. Thought blocking is a disordered thought process in which thoughts seem to flow slowly or haltingly in a delayed manner, with a delay between the question and the response.

14. A   (displacement) is correct. This patient is angry and frustrated with her physician but is displacing or redirecting her feelings to the medical student, who is a less formidable target than her physician.

B   (identification) is incorrect. Identification involves imitating the behavior of a more powerful person (e.g., a young boy who has witnessed his father hitting his mother on several occasions becomes physically aggressive with other children).

C   (projection) is incorrect. Projection involves attributing one's own unacceptable feelings to others (e.g., a married man who is attracted to a female friend suspects that his wife may be having an affair).

D   (rationalization) is incorrect. Rationalization involves justifying unreasonable feelings or behavior with logical explanations (e.g., a mother who dipped her son in scalding water as a punishment says that the boy needs to learn to respect authority).

E   (reaction formation) is incorrect. Reaction formation involves behaving in a way that is opposite to one's own unacceptable impulses (e.g., a woman who has strong unconscious feelings of anger and aggression is always nice to everyone and never loses her temper).

15. A (attention-deficit/hyperactivity disorder) is correct. ADHD is characterized by symptoms of inattention (making careless mistakes in school work) and hyperactivity-impulsivity (interfering with other students' learning, acting before thinking). Common associated features exhibited by this boy include academic underachievement, frequent accidents, and difficulty sleeping.

B (conduct disorder) is incorrect. Conduct disorder involves serious violations of others' rights or societal rules. There may be physical aggression toward people or animals, destruction of property, and deceitfulness or theft.

C (learning disorder) is incorrect. Learning disorders are characterized by performance on standardized achievement tests that is substantially below expected levels for a child's IQ, age, and education.

D (mental retardation) is incorrect. In mental retardation, intellectual and adaptive functioning are significantly below average.

E (oppositional defiant disorder) is incorrect. Oppositional defiant disorder is characterized by a pattern of negativistic, hostile, defiant behavior.

16. D (mental status examination) is correct. The mental status examination includes a component assessing thought content, during which the presence or absence of delusional thinking (i.e., a fixed system of non–reality-based thought, often of a paranoid nature) is an area that is explored.

A (family history) is incorrect. The family history includes information about the disease history of immediate family members and family of origin.

B (global assessment of functioning) is incorrect. The global assessment of functioning score is a subjective assessment of a patient's ability to function socially and occupationally and to have goal-directed activity and thought. The value of the score is influenced by whether the patient is suicidal or homicidal. The presence of delusions would decrease this score.

C (identifying information) is incorrect. The section on identifying information consists of descriptors such as the patient's name, age, sex, marital status, ethnicity, and occupation.

E (strengths and weaknesses) is incorrect. Delusions are a symptom of mental illness and do not add to a patient's coping or mental health. This section of the psychiatric evaluation records innate or social qualities of the patient unrelated to mental illness (e.g., state of health, employment status, relationship or estrangement from family or friends).

17. A (continuous) is correct. A continuous reinforcement schedule involves providing a reward after each desired response. In this example, the boy is rewarded extra play time with a parent each time he puts away his toys. This schedule helps establish new behaviors.

B (fixed-interval) is incorrect. In fixed-interval schedules, reinforcement occurs after a fixed interval of time. The response being reinforced tends to increase immediately before the end of the interval. For example, a mother tells her son that she will check on him every 15 minutes to see if he is doing his homework. If he is working, he receives a star on a chart, which can be accumulated and exchanged for a reward.

C (fixed-ratio) is incorrect. In a fixed-ratio schedule, reinforcement is given after a behavior has occurred a specific number of times. This reinforced schedule produces a high response rate. For example, a word processor receives a certain amount of money for each printed page that she completes.

D (variable-interval) is incorrect. In a variable-interval schedule, reinforcement is given at variable time intervals. This reinforcement schedule produces a slow, steady response rate. For example, a mother tells her son that she will check on him at undetermined time intervals to see if he is working on his homework.

E (variable-ratio) is incorrect. In a variable-ratio schedule, reinforcement is given after a specified average number of responses. This schedule produces a high response rate and is resistant to extinction because it is difficult to determine if reinforcement was stopped. For example, slot machines are set to pay off on an average of a certain number of plays.

18. A (encourage the parents to be present at the hospital as much as possible) is correct. For children younger than 7 years of age, the presence of their parents is a significant factor in helping them cope with hospitalization and medical procedures. The need for attachment figures is extremely strong in young children and increases in response to physical discomfort and fear.

B (instruct the parents to offer rewards for good behavior in the hospital) is incorrect. Rewards are effective in increasing developmentally appropriate behaviors and may be helpful with some aspects of hospitalization (e.g., in promoting cooperation with medical personnel). However, separation from parents tends to be the most difficult aspect of hospitalization for children younger than age 7, and the presence of parents will have a greater positive effect than providing rewards.

C (recommend that the parents read information about hospitals to the child before admission) is incorrect. For children younger than age 7, play with puppets or dolls or role-playing medical procedures is more effective than verbal descriptions in preparing them for hospitalization. Because they are in the preoperational stage of cognitive development, children in this age group have limited ability to use language in understanding a future event.

D (suggest that the child bring favorite toys from home) is incorrect. Bringing favorite toys and other transitional objects will help comfort hospitalized children younger than age 7, but not as much as having their parents present.

19. B (decreased 5-hydroxyindoleacetic acid) is correct. 5-HIAA is the breakdown product of serotonin, and levels lower than normal are found in the body fluids of individuals displaying aggressive and suicidal behavior.

A (decreased choline and acetic acid) is incorrect. These breakdown products of acetylcholine are reduced in patients with Alzheimer's dementia.

C (increased homovanillic acid) is incorrect. HVA, the breakdown product of dopamine, is associated with increased dopaminergic production or activity, as occurs in schizophrenia or psychosis.

D (increased 3-methoxy-4-hydroxyphenylglycol) and E (increased norepinephrine) are incorrect. Levels of norepinephrine are not easily or accurately measurable. Increased levels of MHPG, the breakdown product of norepinephrine, are associated with anxiety.

20. A (alcohol) is correct. The findings described represent fetal alcohol syndrome (FAS). As the child develops through infancy and childhood, mild mental retardation and behavioral problems are likely to be diagnosed.

B (cocaine) and D (methamphetamine) are incorrect. Infants born to mothers who abuse stimulants are likely to have a low birth weight, but they will not have the teratogenic signs seen in FAS. These infants are likely to be jittery and may initially fail to eat well and thrive. As the child ages, conduct and attentional problems are frequently observed.

C (marijuana) and E (nicotine) are incorrect. Infants born to mothers who smoke either tobacco or marijuana are more likely to have low birth weights and respiratory problems. However, no specific teratogenic effects have consistently been observed with use of either substance.

21. D ("it sounds like you miss your wife very much. Losing her has had an enormous impact on your life") is correct. The physician shows empathy by attempting to recognize and understand the patient's feelings regarding the death of his wife.

A ("have you thought about starting a new hobby? Staying busy helps") is incorrect. The physician is suggesting a possible method of coping with grief.

B ("I know how you feel. My mother died when I was a kid, and it was really hard for me") is incorrect. The statement, "I know how you feel," is rarely beneficial, because it disregards the uniqueness of the patient's experience. The disclosure of personal information and feelings in the second sentence may help the physician develop rapport with the patient, but it is not a direct way of recognizing and understanding the patient's feelings.

C ("I'll give you a prescription that will help you get to sleep and sleep well through the night") is incorrect. Prescribing medication is a constructive response to the patient's complaint about lack of sleep but does not demonstrate understanding of the patient's feelings.

E ("you still have many good years to look forward to. You'll feel better soon") is incorrect. This statement offers encouragement but not empathy.

22. A (concentration) is correct. Serial 7s and other tests of simple calculation assess concentration, as does asking the patient to spell the word "world" backward. A poor performance on such a task could be observed in persons with low intelligence or with a learning disability; however, in this case, the individual's profession (accountant) makes it unlikely that these factors are responsible for her performance. The most likely reason for her poor concentration is her depression.

B (immediate recall) is incorrect. Immediate recall is tested by asking the patient to repeat three words immediately back to the examiner. Asking the patient to restate the words after a 5-minute delay tests short-term memory.

C (intelligence) is incorrect. Intelligence is roughly estimated by the patient's fund of knowledge and vocabulary. It can be assessed through the use of formal intelligence tests.

D (judgment) is incorrect. Judgment can be assessed by the patient's general behavior and recent decisions.

E (long-term memory) is incorrect. Long-term memory is assessed by observing the patient's memory of long-term personal events (e.g., birth date, place of birth) or by asking about historical events, such as naming several past presidents.

23. B (borderline personality disorder) is correct. This disorder is characterized by unstable relationships with others, fluctuating self-image, volatile affect, and self-damaging impulsivity, as seen in this patient.

A (antisocial personality disorder) is incorrect. Antisocial personality disorder involves a pattern of disregard for and violation of the rights of others.

C (histrionic personality disorder) is incorrect. Histrionic personality disorder features attention seeking and excessively emotional behavior.

D (narcissistic personality disorder) is incorrect. Narcissistic personality disorder involves a pattern of pretense, boasting, and seeking the admiration of other people, but with insensitivity to the thoughts and feelings of others.

24. A (the child has been enacting sexual behavior with her dolls) is correct. Developmentally unusual sexual behavior is a significant indicator of child sexual abuse. This child most likely is recreating with her dolls the sexual activities that she has experienced or witnessed. The abuser was most likely her father or another male relative.

B (the child has been stealing food) is incorrect. Stealing food is a behavioral sign of neglect, but not a common sign of sexual abuse.

C (the child has no friends) is incorrect. Difficulty with peer relationships is not a common feature of sexual abuse, but it is often associated with emotional abuse.

D (the child has physical developmental delays) is incorrect. Delays in physical development typically are not associated with sexual abuse but may be associated with neglect.

E (the child has recently developed a tic) is incorrect. The development of tics is not associated with any form of child abuse. Tics have a genetic etiology, although they may be exacerbated by stress.

25. A (denial) is correct. In Kübler-Ross's stages of dying, denial is the stage in which the patient does not believe that the diagnosis and prognosis are true. This patient expects to regain her health, travel, and have a child and does not acknowledge that she has a terminal illness.

B (anger) is incorrect. In this stage of dying, the patient asks "Why me?" and is angry about her fate. Physicians and family members often bear the brunt of this anger.

C (bargaining) is incorrect. In this stage, the patient usually bargains with a higher power or fate and wants to trade good behavior for good health or at least a postponement of death.

D (depression) is incorrect. In this stage, the patient believes the diagnosis and prognosis, experiences sadness and distress, and stops fighting to survive.

E (acceptance) is incorrect. This is the stage of dying in which the patient accepts the inevitable, is generally more calm and peaceful, and takes care of unfinished business.

26. B (learning) is correct. Learning theory includes learning through classical conditioning and learning through operant conditioning. Increased adherence to medication that has few side effects and positive outcomes is explained by operant conditioning, which is based on the principle that behavior is a function of its consequences. Responses that are followed by positive consequences will increase in frequency, and responses followed by adverse consequences will decrease in frequency.

  A (cognitive) is incorrect. Cognitive theory focuses on the importance of thoughts in influencing mood and behavior. For example, when applying this theory to medication adherence, a patient may examine his or her beliefs or expectations regarding the effectiveness of the medication.

  C (psychoanalytic) is incorrect. Psychoanalytic theory focuses on the unconscious influence of early experiences on current behavior. Defense mechanisms are a key concept of this theory. For example, when applying psychoanalytic theory to medication adherence, a patient who is frightened by her illness may use denial as a defense mechanism to cope with her anxiety. If she denies the seriousness of her illness, she is less likely to adhere to her medication regimen.

  D (social cognitive) is incorrect. One of the fundamental concepts of social cognitive theory is self-efficacy, or a person's confidence in his or her ability to carry out a behavior. Self-efficacy is an important factor in adherence to medical advice.

27. C (she is unwilling to allow her father to be interviewed alone) is correct. Abusive caregivers want to stay with their dependents during interviews, which allows them to monitor the patient's answers and keep the patient from talking about the abuse.

  A (she brought her father to the emergency department immediately after he broke his arm) is incorrect. Abusers tend to delay seeking help for the victim's injuries.

  B (she is attentive to her father) is incorrect. Often, there will be indifference or tension between the abusive caregiver and the patient, rather than an attentive attitude on the part of the abuser.

  D (she provides information that indicates that she is knowledgeable about her father's medical condition) is incorrect. Often, abusive caregivers do not have adequate knowledge of the patient's medical problems.

  E (she provides specific details about her father's injuries) is incorrect. Abusive caregiver explanations of injuries and how they occur tend to be vague and sometimes implausible. For example, the daughter may say that she really is not sure how her father's arm was broken, but it may have broken when he transferred himself from his bed to a wheelchair.

28. A (Mini-Mental State Examination) is correct. The MMSE is a screening test that is sensitive to the presence of moderate to severe dementia and is used to measure changes in cognitive function over time. The dementia caused by Alzheimer's disease involves impaired memory and other cognitive functions that may be detected by the MMSE.

B (Minnesota Multiphasic Personality Inventory) is incorrect. The MMPI is a self-report test that measures personality and psychopathology. It is sensitive to measuring emotional disorders such as depression and psychosis. The MMPI does not measure the cognitive changes that characterize dementia.

C (Rorschach test) is incorrect. The Rorschach test (also known as the "inkblot test") requires that the patient imagine and explain what each inkblot represents to him or her. The descriptions are systematically analyzed to delineate key features of the patient's personality.

D (Thematic Apperception Test) is incorrect. In this test, patients are asked to make up stories describing what might be happening in ambiguous drawings that they are shown. Analysis of the stories yields descriptions of the patient's dominant personality characteristics.

29. B (2.50%) is correct. The value 105 mm Hg is 2 SD (2 × 10 mm Hg) greater than the mean of 85 mm Hg. Because the data are distributed according to the normal distribution, 95% of blood pressure values fall within the mean ± 2SD. Therefore, the remaining 5% of values fall outside this range, with half of those values (i.e., 2.5%) falling above the upper limit and half falling below the lower limit. In the figure below, the shaded area under the curve represents the area that is 2 SD greater than the mean.

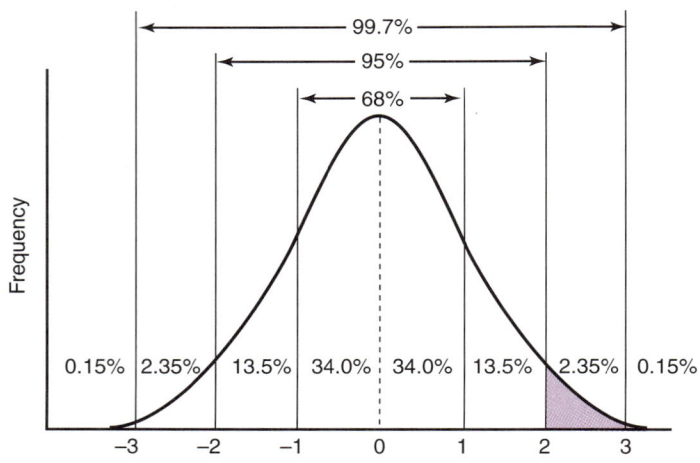

Number of standard deviations from the mean

A   (2.35%) is incorrect. This is the probability that a patient selected randomly from the sample has a diastolic blood pressure between 2 SD above the mean (105 mm Hg) and 3 SD above the mean (115 mm Hg).

C   (5.0%) is incorrect. This option represents the most common error in this type of question. This is the probability that a patient selected randomly from the sample has a diastolic pressure greater than 2 SD above the mean (105 mm Hg) or less than 2 SD below the mean (65 mm Hg). In other words, although 5% of the data values lie outside of the mean ± 2SD, half of those values (2.5%) lie above the upper limit and the other half lie below the lower limit.

D   (16%) is incorrect. This is the probability that a patient selected randomly from the sample has a diastolic blood pressure greater than 1 SD above the mean (95 mm Hg).

E   (32%) is incorrect. This is the probability that a patient selected randomly from the sample has a diastolic blood pressure greater than 1 SD above the mean (95 mm Hg) or less than 1 SD below the mean (75 mm Hg). In other words, 32% of the data values will lie outside of the mean ± 1SD, with half of those values (16%) above the upper limit and the other half below the lower limit.

30. C   (what medical care she wants to receive at the end of her life if she is no longer able to make decisions for herself) is correct. Living wills can include instructions about use of a variety of medical treatments, including ventilators, antibiotics, artificial nutrition, and artificial hydration.

A   (how she wants her property and assets to be disposed of when she dies) is incorrect. A document that states how a person wants his or her property and assets to be disposed of when the person dies is called a will. It is not the same as a living will and does not give instructions about medical care.

B   (what kind of funeral she wants when she dies) is incorrect. A preneed funeral contract can be executed to establish funeral arrangements and payment mechanisms for the arrangements in advance of the person's death. It does not give instructions about medical care.

D   (whether she wants the physician to perform euthanasia if she becomes terminally ill) is incorrect. Euthanasia is illegal in every state; requests for it would not be included in a living will.

E   (who should be appointed to make medical decisions for her in the event that she loses decisional capacity) is incorrect. A durable power of attorney for health care (sometimes called a health care proxy) appoints an individual to make medical decisions for another person in the event that person loses decisional capacity.

31. B (dissociative amnesia) is correct. Dissociative amnesia is characterized by impaired memory for information associated with a traumatic or stressful event that is too extensive to be explained by ordinary forgetfulness. This patient was unable to remember events surrounding his being threatened by an armed robber, an event that was very traumatic for him.

A (depersonalization disorder) is incorrect. In depersonalization disorder, the patient has persistent or recurrent feelings of being detached from his or her body or mental processes, although reality testing remains intact. This patient does not have feelings of detachment, only a gap in his memory associated with a traumatic event.

C (dissociative fugue) is incorrect. Dissociative fugue involves abrupt, unexplained travel out of the individual's usual environment, inability to recall the past, and confusion about personal identity or assumption of a new identity. This patient could not remember events associated with a traumatic incident, but there is no evidence of abrupt, unexplained travel, confusion about his identity, or assumption of a new identity.

D (dissociative identity disorder) is incorrect. Dissociative identity disorder is characterized by the presence of two or more distinct identities that alternately control the individual's awareness and behavior. Some of these identities are unaware of the presence of the other personalities and are amnestic for events that occur while the other identities are in control. There is no evidence of such multiple identities in this patient.

32. A (the daughter has a greater risk of developing a bipolar disorder during the next 10 years than at any other time in her life) is correct. The daughter, now 17 years of age, has not developed a bipolar disorder through childhood and adolescence. Early adulthood remains a time of risk for developing cyclothymic disorder, and it is also the time of greatest risk for developing bipolar I and bipolar II disorders.

B (the daughter has a greater risk of developing bipolar I disorder than bipolar II disorder) is incorrect. Bipolar I disorder is equally common among males and females, whereas bipolar II disorder is more common among females. Therefore, the daughter has a higher risk for developing bipolar II disorder than bipolar I disorder.

C (the daughter has a greater risk of developing a cyclothymic disorder than does the son) is incorrect. Cyclothymic disorder is equally common in males and females; each child has the same risk for this disorder.

D (the son has a greater risk of developing a depressive disorder than does the daughter) is incorrect. Females are twice as likely as males to develop a major depressive disorder and two to three times as likely to develop dysthymic disorder.

E   (the husband's diagnosis has no bearing on his children's risk of developing a mood disorder) is incorrect. Biological relatives of individuals with bipolar I disorder are at greater risk than others for development of a mood disorder.

33. A   (denial) is correct. Denial is a refusal to acknowledge threatening or anxiety-provoking events. Because the patient has symptoms that may be caused by cervical cancer and knows that her mother died of cervical cancer, she is most likely frightened. Denial is a way of coping with intense anxiety, although it is not very constructive for this patient.

B   (isolation) is incorrect. Isolation involves separating painful feelings from stressful situations (e.g., a patient describes her history of childhood sexual abuse in an objective, unemotional manner).

C   (reaction formation) is incorrect. Reaction formation involves behaving in a way that is the opposite of one's own unacceptable impulses (e.g., a woman who has strong unconscious feelings of anger and aggression is always nice to everyone and never loses her temper).

D   (regression) is incorrect. Regression involves returning to earlier patterns of behavior in response to stress (e.g., a hospitalized 5-year-old boy sucks his thumb and wets the bed).

E   (suppression) is incorrect. Suppression is voluntarily postponing attention to unwanted thoughts or feelings (e.g., a physician feels sexually attracted to a patient but consciously directs his attention back to the medical interview).

34. B   (health status of a newborn infant immediately after birth) is correct. An Apgar score lists five characteristics, each rated from 0 to 2: appearance, pulse, grimace, activity, and respiration. An Apgar score of 9 would indicate that an infant is in excellent condition.

A   (developmental milestones in children younger than 6 years of age) is incorrect. The Denver II Developmental Screening Test assesses motor, language, and social development in children younger than age 6.

C   (quality of attachment between an infant and its caregiver) is incorrect. There is no quantitative method for assessing quality of attachment that is commonly used in medical settings.

D   (stage of development of secondary sex characteristics) is incorrect. Tanner stages rate the level of development of secondary sex characteristics.

35. E (major depressive disorder) is correct. The patient has been experiencing a major depressive episode for 3 weeks. This diagnosis requires the presence of depressed mood or loss of interest in almost all activities plus at least four of the SIG E CAPS symptoms (i.e., sleep disturbance, loss of interest, guilt, loss of energy, impaired concentration, changed appetite, psychomotor agitation or retardation, and suicidal ideation). She has had a severely depressed mood (i.e., "in a black hole"). In addition, she has been experiencing sleep disturbance, loss of energy, impaired memory abilities (presumably due to difficulty concentrating), and decreased appetite with significant weight loss. This combination of symptoms qualifies the patient for a diagnosis of major depressive disorder.

A (adjustment disorder with depressed mood) is incorrect. Adjustment disorder with depressed mood is characterized by the development of clinically significant symptoms of depression in response to one or more identifiable psychosocial stressors. There is no evidence of such a stressor in this patient. In addition, a diagnosis of major depressive disorder takes precedence if the presenting symptoms meet the criteria for major depression.

B (bipolar I disorder) is incorrect. A diagnosis of bipolar I disorder requires a pattern of either manic or mixed episodes (usually alternating with some kind of depressive episode). There is no evidence of such a pattern in this patient.

C (bipolar II disorder) is incorrect. In bipolar II disorder, there is a pattern of one or more hypomanic episodes and recurrent major depressive episodes. There is no evidence of a hypomanic episode in this patient.

D (dysthymic disorder) is incorrect. A diagnosis of dysthymic disorder requires a pattern of depressed mood, on more days than not for a period of at least 2 years, accompanied by at least two of the HE SADe symptoms: hopelessness, low self-esteem, sleep disturbance, poor appetite or overeating, difficulty in making decisions, and low energy. This patient has experienced depressed mood for only 3 weeks.

36. A (anorexia nervosa) is correct. This patient has the essential features of anorexia nervosa, including maintenance of body weight significantly below normal, denial of the seriousness of her low weight, distorted perceptions of her own body size, and amenorrhea for at least 3 consecutive months.

B (bulimia nervosa) is incorrect. Bulimia nervosa involves repeated binge eating and use of inappropriate methods to prevent weight gain.

C (eating disorder not otherwise specified) is incorrect. Eating disorder not otherwise specified is the presence of clinically significant disordered eating behavior that does not meet the criteria for anorexia nervosa or bulimia nervosa. For example, this diagnosis would be appropriate if the patient had regular menstrual periods and, thus, did not meet all the criteria for anorexia nervosa.

D (major depressive disorder) is incorrect. Significant weight loss may occur in major depressive disorder, but patients usually do not want to lose an excessive amount of weight and do not have a strong fear of gaining weight.

E (obsessive-compulsive disorder) is incorrect. The patient does not have obsessions and compulsions. Obsessive-compulsive behavior related to food is common in patients with anorexia nervosa. However, an additional diagnosis of obsessive-compulsive disorder is not appropriate unless there are obsessions and compulsions unrelated to food.

37. B (nocturnal myoclonus) is correct. This patient has nocturnal myoclonus (periodic limb movement disorder), which is characterized by repetitive movements of the legs at 20- to 40-second intervals during sleep.

A (narcolepsy) is incorrect. Narcolepsy is characterized by daily episodes of suddenly falling asleep with cataplexy and sleep paralysis. Onset of narcolepsy typically occurs in the teens or young adulthood.

C (obstructive sleep apnea) is incorrect. Obstructive sleep apnea is characterized by episodic pauses in breathing during sleep.

D (restless leg syndrome) is incorrect. Restless leg syndrome is associated with difficulty falling asleep and daytime sleepiness, which is more common with aging. It is characterized by crawling sensations in the leg and irresistible urges to move the leg.

38. A (ego) is correct. According to Freud's structural model of the mind, the id pursues pleasure without consideration of consequences, whereas the ego moderates the impulses of the id and solves problems by examining the realistic consequences of an action. In this case, the man wanted the pleasure of drinking a glass of wine (an impulse of the id), but after thinking about the potential negative outcomes, he resisted the urge to drink. His decision was a function of the ego, which moderates the drives of the id so that its expression is appropriate for external circumstances.

B (id) is incorrect. The id operates under the pleasure principle; that is, pursuing pleasure without consideration of consequences. In this example, the urge to have a glass of wine is a function of the id.

C (superego) is incorrect. The superego represents an individual's moral values and standards of behavior. It influences the individual's determination of right and wrong. A scenario that is an example of the role of the superego might involve the man thinking about the shame he would experience by drinking and thus falling short of his own aspiration of abstinence. The superego offers approval or disapproval of behavior, but the decision to engage in a particular behavior is a function of the ego.

D (unconscious mind) is incorrect. The unconscious mind contains thoughts that are outside of awareness. In this example, the man's decision to abstain from drinking a glass of wine was purposeful and made with an awareness of the potential consequences of drinking.

39. D (dysthymic disorder) is correct. The diagnosis of dysthymic disorder requires a pattern of depressed mood that occurs more days than not for at least 2 years and is accompanied by at least two of the HE SADe symptoms: hopelessness, low self-esteem, sleep disturbance, poor appetite or overeating, difficulty in making decisions, and low energy. This patient's depressed mood fits this pattern; she has two of the HE SADe symptoms: sleep disturbance and worthlessness (i.e., thinks that she is hopelessly incompetent).

A (adjustment disorder with depressed mood) is incorrect. Adjustment disorder with depressed mood is characterized by onset of symptoms of depression within 3 months after the occurrence of an identifiable stressor. In this case, the symptoms began many years ago, ruling out adjustment disorder with depressed mood.

B (bipolar II disorder) is incorrect. A major feature of bipolar II disorder is recurrent major depressive episodes. The symptoms of depression described in this case *do not* involve at least four SIG E CAPS symptoms: sleep disturbance, loss of interest in most activities, excessive guilt, loss of energy, impaired concentration, appetite change, psychomotor agitation or retardation, or suicidal ideation. Therefore, bipolar II disorder is ruled out.

C (cyclothymic disorder) is incorrect. Cyclothymic disorder involves periods of depression and hypomania that are not severe enough to meet the criteria for major depressive and manic episodes. Because this case involves depression only, cyclothymic disorder is ruled out.

E (major depressive disorder) is incorrect. The depression described in this case *does not* involve enough SIG E CAPS symptoms to qualify as a major depressive episode; therefore, major depressive disorder is ruled out. Refer to the discussion for B.

40. A (bias and confounding have not been excluded as likely explanations of the results) is correct. Statistical significance means only that the observed association is unlikely to have occurred by chance. Results that are not due to chance might be due to bias or confounding, rather than to a causal relationship between the exposure and outcome. Bias is systematic error and is avoided through proper study design and execution. Confounding occurs when an extraneous factor confuses, or confounds, understanding of the association between an exposure and an outcome.

   B (the result does not focus on mortality associated with a specific medical disorder) is incorrect. The concept of risk factor can be applied to any medical outcome, including mortality in general or mortality associated with specific medical conditions.

   C (the result may not be clinically important) is incorrect. Not all statistically significant associations have clinical importance, but clinical importance is irrelevant to the issue here.

   D (the sample size is too small) is incorrect. As sample size increases, statistical power or ability to detect an association increases. Thus, small sample size resulting in low statistical power could explain why a study failed to find that an association was statistically significant. However, if a study finds an association to be statistically significant, small sample size does not negate this conclusion.

41. A (Babinski reflex) is correct. The Babinski, or plantar, reflex is present in young infants. It normally disappears by 2–14 months of age.

   B (grasp reflex) is incorrect. The grasp, or palmar, reflex is elicited by placing an object in the palm of the infant's hand. The reflex usually disappears by 5–6 months of age.

   C (Moro reflex) is incorrect. When an infant is startled or feels as though she is falling, she will throw out both arms symmetrically (Moro, or startle, reflex). This reflex should disappear by 3–6 months of age.

   D (rooting reflex) is incorrect. The rooting reflex is seen when the infant turns her head and opens her mouth as her cheek is being stroked. The rooting reflex normally disappears by 3–4 months of age.

   E (stepping reflex) is incorrect. The stepping reflex is the infant's walking movements when she is being held upright. The reflex usually disappears by 2–3 months of age.

42. A (arrange to have a psychiatric consultation to assess the patient's decisional capacity) is correct. In this case, the physician is questioning whether the patient has decisional capacity. In the absence of a life-threatening emergency, requesting a psychiatric consultation to assist in this determination is an appropriate step.

B (declare the patient legally incompetent to make health care decisions) is incorrect. Competence is a legal term, and only a court can determine whether a patient is incompetent. The physician cannot legally declare the patient incompetent, even if the physician is correct in assuming that the patient lacks decisional capacity.

C (determine whether there is family consensus to proceed with surgery) is incorrect. In certain situations, family representatives may be consulted about the care of a patient. In this case, it appears that there is time for the physician to gather additional information about the patient's decisional capacity without obvious risk to the patient and prior to involving the family in decisions about the patient's medical care.

D (proceed with surgery without the patient's express consent) is incorrect. Patient autonomy refers to a patient's right to make decisions about his or her medical care, and informed consent is the process by which an individual gives consent for medical treatment. In this case, proceeding without the patient's consent is not warranted.

43. A (alcohol) is correct. Alcohol use may lead to cerebellar degeneration and subsequent ataxia. Unsteadiness on the feet may be noted during intoxication with other drugs, but not as a residual effect.

B (amphetamines) is incorrect. Amphetamines generally are not associated with CT findings. They are more likely to cause hyperactivity and possibly paranoia.

C (benzodiazepines) is incorrect. Although benzodiazepines may produce an unsteady gait, particularly in the elderly, they are not associated with anatomic pathologic changes such as cerebellar degeneration.

D (cocaine) is incorrect. Cocaine use can produce lacunar ischemia that can be visualized on CT, MRI, and functional imaging scans, but these findings are more widespread and are not confined to a particular portion of the brain.

E (opiates) is incorrect. Opiate intoxication may cause unsteadiness but not the long-term anatomic changes in the cerebellum seen on this patient's CT scan.

44. D (norepinephrine in the sympathetic system) is correct. The noradrenergic response of sympathetic nervous system fibers causes elevated blood pressure and elevated heart rate with increased anxiety.

A (acetylcholine in the parasympathetic system) and B (acetylcholine in the sympathetic system) are incorrect. Although there are some cholinergic fibers in the sympathetic nervous system, most are in the parasympathetic system, where they act in an inhibitory fashion, or in the central nervous system, with broad projections from the nucleus basalis of Meynert to the cerebral cortex and limbic system, where they are associated with memory function.

C (dopamine in the reticular activating system) is incorrect. Dopamine is found in the striatal tracts of the brain and plays a role in mood, emotion, and thought disorders.

E (serotonin in the limbic system) is incorrect. Serotonin is widely distributed throughout the brain, but limbic system responses involve memory and attachment of emotion to perceptions and memories, not peripheral or visceral responses.

45. D (increase in sleep stages 1 and 2) is correct. Sleep becomes increasingly fragmented and lighter with advancing age. As individuals age, less time is spent in the deepest stages of sleep (stages 3 and 4) and more time is spent in the lighter stages of sleep (stages 1 and 2). Although variable among individuals, deep or delta sleep may be virtually nonexistent by the elderly years.

A (decrease in nighttime awakenings) is incorrect. An increase in the number of awakenings during the sleep period is common as one ages. Multiple awakenings can reduce the quality of a night's sleep.

B (increase in delta sleep) is incorrect. A healthy young adult spends about 25% of sleep time in delta sleep. The proportion of time spent in delta sleep diminishes with advancing age.

C (increase in rapid eye movement sleep) is incorrect. Advancing age is associated with a decrease in REM sleep. Newborns, on the other hand, spend about 50% of sleep time in REM sleep.

46. C (proceed with surgery while continuing efforts are made to contact the parents for consent) is correct. Emergency medical care may be given to a minor if attempts to contact the parents or legal guardian are unsuccessful and delaying treatment would endanger the patient's life or health. In this case, the physician is justified in providing treatment without parental consent.

A (ask the dance instructor to provide consent in lieu of the parents) is incorrect. The girl's parents hold the right to authorize treatment for their child.

B (keep the patient comfortable until the parents can be reached) is incorrect. This might be an appropriate course of action in a nonemergency situation.

D (seek emergency authorization from the court to proceed with surgery) is incorrect. In certain circumstances, when parents refuse to consent to treatment for their child, seeking court authorization for care may be warranted. In the case described, the parents have not specifically refused treatment.

---

47. E (memory) is correct. This test is designed to assess the patient's immediate recall and the ability to retain information over a brief period of time.

A (abstract thought) is incorrect. Abstract thought is assessed by asking the patient to interpret proverbs. For example, a patient might be asked to interpret the meaning of the expression, "No use crying over spilled milk."

B (concentration) is incorrect. The patient's ability to concentrate is examined by asking him or her to spell the word "world" backward or to subtract serial 7s starting from 100 (i.e., 100, 93, 86, and so on).

C (fund of knowledge) is incorrect. Fund of knowledge is assessed in general conversation with the patient and provides a rough estimate of the patient's intelligence and educational level.

D (judgment) is incorrect. Judgment is assessed by evaluating the patient's thought and behavior as reflected in the general history (e.g., rational versus impulsive or harmful behavior). It is also formally tested with such questions as, "What would you do if you found a stamped, addressed envelope lying by a mailbox?"

---

48. A (akathisia) is correct. Akathisia, the inability to rest or remain still, is an adverse effect seen with antipsychotic drugs. Had the symptoms been due to the primary illness, an increased dose of the drug might have been helpful. This acute extrapyramidal effect is more pronounced in antipsychotics that work primarily by blockade of dopamine receptors.

B (akinesia) is incorrect. Akinesia, difficulty initiating movements, is a possible side effect of antipsychotic drugs.

C (dystonia) is incorrect. Dystonia is an acute extrapyramidal effect that occurs with the use of many antipsychotic drugs, and is a state of abnormal muscle tension that often affects the neck and facial muscles. It may be seen as oculogyric crisis, in which the eyeballs become fixed in one position, or as torticollis, a painful twisting of the neck and unnatural head position.

D (neuroleptic malignant syndrome) is incorrect. In NMS, muscle rigidity develops in the presence of hyperthermia, elevated creatine kinase levels, elevated blood pressure and heart rate, and delirium.

E (tardive dyskinesia) is incorrect. Tardive dyskinesia is an irregular, choreoathetotic movement disorder that affects the head, limbs, and trunk. It usually develops after months or years of antipsychotic treatment.

49. C (marital relationship) is correct. The factor that appears to be a significant precipitant to this patient's erectile dysfunction is the recent discord in his marital relationship. Although stress and fatigue may contribute to erectile difficulties, these factors are essentially stable and are therefore less likely to be significant contributors to his problem. Because the difficulties began following marital distress, the distress is likely a primary contributor.

A (age) is incorrect. Although certain changes in sexual function occur with aging (e.g., an increased need for stimulation to facilitate erection, an increase in the refractory period), erectile dysfunction itself is not a result of aging. Thus, aging is not a likely factor contributing to this patient's erectile difficulties.

B (long work hours) is incorrect. If this patient's long work hours are associated with stress or fatigue, these factors could contribute to erectile problems. However, in this case, the patient reports a stable work history, with no specific changes in hours or stress level. Thus, these factors are not likely to be primarily contributing to his erectile difficulties.

D (stress level) is incorrect. Stress can contribute to erectile problems, but in this case, the patient reports that his stress level has not changed. His erectile problem is acute and coincides with marital tension. Thus, it is unlikely that his stress level is a primary contributor to his erectile difficulties.

50. D (Native Americans) is correct. Suicide rates for Native Americans (American Indians and Alaska Natives) are higher than suicide rates for all racial and ethnic minority populations and the general population in the United States. Native-American adolescent and young adult males have especially high rates of suicide.

A (African Americans) is incorrect. African Americans have the lowest suicide rate of all racial and ethnic minority populations, although they have higher rates for many other causes of death (e.g., cardiovascular disease, cancer, stroke, and homicide).

B (Asian Americans) and C (Hispanic Americans) are incorrect. Asian Americans and Hispanic Americans have low rates of suicide. Refer to the discussions for A and D.

TEST 2

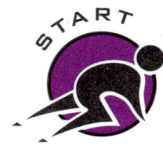

DIRECTIONS: Each numbered item or incomplete statement is followed by options arranged in alphabetical or logical order. Select the best answer to each question. Some options may be partially correct, but there is only **ONE BEST** answer.

1. A 25-year-old woman comes to the emergency department for the third time in the past month complaining of rapid heart rate, weakness, and shortness of breath. Results of the physical examination, laboratory screening including thyroid indices, and ECG are negative. Which drug would be the best choice for providing appropriate and immediate symptom relief for this patient?

○ A. Alprazolam
○ B. Bupropion
○ C. Carbamazepine
○ D. Haloperidol
○ E. Imipramine

2. A physician asks a new patient what caused the scar on his forehead. The patient says that a few months ago he, his wife, and their son were in an automobile accident in which he was injured and his wife and son were killed. He describes the accident without any noticeable emotion. Which of the following defense mechanisms most likely explains this patient's response?

○ A. Altruism
○ B. Displacement
○ C. Isolation
○ D. Rationalization
○ E. Splitting

3. A 59-year-old man sees his physician because he is having intermittent heart palpitations and difficulty sleeping. He has lost 2.2 kg (5 lb) since his wife died in an automobile accident 1 month ago. The patient tells the physician that he is unable to concentrate at work, frequently dreams about his wife, and sometimes thinks he sees her, momentarily, sitting in her favorite chair. This patient is most likely experiencing

○ A. clinical depression
○ B. complicated grief
○ C. delusions
○ D. normal grief

4. Investigators conduct a study comparing mortality risks in men and women 1 year after acute myocardial infarction (MI). The study finds the relative risk for mortality in women compared with men to be 1.33 (95% CI: 0.85–2.48). What can be concluded about the difference in mortality risks between women and men 1 year after an acute MI?

○ A. The higher mortality risk in women may be due to chance
○ B. Men experience higher mortality risk than women
○ C. Mortality risk in women is equal to mortality risk in men
○ D. Mortality risk in women is significantly higher than in men
○ E. Women do not experience higher mortality risk than men

5. The mother of a teenage girl who was killed by a drunken driver initially fantasizes about ways to kill the driver. She then begins to focus her energy on working to strengthen the legal consequences of driving under the influence of alcohol. This mother's behavior is an example of which of the following defense mechanisms?

○ A. Denial
○ B. Displacement
○ C. Intellectualization
○ D. Reaction formation
○ E. Sublimation

6. A physician orders a hospital bed for a 74-year-old woman with emphysema who is being discharged from the hospital and is going home. In addition to her monthly Social Security check, the patient receives a modest income from financial investments and has a savings account. Which of the following sources will pay the largest portion of the charge for the hospital bed?

○ A. Medicaid
○ B. Medicare Part A
○ C. Medicare Part B
○ D. The patient and her family

7. Which of the following sleep findings can be observed in a patient with major depression?

○ A. Increased delta sleep
○ B. Increased total sleep time
○ C. Predominance of rapid eye movement (REM) sleep in later part of night
○ D. Shortened REM latency

8. A 44-year-old man has been irritable and unable to concentrate, and has not slept well for the past 5 weeks. His medical workup is normal. His symptoms began after he was held up by a robber at the store where he works. He feels nauseated when he goes to work each day and refuses to talk about the incident. Which of the following is the most likely diagnosis?

○ A. Acute stress disorder
○ B. Adjustment disorder with anxiety
○ C. Generalized anxiety disorder
○ D. Posttraumatic stress disorder (PTSD)
○ E. Social phobia

9. A physician is taking a history from a patient and says, "I'm not sure if I have this right. You said that you have not been treated for depression before, but you recently have used fluoxetine. Was the fluoxetine for depression or for something else?" The physician's effort to clarify the patient's history is known as

○ A. confrontation
○ B. empathy
○ C. facilitating
○ D. reflecting
○ E. validation

10. A 25-year-old married woman tells the young physician who is taking her medical history that he is very handsome. During the interview, the patient is flirtatious and makes other sexually oriented comments. Which of the following approaches is most appropriate for the physician to use in this situation?

○ A. He should ask a nurse to be present during the examination
○ B. He should ask the patient how things are going in her marriage
○ C. He should ignore the patient's sexual behavior to avoid reinforcing it
○ D. He should respond flirtatiously to establish a positive rapport with the patient

11. Disinhibition of behavior is most closely associated with injury to which area of the brain?

○ A. Basal ganglia
○ B. Frontal lobes
○ C. Parietal lobes
○ D. Reticular activating system
○ E. Temporal lobes

12. A 9-year-old girl whose family recently immigrated to the United States from Cambodia is brought to the physician's office with symptoms of fever, dizziness, and tightness in her chest. While conducting the physical examination, the physician notices bruises on the girl's back that form striped patterns. Which of the following is the most likely cause of the bruises?

○ A. Accidental injury
○ B. Child abuse
○ C. Coining
○ D. Cupping

13. A 72-year-old woman says that she began feeling depressed shortly after the death of her husband 3 months ago. She adds that she cannot sleep or eat, is tired all the time, is forgetful, feels like she is "no good to anybody," and often stays in bed all day without dressing or eating. Which of the following is the most likely diagnosis?

○ A. Bereavement
○ B. Bipolar II disorder
○ C. Dysthymic disorder
○ D. Major depressive disorder

14. A young girl has established her gender identity, knows how old she is, has achieved bladder and bowel control, uses complete sentences, and can ride a tricycle. The age of this child is most likely

○ A. 18 months
○ B. 2 years
○ C. 3 years
○ D. 4 years
○ E. 5 years

15. A man grew up feeling sad and helpless because his younger brother was severely mentally retarded. For the past 20 years, he has been a volunteer in the Special Olympics. This type of volunteer service is an example of which of the following defense mechanisms?

○ A. Altruism
○ B. Displacement
○ C. Rationalization
○ D. Reaction formation
○ E. Sublimation

16. Several weeks after beginning paroxetine treatment for depression, a 30-year-old woman experiences racing thoughts, is unable to sleep, and yells at family members over trivial conflicts. She reports that she has been called as a special envoy for world peace and has created an internet site to receive messages regarding her mission. Which drug would be the best choice to add to her treatment regimen?

○ A. Diazepam
○ B. Imipramine
○ C. Lithium
○ D. Methylphenidate
○ E. Phenelzine

17. A 55-year-old man has metastatic lung cancer and is expected to die within 2 months. He has asked to see his sister, with whom he has not spoken in 10 years. He seems calm and peaceful. According to Elisabeth Kübler-Ross, the patient is in which stage of dying?

○ A. Acceptance
○ B. Anger
○ C. Bargaining
○ D. Denial
○ E. Depression

18. A 12-year-old girl is diagnosed with a sexually transmitted disease. During the evaluation, the girl discloses that a family friend has been sexually abusing her. The mother does not believe her daughter's accusations and tells the physician that her daughter has a boyfriend with whom she must be sexually active. The physician is mandated by law to

○ A. admit the patient to the hospital
○ B. ask the mother to agree to supervised visits with the friend
○ C. contact the family friend and recommend that he get psychological help
○ D. report the abuse to child protective services

19. For the past 2 months, a 35-year-old critical care nurse who has worked the night shift for many years tosses and turns in bed for over an hour each day before falling asleep. The problem began during a stressful period at her job, which has improved. She does not drink caffeinated beverages or alcohol, is taking no medications, and does not use illicit drugs. She is in otherwise good health but frustrated by her sleep problems. She falls asleep easily when she stays overnight with friends on weekends. Which of the following is the most likely diagnosis?

○ A. Adjustment disorder with anxiety
○ B. Circadian rhythm sleep disorder
○ C. Psychophysiologic insomnia
○ D. Substance-induced sleep disorder

20. A 38-year-old woman, who is overweight, seeks help from her physician in planning a regular exercise program. The physician suggests that the patient walk 15 minutes three times a week. At her next appointment, the physician congratulates her for maintaining the walking regimen and suggests that she increase her program to eventually walk 30 minutes five times a week. Which of the following behavioral principles is the physician using in this exercise program?

○ A. Cognitive restructuring
○ B. Reinforcement
○ C. Self-monitoring
○ D. Shaping

21. The news anchor of a local television station slips on ice and goes to the emergency department. He is taken to a private curtained area and while the nurse takes his blood pressure and pulse rate, he recounts the story of his climb to "the top" in the news industry. When the physician arrives, the patient becomes irate and demands to be seen by the "chief of staff." This patient's personality style is best described as

○ A. dependent
○ B. histrionic
○ C. narcissistic
○ D. paranoid

22. A 50-year-old man is most likely to have experienced which of the following normal changes in sexual functioning as he has aged?

○ A. Decreased duration of the refractory period following orgasm
○ B. Increased force of ejaculation
○ C. Need for more direct stimulation to facilitate erection
○ D. Significant decrease in interest in sexual relations

23. A 45-year-old man visits his primary care physician because he has a severe rash on his back. The physician refers the patient to a dermatologist who is associated with the patient's health care plan. However, the patient wants to see the dermatologist who treated his sister but who is not associated with his health care plan. The patient knows that if he sees his sister's dermatologist, his insurance will not cover any of the cost of the visit. This patient is most likely insured through which of the following plans?

○ A. Fee-for-service plan
○ B. Health maintenance organization (HMO)
○ C. HMO with a point of service option (POS)
○ D. Preferred provider organization (PPO)

24. A 28-year-old man with obsessive-compulsive disorder (OCD) is asked by his therapist to touch a doorknob that he feels is contaminated with germs and then to refrain from washing his hands immediately afterward. After about an hour has passed without handwashing, the patient notices that his anxiety about being contaminated has decreased. Which of the following treatments is the therapist using?

○ A. Cognitive restructuring
○ B. Exposure and response prevention
○ C. Flooding
○ D. Imaginal exposure
○ E. Relapse prevention

25. A 37-year-old man who is about to be discharged from the hospital pleads with his physician to continue testing until his unexplained tachycardia, hypertension, and face flushing can be diagnosed. The physician is aware that the nursing staff discovered a half-full box of pseudoephedrine under the patient's mattress. Which of the following is the most likely diagnosis?

○ A. Factitious disorder
○ B. Hypochondriasis
○ C. Malingering
○ D. Psychological factors affecting general medical condition

26. The four-stage theory of cognitive development that describes how children understand the world as they grow older is attributed to

○ A. Chess and Thomas
○ B. Erikson
○ C. Freud
○ D. Piaget
○ E. Tanner

27. A physician asks a 30-year-old woman about a history of sexual abuse. The patient denies any abuse and does not remember that when she was 5 years old she was taken to the emergency department and treated for injuries resulting from sexual abuse by her father. Which of the following defense mechanisms most likely accounts for this woman's inability to remember the traumatic events of her childhood?

○ A. Isolation
○ B. Repression
○ C. Splitting
○ D. Sublimation
○ E. Suppression

28. A 45-year-old man has been receiving chlorpromazine to treat symptoms of schizophrenia for 20 years. The physician notes that the patient occasionally grimaces involuntarily. Which of the following adverse effects is this patient experiencing?

○ A. Akathisia
○ B. Dystonia
○ C. Neuroleptic malignant syndrome (NMS)
○ D. Tardive dyskinesia

29. Which of the following is the leading cause of death among young adults?

○ A. HIV/AIDS
○ B. Homicide
○ C. Malignant neoplasm
○ D. Suicide
○ E. Unintentional injury

30. Of 50 patients followed after being diagnosed with cancer, 10 patients survive for 5 years. What is the probability that two randomly selected patients, A and B, survive for 5 years?

○ A. 4%
○ B. 20%
○ C. 36%
○ D. 40%
○ E. 64%

31. The medical director of an outpatient clinic finds an open bottle of alcohol in the back seat of a colleague's automobile. Several days later, the physician comes to work with the smell of alcohol on his breath and has slurred speech. Which of the following is the director's most appropriate response?

○ A. Contact the colleague's wife to plan a family intervention
○ B. Institute a random drug-screening policy for all clinic employees
○ C. Place a brochure about Alcoholics Anonymous on the colleague's desk
○ D. Talk with the colleague about his alcohol use and help him to arrange treatment

32. The neighbors of a 28-year-old man with bipolar disorder tell the police that the man has been talking incessantly and has not eaten or slept for several days. The police find the man naked in his backyard painting a self-portrait that he says he is doing because of instructions he received in a secret message. He is taken to the emergency department and held on an involuntary basis. He is cooperative but refuses to take prescribed medication. Which statement best describes the rights of this patient in refusing treatment?

○ A. The patient can be forced to take the medication because of his involuntary status
○ B. The patient can refuse medication even if involuntarily committed
○ C. The patient is considered incompetent to make treatment decisions
○ D. The patient must be released within 8 hours if he refuses treatment

33. A 32-year-old woman goes to the emergency department because she is having acute upper abdominal pain. Results of a physical examination and laboratory studies fail to explain her symptoms. A review of her medical history indicates that she has a 10-year history of numerous complaints of gastrointestinal, pseudoneurologic, and sexual pain, none of which can be explained by medical findings. Which of the following is the most appropriate diagnosis?

○ A. Conversion disorder
○ B. Factitious disorder
○ C. Hypochondriasis
○ D. Somatization disorder

34. A 26-year-old man has been having spontaneous panic attacks several times a week for the past few months. During these attacks, the patient experiences shortness of breath, feelings of terror, dizziness, and palpitations. His physician diagnoses panic disorder and prescribes medication. Which of the following drugs is preferred for long-term management of panic disorder?

○ A. Alprazolam
○ B. Carbamazepine
○ C. Haloperidol
○ D. Imipramine
○ E. Sertraline

35. Two years ago, a 72-year-old woman had a stroke and is unable to care for herself. She lives with her daughter, son-in-law, and two grandsons. Her daughter, who provides most of her care, frequently yells at her and belittles her. Her grandsons frequently ignore her and sometimes barge into her room without knocking. Which type of elder abuse or neglect is this woman most likely experiencing?

○ A. Abandonment
○ B. Emotional abuse
○ C. Financial and material exploitation
○ D. Neglect
○ E. Physical abuse

36. A physician is interviewing an injured boy and his father and strongly suspects that the father caused the boy's injuries. The physician is angry with the father and has an urge to verbally attack him. She decides to focus her attention on the medical care of the injured child, but later expresses her anger about the boy's father to a colleague. The physician's behavior is an example of which of the following defense mechanisms?

○ A. Denial
○ B. Identification
○ C. Isolation
○ D. Repression
○ E. Suppression

37. Which of the following techniques is a psychoanalyst most likely to use in treating a patient with depression?

○ A. Biofeedback
○ B. In vivo exposure
○ C. Interpretation of transference
○ D. Positive reinforcement
○ E. Systematic desensitization

38. A 50-year-old man who is an alcoholic is given a medication that will cause him to become nauseated if he ingests alcohol. This treatment approach is based on

○ A. aversive conditioning
○ B. biofeedback
○ C. positive reinforcement
○ D. shaping

39. For the past month, a 27-year-old woman has had episodes in which she experiences tightness in the chest, dizziness, sweating, and feelings of terror. The first episode occurred while she was in a movie theater, and she became so frightened that she sought emergency care. Her medical workup was normal, but she continues to have the same acute symptoms. She engages in her normal routine despite symptoms. She reports a high level of stress since moving to a different state to start a new job. Which of the following is the most likely diagnosis?

○ A. Acute stress disorder
○ B. Agoraphobia
○ C. Hypochondriasis
○ D. Panic disorder
○ E. Specific phobia

40. The male sexual response cycle differs from the female sexual response cycle by the presence of which of the following phenomena?

○ A. Excitement phase
○ B. Plateau phase
○ C. Refractory period
○ D. Resolution phase

41. An 8-year-old boy has been worrying about his mother being killed by terrorists while she is at work. He has recently experienced nausea and vomiting and has headaches before going to school. He wants to drop out of his soccer team and Boy Scout troop. Which of the following is the most likely diagnosis?

○ A. Attention-deficit/hyperactivity disorder (ADHD)
○ B. Autistic disorder
○ C. Conduct disorder
○ D. Oppositional defiant disorder
○ E. Separation anxiety disorder

42. A 75-year-old woman with cancer refuses to undergo further chemotherapy, saying that she has had a good life and wishes to "let nature take its course." Her family and physician believe that she is capable of taking care of herself and that she fully understands the risks of discontinuing treatment and the potential benefits of further treatment, but they strongly disagree with her decision. Which of the following is the physician's best course of action?

○ A. Honor the patient's request to discontinue treatment
○ B. Informally appoint another family member to make decisions about her treatment
○ C. Instruct the family to pursue court proceedings to declare her incompetent
○ D. Tell the family to give her the medication without her knowledge

43. Public health officials need to decide whether to devote their resources to reducing two risk factors for asthma in their city: environmental factor A or environmental factor B. The officials seek to know the potential risk reduction in the city if one of the factors is eliminated. Which statistic calculated for each factor would best supply this information?

○ A. Absolute risk
○ B. Attributable risk
○ C. Odds ratio
○ D. Prevalence
○ E. Risk ratio

44. A 24-year-old woman is being evaluated for complaints of suicidal thoughts. She states that she doesn't want to kill herself but sometimes has thoughts of overdosing on her medications. Which of the following drugs would be the best first-line treatment of depression for this patient?

○ A. Clomipramine
○ B. Fluoxetine
○ C. Lithium
○ D. Nortriptyline
○ E. Phenelzine

45. A 45-year-old man who has recently had coronary bypass surgery is nagged incessantly by his wife, who says that she worries about his health when he does not follow the prescribed dietary restrictions. When the man follows his prescribed diet, his wife stops nagging him. Which of the following learning principles best explains this patient's increased adherence to dietary recommendations?

○ A. Extinction
○ B. Negative reinforcement
○ C. Positive reinforcement
○ D. Punishment
○ E. Shaping

46. For the past 2 weeks, a 30-year-old woman has had trouble sleeping and concentrating after witnessing an automobile accident in which a pedestrian was killed. She feels dazed and emotionally detached from her husband and says things seem unreal. She has been unable to drive or return to work since the accident. Which of the following is the most likely diagnosis?

○ A. Acute stress disorder
○ B. Adjustment disorder with anxiety
○ C. Generalized anxiety disorder
○ D. Specific phobia (driving phobia)

47. An accident victim is brought to the emergency department unconscious. The man has no family with him and no personal identification. The physician is unable to obtain the patient's consent for emergency surgery to repair a ruptured spleen and proceeds with the surgery. The physician has acted under which of the following assumptions?

○ A. Implied consent
○ B. Nonmaleficence
○ C. Therapeutic privilege
○ D. Waiver of consent

48. Clinical investigators compare the results of a new diagnostic test for cancer with biopsy results in 100 consecutive patients. Biopsy is the gold standard. The investigators find that 35 of the 40 patients with cancer, as determined by biopsy, test positive on the new diagnostic test, and 45 of the 60 patients without cancer, as determined by biopsy, test negative on the new diagnostic test. Based on this information, what is the specificity of the new diagnostic test?

○ A. 40%
○ B. 70%
○ C. 75%
○ D. 87.5%
○ E. 90%

49. In which of the following clinical situations is it appropriate to disclose confidential information without the patient's consent?

○ A. A 20-year-old man who has suicidal thoughts but denies intent or plan
○ B. A father who punishes his child by locking him in a closet for hours
○ C. A mother who refuses an experimental treatment for her terminally ill 8-year-old daughter
○ D. A patient who is agitated but denies homicidal thoughts

50. A war veteran who has been diagnosed with posttraumatic stress disorder (PTSD) experiences a startle reflex and hears gunshots. Which of the following medications would most likely be prescribed for this patient?

○ A. Buspirone and fluoxetine
○ B. Clonidine and olanzapine
○ C. Lorazepam
○ D. Lorazepam and fluoxetine

ANSWERS AND DISCUSSIONS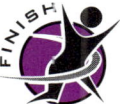

1. A (alprazolam) is correct. This patient has symptoms of a panic attack. Alprazolam will provide the most rapid and appropriate relief in the treatment of panic disorder. This drug increases the amount of GABA binding to receptor sites.

B (bupropion) is incorrect. Bupropion is a dopaminergic antide-pressant without benefit in panic disorder.

C (carbamazepine) is incorrect. The anticonvulsant carbamaze-pine is commonly used as a mood stabilizer in bipolar disor-der, but it is not indicated for panic attacks.

D (haloperidol) is incorrect. Haloperidol is a conventional high-potency antipsychotic used to treat schizophrenia and Tou-rette's disorder. It has no indication for panic disorder.

E (imipramine) is incorrect. Although an effective long-term treatment for panic disorder, the tricyclic antidepressant imipramine requires several weeks to reach therapeutic blood levels. It has been largely replaced as a treatment for anxiety disorders by the safer selective serotonin reuptake inhibitors.

2. C (isolation) is correct. Isolation is the separation of painful feelings from stressful situations. In this example, the loss of his wife and son must have been extremely distressing to this patient. To cope with talking about the traumatic event, the patient has isolated his feelings from his description of the acci-dent to the physician.

A (altruism) is incorrect. Altruism is serving others as a way of dealing with painful feelings. For example, a man who lost a leg in an accident volunteers at camps for children with physi-cal disabilities.

B (displacement) is incorrect. Displacement is redirecting feel-ings about a person or situation to a less intimidating person or situation. For example, a resident feels humiliated by her at-tending physician and then is overly critical of the medical student that she is supervising.

D (rationalization) is incorrect. Rationalization is using logical explanations to justify feelings or behavior that seems unrea-sonable. For example, a mother who dipped her son in scalding water for punishment says that the boy needs to learn to respect authority.

E (splitting) is incorrect. Splitting is the perception of people and situations as either all positive or all negative. For example, a patient is extremely satisfied with her physician. At a recent visit, however, she is diagnosed with hypertension and the physician advises her to lose weight. She becomes extremely angry and tells him that he is the worst doctor she has ever known.

3. D (normal grief) is correct. The physical, psychological, and cognitive responses reported by the patient are all characteristics of normal grief. Other characteristics of normal grief include chest tightness, lack of energy, sadness, anger, guilt, disbelief, and confusion.

A (clinical depression) is incorrect. According to the *Diagnostic and Statistical Manual of Mental Disorders,* 4th edition, text revision (DSM-IV-TR), a diagnosis of clinical depression is usually not assigned until at least 2 months after the loss. Clinical depression also has symptoms that are not usually seen with normal grief. These symptoms include feeling hopeless and worthless; not relating the depressed feelings to any specific event, including the loss; feeling excessive guilt; and having suicidal thoughts.

B (complicated grief) is incorrect. A patient who experiences complicated grief is experiencing grief that is prolonged, intense, postponed, or suppressed. It also may interfere with his or her health or ability to function. This patient's spouse has recently died and although he is experiencing minor health problems and an inability to concentrate at work, these symptoms are not sufficient to be considered complicated grief.

C (delusions) is incorrect. A delusion is a false, fixed belief held by an individual suffering from psychosis. This patient does not have symptoms of psychosis. Individuals who suffer from clinical depression also may have hallucinations and delusions.

4. A (the higher mortality risk in women may be due to chance) is correct. This relative risk is the ratio of risk of acute MI in women compared with men (risk in women/risk in men = 1.33/1). At first glance, it appears that women have a 33% higher risk of acute MI mortality than men; however, this is only a sample-based estimate of the risk of acute MI mortality in all women compared with all men. Thus, although the investigators have little confidence that the actual risk ratio in all women compared with all men is exactly 1.33, the confidence interval (CI) for this risk ratio indicates that they can conclude with 95% confidence that the actual risk ratio is between 0.85 and 2.48 (see figure below). If the risk of acute MI mortality does not differ in women and men, the risk ratio will be 1.0. Because 1.0 is within the 95% CI, the investigators cannot exclude with 95% confidence the possibility that the actual risk ratio is 1.0. Therefore, they cannot exclude with 95% confidence the possibility that risk of acute MI mortality is not different in women and men and that the apparently greater risk in women is due to chance.

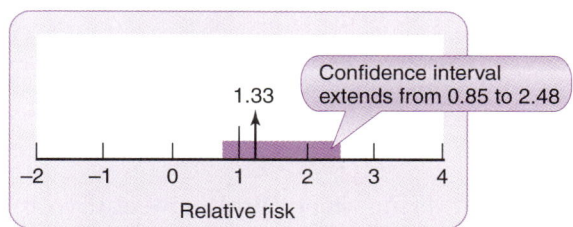

B (men experience higher mortality risk than women) is incorrect. If men experienced greater risk than women, the risk ratio for women compared with men (risk in women/risk in men) would be less than 1.0.

C (mortality risk in women is equal to mortality risk in men) and E (women do not experience higher mortality risk than men) are incorrect. These options state in an unequivocal way that women and men have the same risk of acute MI mortality (i.e., they both accept the null hypothesis). However, the evidence here does not support a statement of such strength. The evidence indicates that the investigators did not find a difference in risk between women and men that could not be attributed to chance; however, the possibility remains that there is an actual difference that the investigators failed to find with this study.

D (mortality risk in women is significantly higher than in men) is incorrect. For mortality risk in women to be significantly higher than in men, the 95% CI must not encompass the value of 1.0.

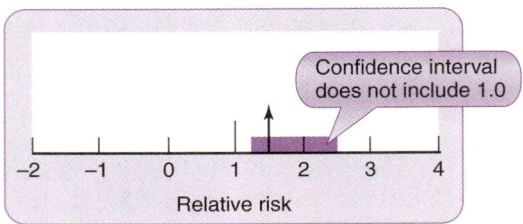

5. E (sublimation) is correct. Sublimation involves channeling unacceptable drives and impulses into socially acceptable activities. Instead of trying to harm the drunken driver who killed her daughter, this mother focuses her efforts on strengthening the penalties for drunken drivers.

A (denial) is incorrect. Denial involves refusing to acknowledge threatening or anxiety-provoking events. For example, a 50-year-old woman with a family history of breast cancer finds a lump in her breast but waits 2 months before seeing her physician.

B (displacement) is incorrect. Displacement involves redirecting feelings from an original source to a more acceptable substitute. For example, a resident feels humiliated by her attending physician and then is overly critical of the medical student under her supervision.

C (intellectualization) is incorrect. Intellectualization involves excessive focus on intellectual aspects of difficult situations to avoid painful feelings. For example, a physician tells a married couple that the woman has lung cancer. When the couple returns home, the husband sits at the computer for several hours, reading about treatments for lung cancer.

D (reaction formation) is incorrect. Reaction formation involves adopting behaviors that are the opposite of one's unacceptable impulses. For example, a woman who has strong unconscious feelings of anger and aggression is always nice to everyone and never loses her temper.

6. C (Medicare Part B) is correct. This patient is older than 65 years of age and is eligible for Medicare benefits. Medicare Part B pays for durable medical equipment, including hospital beds, wheelchairs, and walkers. The patient will be responsible for a coinsurance of about 20% of the approved charge.

  A   (Medicaid) is incorrect. Medicaid is insurance for patients with limited income and resources. A patient with investment income and a savings account, in addition to Social Security benefits, would most likely be ineligible for Medicaid benefits.

  B   (Medicare Part A) is incorrect. Medicare Part A does not pay for durable medical equipment. Medicare Part A benefits include inpatient hospital services, skilled nursing facility care, home health care, and hospice care.

  D   (the patient and her family) is incorrect. The patient and her family will be responsible for about 20% of the approved charges for the hospital bed. However, the largest portion of the cost of the bed will be paid for by Medicare Part B.

7. D (shortened REM latency) is correct. The first REM period occurs about 90 minutes into the sleep cycle; time to the first REM cycle is known as REM latency. In depression, time to the initial REM period is shortened, and REM sleep is reached more quickly.

  A   (increased delta sleep) and B (increased total sleep time) are incorrect. Depression is associated with a decrease in the amount of delta sleep and a decrease in total sleep time.

  C   (predominance of rapid eye movement sleep in later part of night) is incorrect. Normally, most REM sleep occurs in the later part of the night. This pattern is reversed in patients with depression, when REM sleep occurs predominantly in the earlier part of the night.

8. D (posttraumatic stress disorder) is correct. This patient has PTSD, which involves the development of anxiety symptoms (e.g., irritability, poor concentration, restless sleep) following exposure to a severe traumatic stressor (e.g., a robbery). The traumatic stressor also must involve actual or threatened death or serious injury accompanied by feelings of intense fear and helplessness. The patient's refusal to talk about the robbery reflects his efforts to avoid thinking about the trauma, also a characteristic of PTSD.

  A   (acute stress disorder) is incorrect. Acute stress disorder describes an acute anxiety reaction to a severe traumatic stressor that develops within 4 weeks of the stressor. In addition, the reaction persists from 2 days to 4 weeks. This patient describes having symptoms for 5 weeks, thus excluding the diagnosis of acute stress disorder.

B   (adjustment disorder with anxiety) is incorrect. An adjustment disorder with anxiety is characterized by the development of significant anxiety in response to an identifiable psychosocial stressor. However, in this case, the presence of a traumatic stressor, along with the man's accompanying symptoms, suggests the presence of PTSD.

C   (generalized anxiety disorder) is incorrect. Generalized anxiety disorder involves chronic, excessive worry about numerous daily events and persists for at least 6 months.

E   (social phobia) is incorrect. Social phobia is a persistent fear of social or performance situations involving exposure to unfamiliar persons and possible scrutiny. This patient's hesitation to talk about the incident could possibly reflect an underlying discomfort with social situations, but seems more consistent with an effort to avoid recollections of the trauma. In addition, his overall clinical picture is most suggestive of PTSD.

9. A   (confrontation) is correct. Confrontation is an attempt to clarify inconsistencies in patients' statements in general or about their physical presentation.

B   (empathy) is incorrect. Empathy is the attempt to recognize and understand a patient's feelings and experiences; for example, "It sounds like the process of recovering from surgery has been very frustrating for you."

C   (facilitating) is incorrect. A facilitating response is a verbal or nonverbal prompt to encourage the patient to say more; for example, "Tell me more about that."

D   (reflecting) is incorrect. Reflecting, or paraphrasing, involves taking a portion of a patient's statement and repeating it in the form of a question. It encourages the patient to elaborate; for example, "The pain started 5 days ago?"

E   (validation) is incorrect. Validation conveys that a patient's emotional response is understandable for his or her circumstances; for example, "Most people feel worried while waiting for the results of a biopsy."

10. A   (he should ask a nurse to be present during the examination) is correct. Having a nurse or other health care professional present during the medical examination is likely to curtail the patient's sexually provocative behavior. The other health care professional becomes an observer of the interaction between the physician and the patient.

B   (he should ask the patient how things are going in her marriage) is incorrect. Questions about her marriage may be relevant to the patient's clinical problems, but they are not a very constructive immediate response to her sexually provocative behavior.

C   (he should ignore the patient's sexual behavior to avoid reinforcing it) is incorrect. Ignoring sexually oriented comments
may be acceptable early in an interview, particularly if the
comments are quite subtle. However, in this case, the statements have become clearly provocative and are likely to continue if the physician does not deal with them directly.

D   (he should respond flirtatiously to establish a positive rapport
with the patient) is incorrect. Flirting may encourage the patient's sexually provocative remarks and behavior.

11. B   (frontal lobes) is correct. The frontal lobes are associated with
organization, decision-making, and fine-tuning of behavior so
that it is organized and appropriate. Without this control, behavior may become disinhibited. Individuals may become more
aggressive and impulsive after injury to the frontal lobe.

A   (basal ganglia) is incorrect. Damage to the basal ganglia would
result in repetitive movements and behaviors.

C   (parietal lobes) is incorrect. The parietal lobes function in so-
matosensory and symbol perception as well as in motor inte-
gration. Lesions on the right side of the brain would cause
apraxia or neglect, and lesions on the left side would cause
agraphia, acalculia, and no right-left discrimination.

D   (reticular activating system) is incorrect. Malfunction of the
reticular activating system would result in altered mood and
alertness or difficulties in the regulation of the sleep-wake
cycle.

E   (temporal lobes) is incorrect. The temporal lobes determine auditory and language comprehension. They also have some
function in memory.

12. C   (coining) is correct. Coining is a traditional treatment practiced by some Asian Americans, including Cambodians and Viet-
namese. It is used to treat symptoms such as fever and dizziness
and conditions such as "wind illness." A coin is rubbed on the
skin, usually using a lubricant such as tiger balm, which
causes lesions in striped patterns. This practice is believed to
improve circulation and restore balance in the body. Recent immigrants are more likely to use traditional treatments than immigrants who have lived in the United States for a longer time.
When taking the patient's history, the physician should ask
about the family's use of traditional treatments.

A   (accidental injury) is incorrect. Although it is possible that the
patient received the bruises from an accident, it is unlikely
that an accident would causes bruises in a striped pattern.

B   (child abuse) is incorrect. Although it is possible that the
patient received the bruises from child abuse, the pattern of
bruising is not consistent with the usual manifestations of
child abuse. It is more likely that she received them from the
traditional treatment of coining.

D (cupping) is incorrect. Cupping is a traditional healing method practiced by some Asian Americans, including Cambodians. Cups are heated to create a vacuum inside; the cups are then placed on the skin, producing red circular lesions. Cupping is also believed to improve circulation and restore balance in the body.

---

13. **D** (major depressive disorder) is correct. Because many of the symptoms of bereavement and major depressive disorder overlap, the presence of certain symptoms that are not characteristic of normal grieving may help to differentiate the two. The acronym DIP HUG (frequent thoughts of <u>d</u>eath, functional <u>i</u>mpairment, <u>p</u>sychomotor retardation, <u>h</u>allucinations, preoccupation with <u>u</u>nworthiness, excessive <u>g</u>uilt) summarizes the symptoms of major depressive disorder. This patient is probably grieving the loss of her husband. However, two of the persistent symptoms (of more than 2 months' duration)—feeling like she is "no good to anybody" (i.e., feelings of worthlessness) and staying in bed all day without dressing or eating (i.e., functional impairment)—are indicative of major depressive disorder, a diagnosis that takes precedence over normal bereavement.

A (bereavement) is incorrect. As discussed in D, features of both bereavement and major depressive disorder are present in this case. However, major depressive disorder is the more appropriate diagnosis. Nonpathologic bereavement is the context in which this clinical disorder has occurred.

B (bipolar II disorder) is incorrect. Patients with bipolar II disorder have a history of at least one hypomanic episode. Hypomanic episodes feature elevated, expansive, or irritable mood plus at least three FAST PED symptoms: <u>f</u>light of ideas, increased goal-directed <u>a</u>ctivity, markedly decreased need for <u>s</u>leep, <u>t</u>alkativeness, self-defeating <u>p</u>leasure, inflated self-<u>e</u>steem, and <u>d</u>istractibility. This patient's history contains no evidence of a hypomanic episode.

C (dysthymic disorder) is incorrect. Dysthymic disorder is characterized by the presence of at least two HE SADe symptoms on more days than not for at least 2 years. HE SADe symptoms include <u>h</u>opelessness, low self-<u>e</u>steem, <u>s</u>leep disturbance, poor <u>a</u>ppetite or overeating, difficulty in making <u>d</u>ecisions, and low <u>e</u>nergy.

---

14. **C** (3 years) is correct. A typical 3-year-old girl has established her gender identity, knows her age, has achieved both bladder and bowel control, uses complete sentences, and can ride a tricycle.

A (18 months) is incorrect. At 18 months of age, a child usually is able to run, name pictures, use 10–20 words, and engage in pretend play with dolls.

B (2 years) is incorrect. The developmental milestones of a 2-year-old child normally include jumping, walking up and down stairs, using two or three words together, and knowing her full name.

D (4 years) is incorrect. A 4-year-old child usually has surpassed the developmental milestones described above and, typically, the child can hop on one foot, tell a story, and play cooperatively with other children.

E (5 years) is incorrect. A typical 5-year-old child can skip, draw a person, dress and undress herself without help, participate in group games, and understand the concepts of past and future.

15. A (altruism) is correct. Altruism is engaging in service to others to help deal with painful feelings. In this example, the man may have been frustrated by his inability to improve his brother's life. By helping mentally retarded individuals in the Special Olympics program, this man is able to cope with his feelings.

B (displacement) is incorrect. Displacement involves redirecting feelings about a person or situation toward a more acceptable person or situation. For example, a resident feels humiliated by her attending physician and then is overly critical of the medical student under her supervision.

C (rationalization) is incorrect. Rationalization is justification of unreasonable feelings or behaviors by means of a logical explanation. For example, a mother who dipped her son in scalding water for punishment says that the boy needs to learn to respect authority.

D (reaction formation) is incorrect. Reaction formation involves adopting behaviors that are the opposite of one's unacceptable impulses. For example, a woman who has strong unconscious feelings of anger and aggression is always nice to everyone and never loses her temper.

E (sublimation) is incorrect. Sublimation involves channeling unacceptable drives and impulses into socially acceptable activities. For example, a rape victim who initially fantasized about revenge attempts to improve services for other rape victims.

16. C (lithium) is correct. This patient is exhibiting symptoms of mania or hypomania. The mood stabilizer lithium should be added to her treatment regimen. The antidepressant she is currently taking, paroxetine, should be discontinued or its dosage reduced.

A (diazepam) is incorrect. The benzodiazepine diazepam might be a good choice to temporarily manage the patient's agitation, but it is not a long-term treatment for mood stabilization in bipolar disorder.

B   (imipramine) is incorrect. The tricyclic antidepressant imipramine may also lead to manic episodes in a patient with bipolar disorder; it is known to contribute to rapid cycling, particularly if no mood stabilizer is being used. In addition, caution is recommended when combining a tricyclic antidepressant with a selective serotonin reuptake inhibitor (SSRI) such as paroxetine. When combined, tricyclic serum levels must be monitored to prevent toxicity.

D   (methylphenidate) is incorrect. Methylphenidate, a stimulant, would be likely to worsen manic symptoms.

E   (phenelzine) is incorrect. The monoamine oxidase (MAO) inhibitor phenelzine should not be used in combination with an SSRI such as paroxetine. Concurrent use of an MAO inhibitor and an SSRI may precipitate serotonin syndrome, which is an elevated serotonin level that is characterized by agitation, restlessness, insomnia, seizures, and severe hyperthermia.

17. A (acceptance) is correct. In Kübler-Ross's stages of dying, acceptance is the stage of dying in which the patient accepts the inevitable and is more calm and peaceful. The patient may also take care of unfinished business, such as making amends with this sister, whom he has not spoken with in 10 years.

B   (anger) is incorrect. In this stage of dying, the patient asks "Why me?" and is angry about his fate. Physicians and family members often bear the brunt of this anger.

C   (bargaining) is incorrect. In this stage of dying, the patient usually bargains with a higher power or fate and wants to trade good behavior for good health or at least a postponement of death.

D   (denial) is incorrect. Denial is the stage of dying in which the patient does not believe that the diagnosis and prognosis are true. A patient would expect to get better and would not acknowledge that he or she has a terminal illness.

E   (depression) is incorrect. In this stage, the patient believes the diagnosis and prognosis, experiences sadness and distress, and stops fighting to survive.

18. D (report the abuse to child protective services) is correct. Physicians in all states are mandated by law to report suspicions of child abuse to the appropriate child protective agency.

A   (admit the patient to the hospital) is incorrect. Admission to the hospital may be necessary to protect a child from harm. In this case, admission to the hospital does not appear to be warranted.

B   (ask the mother to agree to supervised visits with the friend) is incorrect. Discussing a plan for the mother to never leave the child alone with the friend is appropriate, but it is not a sufficient step. The physician is legally obligated to report suspicions of abuse to the appropriate child protective agency.

C (contact the family friend and recommend that he get psychological help) is incorrect. Physicians are not required to make contact with an individual who has been identified as being an abuser or is suspected of abuse.

19. C (psychophysiologic insomnia) is correct. Psychophysiologic insomnia is a sleep disturbance that has an initial precipitant, however the disturbance persists after the precipitating factor has resolved. Patients with psychophysiologic insomnia have poorly conditioned sleep (i.e., bedtime has become associated with increased arousal and anxiety about being unable to fall asleep). Their sleep may improve when they are in surroundings other than their own bedroom, as is true for this patient when she is visiting friends.

A (adjustment disorder with anxiety) is incorrect. Adjustment disorder with anxiety is characterized by significant anxiety symptoms that develop following an identifiable stressor. Although this patient has had recent work stress, it has resolved, and there is no mention of other symptoms of adjustment disorder with anxiety (e.g., anxious mood or restlessness).

B (circadian rhythm sleep disorder) is incorrect. Circadian rhythm sleep disorder is associated with shift work. However, this patient's work schedule does not seem to be associated with her sleep disorder, because she has had a stable sleep history for many years. Her recent sleep difficulties are associated with work stress. Her clinical presentation fits a pattern of psychophysiologic insomnia.

D (substance-induced sleep disorder) is incorrect. Use of caffeine or amphetamines may be associated with substance-induced sleep disorder. This patient denies use of caffeine or other chemical substances.

20. D (shaping) is correct. Shaping is a process in which small steps toward a goal are identified and rewarded. This patient is rewarded with praise by the physician for reaching her first goal. The physician then suggests the next step needed to reach the goal, walking 30 minutes five times a week.

A (cognitive restructuring) is incorrect. Cognitive restructuring helps a patient learn to modify maladaptive thoughts. If this patient had had reasonable success in meeting her exercise goals but had nonetheless felt "like a failure at exercising," her physician could help her to examine and objectively challenge this thought through the use of cognitive restructuring techniques.

B (reinforcement) is incorrect. Although the physician is using reinforcement in his praise of the patient, the overall process being employed is shaping.

C (self-monitoring) is incorrect. Self-monitoring is a technique in which an individual records his or her behavior to increase awareness of the behavior and more accurately assess it. This patient could use self-monitoring by keeping an exercise diary.

21. **C** (narcissistic) is correct. This patient has a narcissistic personality style, which is characterized by his need for admiration and sense of entitlement (e.g., being cared for only by the best). Despite an attitude of superiority, individuals with a narcissistic style often experience underlying feelings of inferiority.

A (dependent) is incorrect. Individuals with a dependent personality style rely on others for advice and tend to subordinate their own needs to maintain an emotional connection with and the approval of others. This patient does not have these features.

B (histrionic) is incorrect. Individuals with a histrionic personality style also have a need for admiration. If this patient were histrionic, he would be likely to enjoy the attention of any member of the medical staff rather than demand the attention of the chief physician.

D (paranoid) is incorrect. Individuals with a paranoid personality style are mistrustful and suspicious of the motives of others. These qualities are not reflected in this patient.

22. **C** (need for more direct stimulation to facilitate erection) is correct. As men age, they typically require more direct stimulation to facilitate erection.

A (decreased duration of the refractory period following orgasm) is incorrect. As men age, the time spent in the refractory period lengthens.

B (increased force of ejaculation) is incorrect. With aging, there is typically a decrease in the force of ejaculation.

D (significant decrease in interest in sexual relations) is incorrect. Aging itself is not associated with a decrease in sexual interest. However, aging is associated with various factors (e.g., illness, loss of spouse) that may result in changes in sexual desire or the opportunity for sexual relations.

23. B (health maintenance organization) is correct. HMOs generally require that enrollees use physicians who are on the provider panel of the plan. If the dermatologist chosen by the patient is not on the provider panel, the HMO will not pay for the visit.

  A (fee-for-service plan) is incorrect. Patients insured by a fee-for-service plan are free to choose any health care provider for services covered under the plan, and their insurance will pay for a portion of the cost of the visit.

  C (HMO with a point of service option) is incorrect. Patients who have a POS option can choose providers who are not on an HMO panel and a portion of the visit will be paid for by their insurance. However, if this patient decides to see a dermatologist who is not on his provider panel, he will have to pay more out of pocket. Sometimes this type of managed care plan is referred to simply as a POS plan.

  D (preferred provider organization) is incorrect. Patients insured by a PPO may choose physicians who are in-network or out-of-network. If this patient chooses an in-network dermatologist, he will have lower out-of-pocket expenses than if he chooses a dermatologist who is out-of-network.

24. B (exposure and response prevention) is correct. This patient has OCD and is being treated with exposure and response prevention. In this treatment, patients are exposed to feared stimuli (exposure) and then encouraged to avoid ritualizing (response prevention). By doing so, patients have an opportunity to learn that ritualizing is unnecessary to reduce their anxiety, which typically lessens over time and with repeated exposure to the feared item. Exposure and response prevention has been shown to be an effective treatment for OCD.

  A (cognitive restructuring) is incorrect. Cognitive restructuring addresses maladaptive thoughts that can contribute to emotional distress. This treatment approach is not described in this case.

  C (flooding) is incorrect. In flooding, patients are exposed to their most feared stimuli at the start of treatment. There is no mention in this case that the patient is beginning treatment by facing his most feared situation.

  D (imaginal exposure) is incorrect. In imaginal exposure, patients imagine being exposed to feared stimuli. "Real-life" exposure to actual stimuli is not part of this treatment.

  E (relapse prevention) is incorrect. Relapse prevention training is employed in the treatment of addictive disorders. Individuals learn to become aware of high-risk situations in which they may lapse (i.e., resume undesirable behavior) and develop a plan for coping with them.

25. A (factitious disorder) is correct. This disorder features the intentional production of symptoms that cannot be adequately explained by a known medical condition. The motivation for such symptom fabrication is unknown but is presumed to be an effort to gain the attention of health care providers. The tachycardia, hypertension, and face flushing exhibited by this patient appear to have been stimulated by the pseudoephedrine that had been surreptitiously placed under the patient's mattress, suggesting that the symptoms had been intentionally produced.

  B (hypochondriasis) is incorrect. Patients with hypochondriasis fear that they have a serious disease; the fear persists in spite of medical reassurance to the contrary. The patient in this case did not fear having a disease, but instead tried to stimulate disease symptoms to gain medical attention.

  C (malingering) is incorrect. Malingering involves the intentional feigning of symptoms in an attempt to obtain external incentives (e.g., financial payments, drugs). This case contains no evidence of external incentives, only the presumption that symptom feigning was motivated by the desire to gain attention from health care personnel.

  D (psychological factors affecting general medical condition) is incorrect. The hallmark feature of this disorder is the impact that one or more psychological or behavioral factors (e.g., another mental disorder, personality traits, maladaptive habits) have on a known physical condition. There is no verified medical problem nor is there evidence of such a factor in this case.

26. D (Piaget) is correct. Jean Piaget developed the four-stage theoretical model of cognitive development in children and adolescents. The four stages are sensorimotor, preoperational, concrete operational, and formal operational.

  A (Chess and Thomas) is incorrect. Chess and Thomas developed the concept of temperament. They theorized that individual differences in behavioral style are evident early in life, remain relatively stable, and influence development.

  B (Erikson) is incorrect. Erikson developed an eight-stage theoretical model of psychosocial development across the lifespan, with a specific task to accomplish during each stage. The eight stages are trust vs. mistrust, autonomy vs. shame and doubt, initiative vs. guilt, industry vs. inferiority, identity vs. role confusion, intimacy vs. isolation, generativity vs. self-absorption, and ego integrity vs. despair.

  C (Freud) is incorrect. Freud developed a five-stage theoretical model of psychosexual development during childhood. Each stage corresponds with an area of the body where pleasurable sensations primarily occur. The five stages are oral, anal, phallic or oedipal, latency, and genital.

E (Tanner) is incorrect. Tanner developed a five-stage classification of the development of secondary sex characteristics in girls and boys during puberty. The stages are not named. For each stage, a description is given for phase of development of secondary sex characteristics.

27. B (repression) is correct. Repression is blocking unacceptable impulses and painful feelings from conscious awareness. In this case, memories of the sexual abuse and associated injuries likely were extremely distressing to the patient and were unconsciously repressed or "forgotten."

A (isolation) is incorrect. Isolation involves separating painful feelings from stressful situations. For example, a patient describes her history of childhood physical abuse in an objective, unemotional manner.

C (splitting) is incorrect. When the defense mechanism of splitting is employed, an individual's feelings about people and situations are either all positive or all negative. For example, a patient might be extremely satisfied with her physician. However, during one visit, he advises her to lose weight because of her hypertension. She becomes very angry and tells him that he is the worst doctor she has ever known.

D (sublimation) is incorrect. Sublimation involves channeling unacceptable drives and impulses into socially acceptable activities. For example, a rape victim who initially fantasized about revenge attempts to improve services for other rape victims.

E (suppression) is incorrect. Suppression involves voluntarily postponing attention to unwanted thoughts or feelings. For example, a physician who feels sexually attracted to a patient would consciously direct his attention to the medical interview.

28. D (tardive dyskinesia) is correct. Grimacing, along with other abnormal and irregular movements of the face, trunk, and limbs, is characteristic of tardive dyskinesia. This is a common side effect that develops after months to years of treatment with antipsychotic drugs. It is believed to be related to long-term dopamine receptor blockade.

A (akathisia) is incorrect. Akathisia, a sensation of inner restlessness, is a common acute extrapyramidal effect seen with antipsychotic drug use. It would more likely have become apparent much earlier in the course of treatment.

B (dystonia) is incorrect. Dystonia is an acute extrapyramidal effect that is associated with the use of antipsychotic drugs. It is a state of abnormal muscle tension that often affects the neck and facial muscles. Oculogyric crises, in which the eyes become fixed in position, glossospasm, and torticollis, are common. Like akathisia, dystonia would more likely have become apparent much earlier in the course of treatment.

C (neuroleptic malignant syndrome) is incorrect. In NMS, a severe form of drug toxicity, the patient develops high fever, muscle rigidity, delirium, elevated creatine phosphokinase level, and elevated blood pressure and heart rate. This potentially lethal complication of antipsychotic use is usually associated with typical antipsychotics, but it also has been described with clozapine use.

29. E (unintentional injury) is correct. The death rate due to unintentional injury among young adults aged 22–44 years is 32.8 deaths per 100,000 population. This is about 20% of deaths among young adults, making unintentional injury the leading cause of death among this age group. Motor vehicle crashes are the leading cause of injurious death among this group.

A (HIV/AIDS) is incorrect. During the mid-1990s, HIV/AIDS was the leading cause of death among young adults, with 37.4 deaths per 100,000 population. However, by 1999, it had dropped to fifth place, with 10.9 deaths per 100,000 population.

B (homicide) is incorrect. Homicide, or assault, is the third leading cause of death (11.2 deaths per 100,000 population) among adults younger than age 35 years, but only the seventh leading cause in adults aged 35–44 years (7.2 deaths per 100,000 population). When data for these two groups are combined, homicide is not among the top five leading causes of death.

C (malignant neoplasm) is incorrect. Malignant neoplasm is the second leading cause of death among young adults, with 15.9 deaths per 100,000 population. This is about 16% of deaths among young adults.

D (suicide) is incorrect. Suicide is the fourth leading cause of death among young adults, with 8.9 deaths per 100,000 population. This is about 9% of deaths among young adults.

30. A (4%) is correct. The probability of any randomly selected patient surviving for 5 years is 20% (10/50). Therefore, the probability of two randomly selected patients surviving for 5 years (i.e., A survives *and* B survives) is the probability that A survives (20%) *multiplied* by the probability that B survives (20%). This is equal to 4%.

B (20%) is incorrect. This is the probability of any *one* patient surviving for 5 years.

C (36%) is incorrect. This is the probability that A *or* B survives for 5 years. It is calculated as the *sum* of the probability that A survives (20%) and that B survives (20%) minus the probabil-ity that both survive (4%).

   D (40%) is incorrect. This is the probability that A or B survives for 5 years, calculated *incorrectly* without adjustment for the probability that both survive.

   E (64%) is incorrect. This is the probability that *neither* A *nor* B survives for 5 years. It is calculated as the probability that A does not survive (80%) multiplied by the probability that B does not survive (80%).

31. D (talk with the colleague about his alcohol use and help him to arrange treatment) is correct. Physicians have an ethical obli-gation to protect patients from harm, as well as to intervene with physicians who are impaired in their ability to practice medicine. In this case, a responsible action by the medical direc-tor is to directly address the alcohol use with the colleague and help him access help. The director should also take steps to ensure the safety of the colleague's patients.

   A (contact the colleague's wife to plan a family intervention) is incorrect. Although notifying the colleague's wife may be an option, the medical director also needs to discuss the problem directly with the physician and take steps to ensure the safety of his patients.

   B (institute a random drug-screening policy for all clinic employ-ees) is incorrect. Instituting a clinic-wide drug screening pol-icy is not a specific action that addresses the colleague's alcohol use.

   C (place a brochure about Alcoholics Anonymous on the col-league's desk) is incorrect. This approach is indirect and does not involve specific, concrete steps to facilitate the colleague's getting help and to protect his patients from potential harm.

32. B (the patient can refuse medication even if involuntarily com-mitted) is correct. Individuals who are involuntarily committed can refuse treatment, unless such treatment has been ordered by the court. However, if emergency treatment becomes neces-sary to protect the patient or others from harm, the psychia-trist can override the patient's refusal to take medication.

   A (the patient can be forced to take the medication because of his involuntary status) is incorrect. Patients cannot be forced to take medication, even if involuntarily committed, unless the treatment is court ordered or the patient presents a danger to self or others.

   C (the patient is considered incompetent to make treatment de-cisions) is incorrect. Involuntary commitment does not auto-matically result in a determination that an individual is incompetent to make decisions about health care.

D   (the patient must be released within 8 hours if he refuses treatment) is incorrect. Patients who are committed involuntarily have the right to refuse treatment, but this does not directly affect their court-ordered confinement.

---

33. D   (somatization disorder) is correct. Somatization disorder involves at least four pain symptoms, two gastrointestinal symptoms, one sexual symptom, and one pseudoneurologic symptom. The description of many such symptoms over a 10-year period is consistent with the features of this disorder.

A   (conversion disorder) is incorrect. Conversion disorder is characterized by unexplained sensory or motor dysfunction that cannot be adequately explained by a neurologic or general medical condition. There is no evidence of such dysfunction in this case.

B   (factitious disorder) is incorrect. Factitious disorder involves feigning of symptoms, presumably to gain the attention of health care providers. There is no evidence of symptom fabrication in this case.

C   (hypochondriasis) is incorrect. Hypochondriasis involves a preoccupation with the fear or belief that one has a serious disease, based on misinterpretation of one's symptoms. There is no evidence of such a fear or belief in this case.

---

34. E   (sertraline) is correct. Sertraline is a selective serotonin reuptake inhibitor (SSRI) that has been approved by the FDA for the treatment of panic disorder. The SSRIs have fewer side effects, such as the anticholinergic properties of the tricyclic antidepressants (e.g., imipramine); thus, sertraline is the best choice for long-term management of panic disorder.

A   (alprazolam) is incorrect. Alprazolam is a benzodiazepine with rapid anxiolytic effects. It may be used as an adjunctive treatment in panic disorder. Benzodiazepines carry a risk of abuse and dependence. Although patients with panic disorder are unlikely to abuse this drug, the potential for abuse makes it less appropriate for long-term treatment.

B   (carbamazepine) is incorrect. Carbamazepine is an antiepileptic drug that is also used as a mood stabilizer in the treatment of bipolar disorder.

C   (haloperidol) is incorrect. Haloperidol is an antipsychotic drug that is also used for rapid tranquilization. As with other older-generation antipsychotics, there is a risk of developing tardive dyskinesia. Other treatment alternatives have been effective and are more appropriate.

D   (imipramine) is incorrect. Imipramine is a tricyclic antidepressant that was once widely used in the treatment of panic disorder. Although it is effective, it has more side effects (e.g., anticholinergic effects) and is more likely to be lethal in overdose than SSRIs (e.g., sertraline). Imipramine remains a treatment alternative, but it is not considered a first-line treatment choice when other options are available.

35. B (emotional abuse) is correct. The woman is suffering from emotional abuse, evidenced by the daughter's and the grandsons' abusive behavior. Other examples of emotional abuse include isolating an elder, treating an elder like an infant, and denying an elder the right to make his or her own health care decisions.

A (abandonment) is incorrect. There is no indication that the daughter, who provides most of the woman's care, has abandoned her mother.

C (financial and material exploitation) is incorrect. There is no indication that the daughter is improperly attempting to take control of her mother's financial assets or property, or to have her change her will, which would constitute financial and material exploitation.

D (neglect) is incorrect. There is no indication that the daughter is failing to meet her mother's physical needs or financial obligations. Although the daughter and her family clearly are not meeting the woman's emotional needs, the extent of their actions constitutes emotional abuse, not neglect.

E (physical abuse) is incorrect. The woman has not sustained physical injuries. Other acts of physical abuse would be a caretaker overdosing or underdosing the patient's medications.

36. E (suppression) is correct. Suppression involves voluntarily postponing attention to unwanted thoughts or feelings. A verbal attack on the father would have been inappropriate for the physician providing medical care. Recognizing this urge and deciding to postpone the expression of her feelings to a later discussion with a colleague is an example of suppression.

A (denial) is incorrect. Denial involves refusing to acknowledge threatening or anxiety-provoking events. For example, a 50-year-old woman with a family history of breast cancer finds a lump in her breast but waits 2 months before seeing her physician.

B (identification) is incorrect. Identification involves imitating the behavior of a more powerful person. For example, a young boy who has witnessed his father hitting his mother on several occasions becomes physically aggressive with other children.

C (isolation) is incorrect. Isolation involves separating painful feelings from stressful situations. For example, a patient describes her history of childhood sexual abuse in an objective, unemotional manner.

D (repression) is incorrect. Repression involves blocking unacceptable impulses and painful feelings from conscious awareness. For example, a young girl witnesses a playmate being struck and killed by a car. As an adult, she has no memory of the event.

37. C (interpretation of transference) is correct. Interpretation of transference involves helping patients to understand their reactions to their analyst. These reactions have been influenced by experiences with individuals who were important in the patients' early development. The process leads to insight regarding relationship patterns with others.

A (biofeedback) is incorrect. Biofeedback measures involuntary physiologic processes to give a patient feedback about a physiologic function. From this feedback, the patient learns to modify the function and reduce unpleasant symptoms. For example, in the treatment of tension headaches, electrodes are placed on the forehead and visual or auditory feedback informs the patient about the level of muscle tension. With this feedback, the patient learns to reduce muscle tension and, consequently, headaches.

B (in vivo exposure) is incorrect. In vivo exposure is a behavior therapy technique that involves gradually exposing a patient to feared situations. For example, an agoraphobic woman who is afraid to drive out of her neighborhood drives on a local highway and gets off at the first exit. Once she can drive this route with minimal anxiety, she drives to the next exit, progressively increasing her distance from home.

D (positive reinforcement) is incorrect. Positive reinforcement is a behavior therapy technique in which positive rewards are given following desired behaviors. For example, a young girl might receive a sticker on a chart each time she completes her homework.

E (systematic desensitization) is incorrect. Systematic desensitization is a behavior therapy technique in which the patient relaxes while visualizing being gradually exposed to feared situations. For example, a man who is afraid of flying learns a relaxation procedure. He relaxes and then imagines that he is driving to the airport. Once this image produces anxiety, he relaxes again. This process is repeated until he can keep the feared image in mind and remain relaxed. The procedure is repeated for each situation on the anxiety hierarchy.

38. A (aversive conditioning) is correct. Aversive conditioning involves repeated pairing of an unpleasant stimulus with a response, which leads to a reduction in that response. In this case, the repeated pairing of nausea (the unpleasant stimulus) with alcohol use (the response) leads to a reduction in the man's use of alcohol.

B (biofeedback) is incorrect. Biofeedback uses an auditory or visual signal that provides information to an individual about his or her ability to influence a physiologic process (e.g., muscle tension). The signal acts as a reinforcer when the desired change occurs (e.g., reduction in muscle tension), making it more likely that the individual will repeat the process that led to this change.

C (positive reinforcement) is incorrect. Positive reinforcement refers to the process in which behavior is more likely to be repeated when followed by a positive consequence (reward). In this case, the medication causes the patient to become ill, thus serving as a punishment. It is likely to lead to a reduction in the frequency of the behavior (e.g., drinking alcohol) that preceded the punishment.

D (shaping) is incorrect. Shaping refers to rewarding successive approximations of a desired behavior. For example, the physician asks the patient to reduce his use of alcohol, with the overall goal being to completely eliminate it. The patient returns to see his physician and is praised for reducing his use of alcohol. The physician then suggests further reduction in the patient's alcohol use as a step toward the goal of cessation.

39. D (panic disorder) is correct. Panic disorder involves repeated, unexpected panic attacks. Following an attack(s), patients are concerned about having more attacks or about the significance of the attack, or may change their behavior because of the attack. Patients often seek emergency care because they fear they may be having a heart attack.

A (acute stress disorder) is incorrect. Acute stress disorder is an acute anxiety reaction to a severe traumatic stressor. The reaction develops within 4 weeks of the traumatic event and resolves in 2 days to 4 weeks. This patient has not suffered trauma. Furthermore, her symptoms are consistent with those of panic disorder.

B (agoraphobia) is incorrect. Agoraphobia is anxiety about being in places where escape would be difficult or embarrassing or where help might not be available if panic symptoms occurred. This patient continues to engage in her normal routine, suggesting that she is not avoiding situations. Agoraphobia frequently coexists with panic disorder.

C   (hypochondriasis) is incorrect. Hypochondriasis is a preoccupation with having a disease. Although the patient was initially afraid and sought medical help, she has not shown a persistent fear of having a disease.

E   (specific phobia) is incorrect. Specific phobia is an irrational fear of a specific object or situation. Although individuals with specific phobia may experience a panic attack when exposed to a feared situation (e.g., riding through a tunnel), their primary fear is not related to having a panic attack itself. Rather, their fear is related to the tunnel. This patient is afraid of panic attacks and not a specific stimulus.

40. C   (refractory period) is correct. The refractory period, which occurs during the resolution phase, occurs only in males. It represents the time following orgasm before a male is able to be restimulated to orgasm. The duration of the refractory period varies among males, but generally tends to increase with aging.

A   (excitement phase) is incorrect. Both males and females experience this phase of the sexual response cycle. The excitement phase is characterized by penile erection and elevation of the testes in males, vaginal lubrication and enlargement and breast swelling in females; both males and females experience an increase in heart rate, blood pressure, and respiration.

B   (plateau phase) is incorrect. The plateau phase is characterized by an increase in the size of the testes in males, and significant vasocongestion of the outer third of the vagina in females.

D   (resolution phase) is incorrect. The orgasmic phase is followed by the resolution phase, during which male and female physiology return to baseline.

41. E   (separation anxiety disorder) is correct. This patient is exhibiting several symptoms associated with separation anxiety disorder, including persistent worry about harm occurring to his mother and reluctance to go to school and other activities that require separation from his mother. He also has repeated physical complaints.

A   (attention-deficit/hyperactivity disorder) is incorrect. A diagnosis of ADHD requires symptoms of inattention and hyperactivity or impulsivity.

B   (autistic disorder) is incorrect. Autistic disorder involves significant deficits in social interaction and communication.

C   (conduct disorder) is incorrect. Conduct disorder involves serious violations of the rights of others or societal rules.

D   (oppositional defiant disorder) is incorrect. Oppositional defiant disorder involves a pattern of negativistic, hostile, defiant behavior.

42. A (honor the patient's request to discontinue treatment) is correct. Patients have the right to make decisions about their own health care. In this case, there is no reason to suspect that the patient is impaired in her decisional capacity. She understands the risks of discontinuing treatment and the benefits of further treatment, and she appears sound in her decision-making. Therefore, the physician should honor the patient's request to discontinue treatment.

B (informally appoint another family member to make decisions about her treatment) is incorrect. There is no reason to believe that the patient is impaired in her decisional capacity. Therefore, taking steps to designate another individual to make decisions for the patient is not indicated.

C (instruct the family to pursue court proceedings to declare her incompetent) is incorrect. Because the patient shows no signs of impaired decisional capacity, pursuing a determination by the court regarding her competence is inappropriate.

D (tell the family to give her the medication without her knowledge) is incorrect. This patient shows no evidence of impaired decisional capacity, so there is no justification for not honoring her request to discontinue treatment or for not fully informing her about her treatment.

43. B (attributable risk) is correct. The attributable risk is the proportion of total risk of a disorder attributable to exposure to a certain factor. It is calculated as the additional risk in persons exposed to the factor compared with persons not exposed to the factor. In theory, elimination of exposure will reduce risk by the additional risk attributable to exposure to that factor. A formula for attributable risk is:

Attributable risk =
(risk in exposed group) − (risk in unexposed group)

A (absolute risk) is incorrect. The absolute risk, or just risk, is the probability of a certain outcome in a group of people exposed to a certain factor. In this example, that would be the probability of asthma developing in a person exposed to one of the environmental factors. This risk includes the risk of asthma in persons not exposed to the environmental factor plus the specific risk attributable to this factor.

C (odds ratio) and E (risk ratio) are incorrect. The relative risk is the ratio of risk in exposed and unexposed persons (i.e., divide the risk in the exposed group by the risk in the unexposed group). This is different from the difference in risk between these two groups (i.e., subtract the risk in the unexposed group from the risk in the exposed group). The odds ratio is an estimate of the risk ratio.

D (prevalence) is incorrect. The prevalence of asthma would be the number of cases during a specified time period. Because not all of these cases can be attributed to any one specific factor, prevalence would not indicate the reduction in risk associated with elimination of one factor.

44. B (fluoxetine) is correct. Fluoxetine is a selective serotonin reuptake inhibitor (SSRI) that is an appropriate first-line treatment for depression. Its potential for lethal overdose is minimal when compared with the other drugs listed; the SSRIs have fewer serious side effects than the other categories of drugs.

A (clomipramine) and D (nortriptyline) are incorrect. Clomipramine and nortriptyline, tricyclic antidepressants, can be potentially lethal in overdose and should be used with caution in a patient at risk for suicide. For this reason, neither is a first-line drug for treatment of depression.

C (lithium) is incorrect. The mood stabilizer lithium is sometimes used to augment the response to antidepressants in resistant cases of depression, but it is not a first-line treatment for depression. Because it is potentially lethal, it should be used with caution in any patient with suicidal thoughts.

E (phenelzine) is incorrect. Phenelzine is a monoamine oxidase (MAO) inhibitor. Patients at high risk for suicide must be closely supervised while taking this drug because overdoses may be lethal. In addition, MAO inhibitors interact with many other drugs and foods.

45. B (negative reinforcement) is correct. Negative reinforcement is the removal of an adverse stimulus, which strengthens the behavior that caused the adverse stimulus to cease. In this example, the wife's nagging is the adverse stimulus. Because the nagging is unpleasant to the patient, and it stops when he follows his diet, he receives negative reinforcement, which increases the likelihood that he will continue to adhere to his prescribed diet.

A (extinction) is incorrect. Extinction occurs when a reinforcement is discontinued, resulting in cessation of the previous response. For example, the parents of an 18-month-old girl pick her up each time she cries at night and rock her back to sleep. They seek advice on how to reduce nighttime crying and are instructed by their pediatrician to briefly comfort their daughter when she cries but to not remove her from her crib. After several nights of this routine, the child stops crying during the night. Picking up the child and rocking her reinforced her crying; stopping the reinforcement stopped the crying.

C (positive reinforcement) is incorrect. Positive reinforcement is giving a positive consequence or reward after a person exhibits a certain behavior. The positive consequence causes the behavior to occur more often.

D   (punishment) is incorrect. Punishment is giving an unpleasant consequence or removing a pleasant consequence after an individual exhibits a certain behavior. This causes the behavior to occur less often or stop.

E   (shaping) is incorrect. Shaping is the reinforcement of behaviors that become more and more similar to a desired behavior. For example, a man is encouraged to begin walking 10 minutes a day, 3 days a week. Upon reaching this initial goal, his physician praises him and recommends an increase in his walking time to 30 minutes, 5 days a week.

46. **A**   (acute stress disorder) is correct. Acute stress disorder is an acute anxiety reaction to a severe traumatic stressor. The response occurs within 4 weeks of the stress and persists from 2 days to 4 weeks. This woman witnessed a traumatic event and is having acute symptoms (e.g., feeling dazed, having trouble concentrating and sleeping) that are consistent with acute stress disorder.

B   (adjustment disorder with anxiety) is incorrect. Adjustment disorder with anxiety is characterized by the development of anxiety symptoms after an identifiable psychosocial stressor. The nature of the stressor can influence the diagnosis. This patient experienced a traumatic stressor (an accident in which a pedestrian was killed). This experience, followed by the acute symptoms, is consistent with acute stress disorder rather than adjustment disorder.

C   (generalized anxiety disorder) is incorrect. Generalized anxiety disorder is characterized by chronic, excessive worry about day-to-day events. One diagnostic criterion is the presence of worry for more days than not for at least a 6-month period. This woman's symptoms are acute in nature and specifically related to a traumatic stressor rather than to several concerns.

D   (specific phobia) is incorrect. A person who has witnessed a fatal automobile accident may develop driving phobia. However, this woman's current symptoms are consistent with those of acute stress disorder. If her fear and avoidance of driving continue, a further evaluation for a specific phobia is warranted.

47. A (implied consent) is correct. Implied consent is assumed in emergency circumstances in which the patient cannot provide consent (e.g., the patient is unconscious). Implied consent is based on the notion that reasonable individuals would want care to be given to them in an emergency.

B (nonmaleficence) is incorrect. Nonmaleficence refers to the principle that physicians must "do no harm."
C (therapeutic privilege) is incorrect. Therapeutic privilege is enacted when the physician, believing that informing the patient about treatment might result in harm, forgoes obtaining informed consent from the patient.
D (waiver of consent) is incorrect. A waiver of consent is an exception to obtaining informed consent. A waiver of consent is in effect when the patient waives his or her right to be further informed.

48. C (75%) is correct. Specificity is the proportion of patients without the disorder (60) who test negative (45). This is 45/60, or 75%.

A (40%) is incorrect. This is the proportion of all patients tested (100) who have the disorder (40), as determined by the gold standard. This is 40/100, or 40%.
B (70%) is incorrect. This is the positive predictive value, or the proportion of positive test results (35 + 15) that are correct (35). This is 35/50, or 70%.
D (87.5%) is incorrect. This is the sensitivity, or the proportion of patients with the disorder (40) who test positive (35). This is 35/40, or 87.5%.
E (90%) is incorrect. This is the negative predictive value, or the proportion of negative test results (5 + 45) that are correct (45). This is 45/50, or 90%.

49. B (a father who punishes his child by locking him in a closet for hours) is correct. Physicians are mandated by law to report suspected child abuse to the appropriate child protective agency. In this case, the father admits to abusing his child, and a report to child protective services is indicated.

A (a 20-year-old man who has suicidal thoughts but denies intent or plan) is incorrect. Confidentiality may be broken if there is a significant risk of suicide. In this case, the man reports suicidal thoughts but denies suicidal intent or suicide plans. Based on this information, he most likely is not at imminent risk of suicide, so breaking confidentiality does not appear to be warranted.
C (a mother who refuses an experimental treatment for her terminally ill 8-year-old daughter) is incorrect. The parent's decision not to pursue an experimental treatment for her child is not itself grounds for breaking confidentiality. Breaking confi-

dentiality is warranted if the mother refuses an established medical treatment that carries a high likelihood of benefit to the child and the child is likely to die without the treatment.

D (a patient who is agitated but denies homicidal thoughts) is incorrect. Breaking confidentiality is warranted if a patient has homicidal thoughts directed at an identified individual. In this case, the patient is agitated but denies homicidal ideation. Therefore, breaking confidentiality does not appear to be warranted.

50. B (clonidine and olanzapine) is correct. PTSD symptoms in this patient include the easy startle reflex and the auditory hallucination of hearing gunshots. Clonidine has been noted to reduce the startle reflex; a low dose of an antipsychotic medication (e.g., olanzapine) would be used to treat the auditory hallucination.

A (buspirone and fluoxetine) is incorrect. Buspirone is used for generalized anxiety symptoms, but not for PTSD. A selective serotonin reuptake inhibitor (SSRI), such as fluoxetine, would not relieve psychotic symptoms or the startle reflex.

C (lorazepam) is incorrect. Benzodiazepines (e.g., lorazepam) should not be given to patients with PTSD because they have the potential for abuse. They are not appropriate in long-term treatment of PTSD.

D (lorazepam and fluoxetine) is incorrect. Benzodiazepines (e.g., lorazepam) are not ideal in long-term treatment of PTSD. An SSRI (e.g., fluoxetine) would be beneficial in the treatment of depression but would not reduce the startle reflex or the auditory hallucination (hearing gunshots).

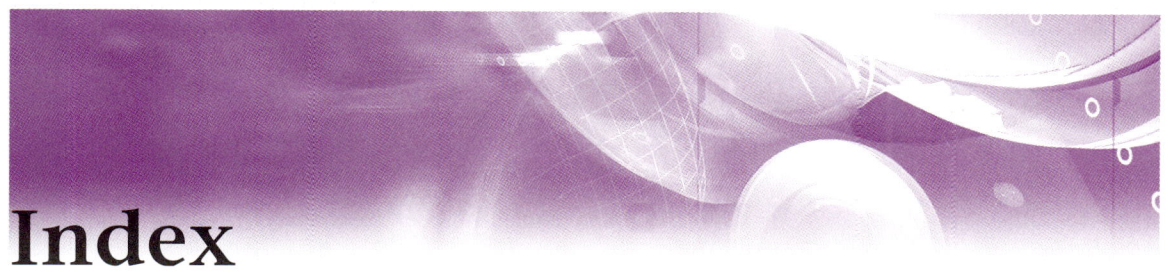

Index

5-HT$_{1A}$ receptors, stimulation. *See* Raphe nucleus
5-hydroxyindoleacetic acid, decrease, 113

A

AA. *See* Alcoholics Anonymous
Abandonment, 175
ABC. *See* Antecedent beliefs consequences
Abdominal fat, association. *See* Mortality
Abnormal findings, 71
Abortion, 57
Abuse. *See* Child abuse; Elder abuse
  evidence. *See* Children
  history, 178
  perpetration, 170
  potential, 91
  reporting, 173
  signs, 176
  victim, risk increase, 170
Abused substances, 130
Abusers, protection, 169
Abuse/violence, 169
  overview, 169-170
  physical/psychological health problems, association,
    169-170
Abusive relationship, characteristics, 173
Academic performance. *See* Children
Acceptance, 67
Acculturation level, 13
Accuracy, 196b. *See also* Medical tests
Acetylcholine, release, 29
Achievement tests, 74t, 75, 184
ACTH. *See* Adrenocorticotropic hormone
Action potentials, 29
Active-phase symptoms, 101
Activities of daily living (ADLs), 63-64. *See also*
    Instrumental activities of daily living
Acute stress disorder (ASD), 122-123
  clinical presentation, 122-123
  differential diagnosis, 123
  epidemiology/etiology, 122
  management, 123
  overview, 122
Adaptation response, 18
Adaptation syndrome. *See* General adaptation
    syndrome

Adaptive emotion, 114
Addiction
  neurotransmitter pathways, 131
  risk, 168
Addition rule. *See* Probability
Adenosine triphosphate (ATP), 29f, 81
Adenyl cyclase, activation, 30
ADHD. *See* Attention-deficit/hyperactivity disorder
Adherence (compliance). *See* Medication;
    Nonadherence; Patients; Treatment regimens
  factors. *See* Medical treatment
  improvement, 22
Adipose tissue, 135
Adjusted mortality rates, 186-187
Adjustment disorders, 110, 115, 167
  clinical presentation, 167
  diagnosis, 167
  management, 167
  overview, 167
  PTSD, contrast, 123
Adolescence (eleven to twenty-one years)
  adoptive families, 59
  cognitive development, 57, 57t
  death, leading causes, 59
  development, 56-59
  health problems, 57-58
  physical changes, 56-57
  physical development, 56-57
  pregnancy, 46
  social development, 57, 57t
  stages, 56
Adolescents
  chronic illness, 58
  depression, chances, 10
  drop out rate. *See* High school
  medical care, developmental issues, 58-59
  medical treatment, nonadherence, 58b
  physical handicaps, 59
  pregnancy, rate, 57
  substance abuse problems, 10
Adopted children, emotional/behavioral
    problems, 11
Adoption, 10-11
  discussion, 54
  stepparents, involvement, 10